WORKING WITH SUBSTANCE MISUSERS

A Guide to Theory and Practice

Edited by Trudi Petersen and Andrew McBride

ROUTLEDGE
Taylor & Francis Group

London and New York

First published 2002
by Routledge
11 New Fetter Lane, London EC4P 4EE

Simultaneously published in the USA and Canada
by Routledge
29 West 35th Street, New York, NY 10001

Routledge is an imprint of the Taylor & Francis Group

Typeset in by Sabon and Futura by
Keystroke, Jacaranda Lodge, Wolverhampton
Printed and bound in Great Britain by
TJ International Ltd, Padstow, Cornwall

British Library Cataloguing in Publication Data
A catalogue record for this book is available from the British Library

Library of Congress Cataloging in Publication Data
A catalog record for this book has been requested.

ISBN 0–415–23567–7 (hbk)
ISBN 0–415–23568–5 (pbk)

WORKING WITH SUBSTANCE MISUSERS

Working with Substance Misusers is a practical handbook for students and those who work with people who misuse drugs or alcohol. Written by experienced teachers and clinicians, the book introduces:

- the substances themselves
- theories relevant to substance use and misuse
- the skills necessary to work with this client group
- the broad range of approaches to treatment
- particular problems of specific groups.

The reader is encouraged to read and reflect on the material in relation to their own practice. To help this process, each topic has an identified set of learning objectives. Activities designed to reinforce learning and include discussion points, case studies, role plays and group exercises.

Working with Substance Misusers makes clear the connection of theory and practice and encourages a skills-based, but reflective, approach to work in this complex field. Cutting across professional boundaries, it provides new and more experienced practitioners with a key text.

Trudi Petersen has worked in acute psychiatric services, substance misuse and health promotion. She currently works as a hepatitis research nurse specialist at Bristol Specialist Drug Service and lectures at the University of Glamorgan in South Wales.

Andrew McBride is a consultant psychiatrist in Oxford. He previously ran services in Cardiff and Mid Glamorgan.

This book is dedicated to the memories of Bleddyn Griffiths and Dylan Hopkins

CONTENTS

FIGURES AND TABLES

FIGURES

TABLES

CONTRIBUTORS

Paul Bennett is a psychologist and senior lecturer at the University of Wales College of Medicine in Cardiff.

Mike Blank is the Executive Director of Surrey Alcohol and Drug Advisory Service.

Jeff Champney-Smith is a lecturer practitioner based at Caerleon and Cardiff and was previously the Clinical Manager of the Community Addictions Unit at Cardiff.

Jane Christian is the Service Manager at Druglink-North Staffordshire, a multi-disciplinary community drug service.

Precilla Choi is a psychologist and senior lecturer at Keele University in Staffordshire.

Ilana Crome is a professor of psychiatry at the University of Wolverhampton.

Meurig Davies works as a community psychiatric nurse with Mid Glamorgan Community Drugs Team.

Ed Day is a specialist registrar in psychiatry at the Queen Elizabeth Psychiatric Hospital in Birmingham.

Edzard Ernst is based at the department of Complementary Medicine at Exeter.

Eilish Gilvarry is a consultant psychiatrist and clinical director of the Alcohol and Drug Service in Newcastle upon Tyne.

Michael Gossop is the Director of the National Addiction Centre in London.

Kim Hager is a researcher, trainer and consultant and lives in Cornwall.

Mary Hepburn is a senior lecturer in women's reproductive health at the University of Glasgow and a consultant obstetrician and gynaecologist at the Royal Maternity Hospital in Glasgow.

Ray Hodgson is the Director of Cardiff Addiction Research Unit and scientific officer for the Alcohol Education Research Council.

Julia Lewis is a Clinical Research Fellow and Honorary Specialist Registrar (psychiatry) at the Institute of Medical Genetics, University of Wales College of Medicine.

Andrew McBride is a consultant psychiatrist in Oxford.

John Merrill is a consultant psychiatrist specialising in Drug Dependence at Drugs North West in Manchester.

Suzanne Midgley trained as a social worker and nurse. She is employed as a drug treatment and testing order manager at Bristol Specialist Drug Service.

Judy Orme is a principal lecturer in health promotion/public health and Director of the Public Health and Primary Care Development Research Centre at the University of the West of England in Bristol.

Richard Pates is a consultant clinical psychologist at the Community Addiction Unit in Cardiff.

Trudi Petersen is a hepatitis research nurse specialist with Bristol Specialist Drug Service and a part-time nurse lecturer on secondment at the University of Glamorgan in South Wales.

Moira Plant is the Deputy Director of the Alcohol & Health Research Centre in Edinburgh, but is now based at the University of the West of England in Bristol.

Duncan Raistrick is a consultant addiction psychiatrist and Clinical Director of Leeds Addiction Unit.

Fenella Starkey is a research associate at the Department of Social Medicine at Bristol University.

Zelda Summers is a consultant psychiatrist with Mid Glamorgan Community Drugs and Alcohol Team in South Wales.

Lorna Templeton is a researcher with the Mental Health Research and Development Unit at Bath University.

Gillian Tober is the Head of Training and Deputy Clinical Director at Leeds Addiction Unit.

Richard Velleman is Director of Research and Development and Professor of Mental Health Research at Bath University.

Adrian White is a senior lecturer at the Department of Complementary Medicine at the University of Exeter

Caroline Williams is a doctor at Broadway Lodge, a 12 step rehabilitation facility. She also works at Bristol Specialist Drug Service as a clinical assistant.

Simon Williams is a locality manager and community psychiatric nurse at Cardiff Addiction Unit.

Kathryn Williamson is a consultant in the care of the elderly at St Cadoc's Hospital in South Wales.

ACKNOWLEDGEMENTS

We would like to thank the authors who contributed to this book. Your contributions and patience have been greatly appreciated, and we are sure that readers will share our enthusiasm for what you have written. We would also like to thank the clients and colleagues from whom we have learnt what little we know.

Trudi Petersen would like to thank her long-suffering husband Aaron and children, Saskia and Pearl who have had to put up with too many missed weekends in the course of the production of the book; colleagues and friends at Bristol Specialist Drug Service and at Mid Glamorgan CDAT, and especially those who read through and commented on the CAT – Kerensa, Raj, Claudi, Caroline, Steve. I promise not to mention the 'B' word for – well a while at least. Special thanks to Suzanne Stone for all the support, phone calls and helpful coercion; Julie Coughlin for being a brick; Dave, Bron, Abi, Tanya and Gid, Ruth and Toby and Elizabeth for helping out with the girls; Suzanne Midgley for changing some of the ways that I think; Thomas Moore for introducing me to my brain; my sister Marian Gill (mature student – hah!) and my brother Johnny (Taff). Hi to Julie L and Lloyd and thank you to my fellow editor for being calm in the face of chaos.

Andrew McBride would like to thank Charlotte and Kate.

INTRODUCTION

Andrew McBride and Trudi Petersen

This book grew out of our experiences as practitioners in the field of substance misuse; conversations with service users, students and trainees, and colleagues in clinical practice, education, research and commissioning. We are well aware that there are many excellent books about substance misuse already available, from those providing basic information on drugs and alcohol through to highly complex, specialist tomes, guaranteed to baffle all but the most academic (McBride *et al.* 2000).

What we cannot find is a straightforward way of giving students and new staff a user-friendly introduction to the sorts of stuff you need to know a bit about straight away to follow what is going on. If you are a student or trainee, mentor or teacher, you will know the sort of questions that crop up: How are services organised? What is motivational interviewing? Why are people worried about 'dual diagnosis'? How do you do harm reduction? Who goes to Alcoholics Anonymous? Where is the best place to get this person sober enough to move on? What is 'maintenance' prescribing? And so on.

Now, a perfectly reasonable response is to hand out a reading list and point people to the library. The problem is that the sheer breadth of questions requires searching and reading that is probably beyond all but the most diligent.

What you have in your hand is our attempt to provide an entry level book offering a basic guide to the practice of working with substance misusers in the UK. We have sought to make explicit the link between theory and practice. We did not want to be remaindered before any reviews come out so we hope to have produced something useful, helpful and in bite-sized chunks so that nobody has the excuse not to read the relevant chapter. There are suggestions for further reading for the interested, references for the enthusiastic and things to think about, talk about and do.

The intended readership includes nursing and medical staff, social workers, psychologists, counsellors and volunteers, lecturers, tutors and trainers. Though aimed at neophyte practitioners the scope and breadth of the book may also offer something of interest for the more experienced (the editors certainly learned a lot).

The contributing authors are 'experts' from as wide a range of backgrounds as we could manage. The one thing they all have in common is that they have their roots in practice and are able to recognise the issues that are important for practitioners. A book like this is only as good as its contributors, and we believe our contributors to be very good indeed.

Having identified what this book is about, it seems sensible to point out what it is *not* about. This is not primarily a book about substances, although some substances of misuse are addressed very briefly in Chapter 1. We have concentrated on illicit drugs and alcohol, touching on prescribed drugs and omitting nicotine completely. We have dealt in most detail with those substances, approaches and difficulties that practitioners in this country are most likely to encounter. As editors we have no axe to grind – we have not sought to give one problem or approach priority over any other, nor do we necessarily agree with everything the contributing authors write. In the field of substance misuse and dependence, problems are big, our understanding is limited and the tools we have to help people tend to seem flimsy by comparison with the difficulties people face. Humility and open-mindedness are free and probably only raise the blood pressure of zealots, which we consider to be a win-win editorial position. Some topics are missing, and some authors have chosen, for reasons of space, to emphasise alcohol or drugs at the expense of the other. We make no apologies: if you want a comprehensive textbook you need something too big and detailed for our purpose (and yours).

HOW TO USE THIS BOOK

The book is split in five parts. Part I concentrates on the basics. It is recommended that you read all of the chapters in this section first. Chapter 3 contains a questionnaire (the Competence Assessment Tool, CAT). It is recommended that you fill this in with a mentor or supervisor. It is intended to help you to direct and shape your own learning with and without this book.

Part II focuses on different approaches to the care and treatment of substance misusers. Part III concentrates on some specific populations. Part IV looks at organisational and policy issues. Part V is a number of stories (case studies) interspersed with questions and debating points. These may be of particular value if you are not currently working in a clinical setting.

Each chapter commences with a set of learning objectives which outline what you should gain from reading the chapter. At the end of each chapter are 'reader input' sections. This is where *you* do the work. These range from simple, text related questions which may be completed by a single individual, to activities, role plays, groupwork exercises and debating points which can be used by individuals or groups / classes with a facilitator. We don't provide model answers to the questions, although some can be found in the text. Once you have read the chapter and completed the 'reader input' go back and re-read the learning objectives. Have you achieved them? Can you demonstrate that you have? If not, you may find it useful to get hold of the recommended reading.

Terminology used in this book

There are a few terms which are used throughout this book which require particular explanation. ***Substance of misuse*** – this term is used to denote any substance which has the potential for misuse and may include both legal and illegal substances. The terms ***misuse and misuser*** are used in preference to use and users, abuse and abuser, addiction and addict, or problem drug user / drinker.

Where there are variations from misuse and misuser, this is because the author of a particular chapter has chosen to use an alternative term, because it fits in with their own beliefs and language systems, or because it ties in with a particular philosophical approach.

Finally, we hope you enjoy your contact with substance misuse education, training and services, and of course that you read, enjoy and benefit from this book. Effective practice is about thinking, questioning and doing. If you think of ways we could improve the book or have questions about it then please do let us know (Mcbrideaj@doctors.org.uk) / (Trudi@tesco.net).

REFERENCE

McBride, A. J., Pates, R., Ball, N. and Arnold, K. (2000) Desert Island Addiction Books. *Journal of Substance Use*, 4(4): 242–7.

PART I

THE BASICS

CHAPTER 1

SOME DRUGS OF MISUSE

Andrew McBride

LEARNING OBJECTIVES

After you have studied this chapter you will understand the basic effects and ill effects of some of the more commonly used substances in the UK.

INTRODUCTION

The drugs described in this chapter, and throughout most of this book, act specifically on the brain and central nervous system and therefore on the mind. They commonly also have effects on many other parts of the body. Drugs not usually considered to be 'psychoactive' (mind altering) also commonly have effects on the metabolism of the brain, and in some circumstances cause psychological effects. There are almost no limits to the drug effects that some people will seek out for pleasure (for example, high doses of aspirin) but only commonly used psychoactive drugs will be considered here.

The number of existing and designable potent psychoactive drugs runs to more than a thousand, and the effects at a chemical and cellular level are incomprehensibly complex for all but the specialist neuro-psycho-pharmacologist. Fortunately, for most practical purposes the psychoactive drugs that people take for pleasure can be classified much more simply, by their effects.

A SIMPLE CLASSIFICATION OF PSYCHOACTIVE DRUGS

The simplest such classification might categorise drugs by their most obvious effect into:

- Stimulants; that wake you up, speed you up and give you energy. This group includes amphetamine and cocaine.
- Depressants; that make you calm, drowsy or put you to sleep. This group includes opioids, benzodiazepines, volatile substances and cannabis.
- Hallucinogens; that change your perception of the world, by distorting what you see and hear, or make you experience things that aren't there at all. This group includes LSD and Magic Mushrooms.
- Others; this group might include drugs with relatively little potential for misuse such as antipsychotic and antidepressant drugs.

With enhanced understanding of the chemical structures, actions and effects of different drugs, more sophisticated classifications are now available, usually based on pharmacological mechanisms. Unfortunately this can lead to confusion for anybody with no basic understanding of pharmacology (such as most drug users). Ultimately all different drugs are unique in some respect, so that the best classification is the most helpful for understanding in the relevant context.

It is worth remembering that the interconnectedness of the brain means that the same subjective and objective effects of any drug may be mediated by the same or very different mechanisms, and that drugs which are chemically very similar may have seemingly very different (even opposite) effects.

DRUG EFFECTS

The effects of any psychoactive drug depend on several factors, including:

- the amount taken (the dose)
- the number and timing of doses
- the route by which the drug is taken
    - by mouth
    - by smoking
    - by injection (subcutaneous, intramuscular, intravenous)
- the speed with which the drug reaches the brain
- the rate at which the drug is broken down (or excreted unchanged)
- the user's past experience with this and similar drugs
    - expectations
    - motivations
    - physiological tolerance to the drug's effects
- whether the drug is taken alone or in combination with other drugs
- the circumstances in which the drug is taken

  - place
  - atmosphere
  - company
- The person
  - inherited biology
  - personality
  - health
  - mood

The same dose of the same drug can have different outcomes

It is important to remember that psychoactive drugs have no intrinsic moral value and few inevitable effects. Consider, for example, the likely effect of 10 units of alcohol on:

1 A sixth-form school student, who has never drunk alcohol before, at a post-exam celebration night out, who drinks lager over 3 hours.
2 A middle-aged, middle-class woman at her weekly bridge club, who drinks gin and tonic over a period of 5 hours.
3 An alcohol dependent serial killer who has been taking amphetamine and high doses of benzodiazepines for two weeks, who injects vodka intravenously in the bathroom of a house he is burgling whilst the residents are asleep.
4 A bishop alone, at home, grieving over the death of his wife, who drinks sherry over 2 hours before going to bed, because he hasn't slept for two nights.

The same drug, the same quantity, but the effects might reasonably be expected to be very different.

Drug effects and drug interactions

Users of psychoactive drugs tend to use more than one type of drug. Heavy drinkers commonly smoke tobacco, amphetamine users frequently take benzodiazepines, methadone users often drink heavily, and for young, non-dependent users of 'recreational' drugs, complex patterns of poly-drug use are commonplace. 'Pure' single drug use or dependence is sometimes seen but it is unusual in clinical populations. What do we understand about the effects of taking combinations of drugs?

Many drugs of misuse are unlicensed for any medical indication, and have therefore never been subject to mandatory testing and monitoring for effects and side effects. Getting ethical approval and funding to research such effects is therefore potentially problematic. When such testing is undertaken, it can only be with 'safe' doses (which may bear no relation to doses taken by misusers) on a small number of occasions (avoiding tolerance and dependence), in healthy volunteers (who will be unlike the 'typical' misuser), in laboratory conditions (an unusual setting for drug taking), without any other psychoactive drugs being taken. Any other approach would be unacceptably risky, but it leaves many real-life questions unanswered. For example, I was once asked in a criminal court for the likely effects, on a teenager, of three litres of 6 per cent ABV cider, four 'ecstasy' tablets, a large but unknown quantity of two different benzodiazepines, some amphetamine and possibly some LSD.

As a general rule, if you take more than one drug in the depressant group the effect will be increased. The majority of deaths from 'heroin' overdoses follow the use of heroin and/or alcohol and/or benzodiazepines and/or other opioid drugs. The use of two or more stimulant drugs will similarly increase stimulant effects. As a rule of thumb, any combination of drugs is more hazardous than any drug taken by itself, and the more complex the cocktail the more unpredictable the effects.

Drug prices

Drugs are commodities, like any other. In a free market, the price of a drug is therefore determined by supply and demand. In the UK the price of alcohol (and tobacco) is inflated by taxation, although this has long been circumvented by smugglers and latterly white-van-man, who import from countries with lower tax rates. Illegal drugs rely entirely on covert manufacture or smuggling, but market forces still apply. Because of the necessarily covert supply chain for illegal drugs, and the difficulty buyers have in checking drugs for purity, unscrupulous sellers adulterate ('cut') the drug with other, cheaper substances, usually inert but sometimes potentially poisonous.

Illegal drug prices and purities can change markedly over time. The following two examples come from my own experience.

1. When pharmaceutical amphetamines effectively disappeared because of controls on prescribing, it was replaced by amphetamine sulphate 'powder' from illegal laboratories. A gram of good quality (probably 70+ per cent) amphetamine cost around £10 in South Wales in the early 1970s, but would fuel two nights out for a couple of people. Twenty years later the price was the same, but the purity had fallen to between 0 (yes, zero) and 10 per cent. The fall in purity more than made up for price inflation. Increased availability and competition from heroin has since pushed the purity up and the price down.
2. In 1991 heroin was effectively unavailable in South Wales. When it was first brought over the Severn Bridge from Bristol it was sold in £10 wraps which contained maybe one fifteenth of a gram of poor quality stuff. By 2001 heroin was widely available, almost uncut from the point of importation, costing as little as £90 for 3.5 grams. The five-fold fall in price could reflect reduced demand, but unfortunately almost certainly highlights increased availability that has managed to outstrip the increase in use.

The law

The law concerns itself with aspects of the production, importation and exportation, supply, and taxation of psychoactive substances.

Alcohol is supplied under the auspices of the licensing laws, which restrict who can sell alcohol, of what type, in what circumstances, between what hours, and only ever to those over the age of 18 years (although younger people may legally drink alcohol). Taxation on all forms of alcohol is high in the UK compared to most other European countries. This combination of controls has exerted downward pressure on per capita alcohol consumption since before the First World War. Licensing laws have been progressively relaxed over recent years and the real price of alcohol is falling (compared to average income) and availability increasing.

Other psychoactive drugs are controlled by a complex network of legislation; designed to limit the availability of illegal drugs and to control supplies of prescribed (Prescription Only Medicines, POM) and over the counter (OTC) drugs. These laws include the Misuse of Drugs Act and the Medicines Act, but only the former will be briefly outlined here.

The Misuse of Drugs Act

Among its many provisions, the Misuse of Drugs Act (1971) ranks drugs (other than alcohol and tobacco) into three classes and gives guidelines for the penalties that courts can impose for possession (for personal use) and supply (or intent to supply) to others. The boundaries make only limited pharmacological or 'health risk' sense. For example, different opioid drugs fall within each of the three categories and some are omitted altogether. The following lists are not exhaustive. The maximum sentences listed cannot be imposed by a Magistrate's Court, only by Crown and higher courts.

Class A drugs

Amphetamine (if prepared for injection), cocaine, ecstasy, heroin, LSD, morphine (Magic Mushrooms if 'prepared for use' but not in their natural state), methadone, opium, and pethidine. The maximum penalties that can be imposed by the courts are: Possession: seven years imprisonment and/or a fine; Supply: life imprisonment and/or a fine.

Class B drugs

Amphetamine (not prepared for injection). Cannabis (in 2001 the Home Secretary announced the intention to reclassify cannabis as class C). The maximum penalties that can be imposed by the courts are: Possession: five years imprisonment and/or a fine; Supply: fourteen years imprisonment and/or a fine.

Class C drugs

Possession of temazepam and flunitrazepam. Supply of anabolic steroids and some hypnosedative drugs. The maximum penalties that can be imposed by the courts are: Possession: two years imprisonment and/or a fine; Supply: five years imprisonment and/or a fine.

Volatile Substances It is an offence to supply solvents to persons under the age of 18 if the supplier has reason to believe that they intend to misuse them (or to an adult who will supply them on).

Alcohol

Introduction

Alcohol has been used by almost every known human culture, and is also popular with other mammals and even insects. It is naturally produced by the action of yeast, and other simple organisms, on sugar, water and air, at warmish temperatures. Our favourite drug is thus revealed as the waste product of bacteria.

Main drug name Alcohol, ethanol and many hundreds of generic, proprietary and slang names.

What it looks like Pure ethanol is a clear colourless liquid, which smells and tastes of – well – alcohol.

Mode of use Alcohol is almost invariably drunk. It is available in a bewildering variety of flavours and strengths. It can be and therefore is injected.

Quantities used A British 'unit' of alcohol is 10 mls, or 8 grams. One litre of 5.2 per cent ABV (alcohol by volume) lager therefore contains 5.2 units of alcohol. One 75 cl bottle of 12 per cent ABV wine contains 9 units. Recommended levels for safer drinking are up to 21 units per week for men and 14 for women, in divided doses. A very heavily dependent drinker with high tolerance may consume 1.5 litres of 40 per cent ABV spirits per day (420 units per week) or more.

Pharmacology Chemical structure and receptor actions: C_2H_5OH, a simple nine atom molecule that affects almost every metabolic activity in the body, and pretty well every transmitter system that has been investigated.

Main effects The effects of alcohol are dose dependent, and vary from the seemingly stimulant, anxiety reducing, socially lubricating disinhibition that is almost universally the object of a few drinks, to unconsciousness, coma and death.

Side effects Alcohol is highly toxic to almost all human organ systems, particularly the nervous system. Single episodes of intoxication greatly increase the likelihood of falls and accidents, because of impaired motor coordination, and slowed reaction times, acts of aggression, and behaviour that will be regretted later because of impaired social judgement. Other acute toxic effects include impaired sexual performance, vomiting, episodes of amnesia, unconsciousness and incontinence. Longer-term health effects are discussed in Chapter 13.

Withdrawal effects These are predominantly symptoms and signs of over-arousal, from mild anxiety to confusional states and seizures (see Chapter 12).

Risks Alcohol is strongly associated with accidental death, violent crime, family discord and physical abuse, absenteeism, deliberate self-harm, suicide and mental health problems. Alcohol is the next most likely drug after nicotine to lead to chronic dependence, ill health and premature death.

Who uses Ninety per cent of the UK population drinks alcohol. At any one time perhaps 5 per cent of men and 1 or 2 per cent of women drink heavily enough to place them at high risk of developing problems.

Cannabis

Introduction

Cannabis has been in use for thousands of years recreationally and as medicine. All preparations of cannabis come from varieties of the plant *Cannabis Sativa*, which grows throughout the world. Cannabis in the UK comes from a variety of sources. Resin from the Indian subcontinent, Lebanon and Morocco. Herbal cannabis is increasingly 'home grown' in the UK and Europe, often using sophisticated growing equipment. Specially bred strains of high potency herbal cannabis are increasingly common.

Main drug name Cannabis, also called: blow, dope, draw, ganja, grass, hashish (hash), marijuana, mary-jane, rocky, wacky-baccy, weed, etc.

What it looks like Hashish is made of the compressed resin of the plant and is brown or black in colour. It is usually imported in 9 ounce 'soap' shaped bars, or 'slates', and sold by weight. Marijuana is the dried flowering tops of the female plant and looks like dried flowers or tea leaves. Hash-oil is concentrated plant extract and looks like treacle.

Mode of use Cannabis is usually smoked. Cannabis resin is usually mixed with tobacco, whereas herbal cannabis is usually smoked as it is. If rolled into a cannabis cigarette this is usually called a 'spliff' or, 'joint'. Alternatively cannabis can be smoked in a variety of smoking devices; pipes, 'water pipes', 'bongs', 'buckets', 'hot knives', etc. Cannabis can also be consumed in a wide variety of foodstuffs: fudge, cakes, biscuits (hash cookies), hot drinks, and even stuffed chicken.

Quantities used Consumption varies very widely, and the majority of British users consume the drug only occasionally. Very heavy users may consume up to around 30 grams per week.

Pharmacology Chemical structure: the main active ingredient is THC (delta 9 tetrahydrocannabinol), but there are many other related chemicals in cannabis, and that could be manufactured. Receptor actions: the body and brain both contain specific receptors for cannabis-like molecules, and one endogenous substance, christened anandemide, has been discovered with cannabis-like effects.

Main effects Smoking cannabis produces almost instant intoxication, the effects lasting from 1 to 4 hours, depending on the amount used. The desired effects are: carefree mood and euphoria, intensified visual and auditory perceptions, an enhanced sense of creative performance, changes in the perception of time and space and muscular relaxation.

Side effects Negative mood states and dysphoria can occur and short-term memory impairment is quite common. Physical ill-effects can include: dry mouth, red eyes, increased heart rate, fatigue, craving for food (the munchies), nausea and vomiting. Hangover effects may occur but are slight.

Withdrawal effects Even after heavy regular use cannabis produces only minimal physical withdrawal symptoms, comparable to a mild upper respiratory virus.

Risks Fatalities from cannabis use are unknown. Transient anxiety, panic and paranoia reactions are common. Psychosis may be precipitated in those at high risk. Individuals with existing serious mental illness may increase their risk of relapse. Cannabis impairs tasks involving concentration and motor coordination

– such as driving a car. The effects persist after the subjective effects of the drug have worn off. The way in which cannabis is smoked increases the likelihood of chest disease compared with tobacco.

Who uses Cannabis is the most widely used illegal drug in the UK. Around half of all teenagers will experiment with the drug. Only a very small proportion of the population use the drug after they reach their mid-twenties.

Stimulants

Introduction

Stimulant drugs vary greatly in potency and duration of effect but are otherwise broadly similar. Coca leaf from the *Erythroxylon coca* bush (derivatives cocaine, and its smokable free-base form 'crack'), khat from the shrub *Catha Edulis Forsk* (principle active ingredient cathinone) and caffeine (in coffee and tea), are all naturally occurring; amphetamine (and its smokable free-base form 'ice') is synthetic. Ecstacy and some other synthetic drugs are closely chemically related to stimulants.

Main drug names Amphetamine, also known as speed, whizz, billy, powder, etc.; Cocaine, also known as coke, Charlie, C, Bolivian marching powder, flake, snow, etc.; Khat, names and spellings vary greatly; Caffeine, also known as tea, coffee, 'Coca Cola', 'Red Bull', etc.

What it looks like In the UK both amphetamine and cocaine are mainly sold as whitish crystalline powders (sometimes dyed). Crack cocaine is sold in small 'rocks' sometimes called bones. These make a popping/cracking noise when smoked, hence the name. Caffeine is sold mainly in a wide range of drinks but can be bought in tablet form. Khat is bought as bunches of fresh leaves and shoots.

Mode of use Amphetamine is either swallowed, snorted or injected. Smokable amphetamine is very unusual in the UK. Cocaine is snorted or rubbed onto mucous membranes (gums or genitalia). Crack cocaine is smoked, usually in small pipes. Khat is chewed and retained in the cheek as a quid.

Quantities used Recreational users of amphetamine and cocaine take them in small quantities (fractions of a gram) to socialise. Heavy dependent users may consume up to 10 grams of amphetamine or cocaine in a day. Khat users in the UK rarely use more than one or two bundles of khat per day. Dependent caffeine users know who they are because they cannot leave the house in the morning without several cups of tea or coffee.

Pharmacology Chemical structure and receptor actions: stimulant drugs are closely related to the brain's naturally occurring monoamines. Increased activity is found in all these systems.

Main effects The onset of effects varies with the route used. The duration of effect is shortest and most intense for crack cocaine – a few minutes' snorted cocaine lasts up to 30 minutes, whereas amphetamine lasts for 6–8 hours. The desired effects are alertness, clarity of thinking, improved concentration, euphoria, self-confidence, talkativeness, increased energy and stamina. The need for food and sleep are suppressed.

Side effects Undesired psychological effects include restlessness, over-excitement, anxiety, suspiciousness, grandiosity, irritability, and aggressive behaviour. Repetitive, sometimes bizarre behaviour may occur, from teeth grinding to complex actions carried out over minutes or hours (stereotypy). Physical effects include increased pulse and rate of breathing, raised blood pressure, dilated pupils, raised body temperature, sweating, headache, blurred vision, dizziness, flushing or pallor, and tremor. Regular high dose use can lead to weight loss, exhaustion, and illnesses related to malnutrition. Cocaine is a local anaesthetic and constricts blood vessels, sometimes to the point of tissue damage. This can cause damage to and perforation of the nasal septum in those who snort the drug.

Withdrawal effects Irritability, depressed mood, headache, fatigue, long but troubled sleep, hunger, depression and violence may also occur.

Risks Unlike opioids, stimulant use is associated with increased sexual risk taking. A dose dependent psychosis can be brought on by stimulant use. The psychosis is similar to paranoid schizophrenia, characterised by persecutory delusions, auditory hallucinations, visual misinterpretations and hallucinations, and more rarely delusions of infestation and tactile hallucinations. The duration of symptoms is typically brief but may persist if the individual is at high risk of psychosis or if drug use persists after psychosis develops. Death can occur as a consequence of cardiovascular disease; stroke, myocardial infarction and the long-term effects of high blood pressure.

Who uses

Amphetamine is the second most widely used drug after cannabis, and use is widespread among the young and not so young intent on a good, late, night out. Cocaine is promoted by the media as the champagne of drugs, seemingly beloved of the rich and famous. As the price falls use is spreading to the many. The short duration of action makes it expensive as fuel for a night's drinking and dancing. Khat use is limited to those with roots in countries where use is endemic.

Anxiolytics and hypnotics

Introduction

Availability of anxiolytics and hypnotics in the UK is effectively limited to diverted supplies of prescribed benzodiazepines. Benzodiazepines replaced barbiturates, which were less effective as anxiolytics, more likely to cause intoxication, dependence and very much more dangerous in overdose. Chloral, chlormethiazole, zimovane and probably every effective agent has the potential for misuse and at least psychological dependence. Benzodiazepines vary in their rate of onset, potency, metabolism and duration of effect, but are otherwise very similar in effects.

Main drug name 'Benzodiazepines': diazepam (Valium), chlordiazepoxide (Librium), oxazepam, lorazepam (Ativan), temazepam, nitrazepam (Mogadon), etc.

What it looks like A wide variety of tablet sizes, shapes and colours.

Mode of use Usually taken orally; tablets are more rarely crushed, dissolved, filtered and injected.

Quantities used The lowest tablet dose of the most widely prescribed anxiolytic (diazepam) is 2 mg. At the height of the craze for injecting temazepam capsules (now unavailable in the UK), daily doses of 1 gram (diazepam equivalent) were sometimes claimed. Daily doses of 100 mg of illicit diazepam are not unusual.

Main effects Benzodiazepines reduce anxiety and help to induce sleep. They can also cause disinhibition, particularly at high doses and in combination with alcohol. They are popular with users of most other drugs as 'second best' and to help with withdrawal symptoms.

Side effects Over-sedation, inappropriate intoxicated and violent disinhibited behaviour, dense amnesia and accidents may all occur particularly in combination with alcohol.

Withdrawal effects Anxiety, panic, insomnia, depression and symptoms of over-arousal are common, but not universal. Epileptic seizures may occur in high dose users and vulnerable groups. Hyperaesthesia and unusual sensory phenomena are rare. Long-term users (including low-dose therapeutic users) may experience long-term anxiety and adjustment problems if withdrawn too quickly and without adequate psychosocial support.

Risks Benzodiazepines are extremely safe drugs. Falls and accidents, particularly in the elderly are more likely. Overdose in combination with alcohol and opiates can be fatal.

Who uses A significant percentage of the population takes prescribed low dose benzodiazepines, with some benefit and no significant problems. High dose illicit users most commonly also take other drugs such as opiates or stimulants.

Volatile substances

Introduction

This range of substances exists as gases or volatile liquids at room temperature. They are found in a large number of household items:

- lighter fuel (butane)
- petrol
- aerosol propellant gases (various)
- some glues (usually toluene)
- some paints, thinners, dry cleaning and correcting fluids (various).

Preparations None of these products are intended for human consumption. Butane gas is dangerously cold when released from its container, room spray is heavily perfumed, and fire extinguishers are highly pressurised. Each carries its own particular risks.

Mode of use

Volatile substances are inhaled, either directly from their container, or transferred to a bag from which they can be inhaled more easily, without waste, and in greater quantity.

Quantities used Many people who try volatile substances use them only experimentally, on one or two occasions and only one or two breaths. Chronic heavy users may consume the contents of a litre tin of glue, or ten tins of lighter fuel per day, over a number of years.

Pharmacology Most volatile substances are complex hydrocarbons, which are highly fat-soluble and rapidly pass through the lungs and blood brain barrier. Onset is very rapid and the duration of action is usually 15–45 minutes.

Main effects Low dose use produces effects similar to alcohol, a sense of dreamy intoxication and drowsiness.

Side effects At higher doses hallucinations (mainly visual) may develop. Pulse and respiratory rate are reduced. Repeated inhalation can lead to disorientation, and unconsciousness. Hangover (headache, nausea and impaired concentration) can last up to 24 hours.

Withdrawal effects Tolerance develops with regular use. Physical dependence and withdrawal symptoms do not.

Risks This is a highly dangerous group of compounds, and there is no strictly safe way to take them. Heart arrhythmias can occur as a direct effect of volatile substances and can be fatal, particularly if the user exercises. There is a risk of accidental injury or death when intoxicated and unaware of risk. (Young people use volatile substances in hazardous places where they will not be identified. Up trees and on windowsills are surprisingly popular.) A combination of vomiting and unconsciousness can also be fatal. Suffocation may follow the use of plastic bags over the head or spasm of the larynx and oedema because of direct squirting of gas into the mouth. Volatile substances are highly flammable, and burns are common. Heavy solvent misuse over years can result in brain damage, affecting cognition and movement. Kidney and liver damage can also follow prolonged use of some products.

Who uses In the UK use fluctuates widely over time, but is largely restricted to 12–16 year olds. Very few present to services for this problem.

Hallucinogens

Introduction

This is the only group of drugs taken in order to produce psychotic experiences, rather than such phenomena arising because of sensitivity or overdose. The use of hallucinogenic drugs is widely believed to have been central to early mystical and spiritual ritual, and the idea that hallucinogens could lead to enlightenment only gave way to the aesthetics of the dance floor during the very late twentieth century. Hallucinogens can be found in plants, fungi, cacti, in the secretions of toads, but most commonly in laboratories. In the UK the two most commonly taken hallucinogens are the synthetic drug LSD (Lysergic Acid Diethylamide) and the autumnal fungus Magic Mushrooms (*Psilocybin Semilanceata*).

Main drug name LSD, also known as acid, trips, blotters, tabs, etc.; Magic Mushrooms, also known as liberty caps, etc.

What it looks like LSD is usually sold as small squares of impregnated paper, with a printed design on it. Magic Mushrooms are approximately 3.5 cm long and 1 cm in diameter if fresh, but shrivel when dried. Accurate identification is always essential to avoid more poisonous fungi of similar appearance.

Mode of use Both drugs are invariably taken orally, but can be processed for injection.

Quantities used One LSD tab (100–200 micrograms) or 40 mushrooms bring on a 'trip'. Hallucinogens very rapidly cause tolerance.

Pharmacology Chemical structure and receptor actions: LSD is similar in structure to the monoamine neurotransmitter. It is thought to act primarily through serotonin pathways. Other hallucinogens have strikingly different modes of action.

Main effects Effects begin ½ to 1 hour after taking LSD, peak after around 6 hours and stop after 12 hours. Experiences are usually mainly visual, but can occur in any modality and may include synaesthesia, the experience of sensing, for example, colour as a sound, or a smell as a sound. Sensual experience may be simply heightened, distorted or misinterpreted, and at higher doses hallucinations may occur. Time may appear to stand still, thinking takes on unusual patterns and ideas, memories may be transformed, and 'spiritual' experiences may arise. Unsurprisingly these experiences vary with the emotional state of the user, and in turn produce further emotional responses.

Side effects The most common ill effect of hallucinogens is the 'Bad Trip', usually the result of taking the drug in the wrong sort of mood and circumstance. Anxiety, panic and fearful experiences, memories and misperceptions may lead to loss of insight, a fear of imminent insanity and acting out. Kind and friendly 'nursing' in a well lit, non-threatening, peaceful environment, with reassurance, 'talking down' and perhaps a benzodiazepine tranquilliser for anxiety, will invariably have the desired effect. Psychotic reactions may persist beyond the duration of the trip in vulnerable users. Flashbacks occur when an LSD experience recurs weeks or years after the drug was last taken. They usually happen when tired or after taking other drugs. Flashbacks are frequently written about but rarely seen in practice or problematic.

Withdrawal effects Hallucinogens are not dependence inducing and have no withdrawal symptoms.

Risks Suicide can occur but is very rare. Death from overdose is almost unknown. Accidents happen to people who have very little correct perception of their environment.

Who uses Most use is probably experimental or aesthetic rather than a search for enlightenment or part of a regular pattern of psychedelic use. Few people who reach drug services have not taken a few trips in their time.

Opioids

Classification Opiates are derived from the exudate of the Asian opium poppy (*Papaver somniferum*) and include opium, morphine and codeine. The wider group of drugs known as opioids includes both opiates and synthetic drugs that have the same mode of action as opiates (e.g. pethidine, methadone and dextropropoxyphene). In this chapter heroin will be used as the example drug, but probably all opioid drugs are misused to some extent.

Heroin (Diacetylmorphine) has many street names including brown, smack, junk and gear.

What it looks like Heroin is either a white powder, or a brownish powder depending on its chemical state. Most heroin imported into the UK is 'brown' hence its popular street name. Pharmaceutical opioid drugs come in a bewildering variety of preparations for administration by every possible route.

Mode of use Heroin is commonly injected, but brown heroin is not readily water soluble and needs acid, usually citric acid or lemon juice to make it dissolve. The alternative is for the drug to be 'smoked'. Brown heroin vaporises when heated on metal foil and can be inhaled through a tube. Pursuing the wisps of smoke in this way gives rise to the description 'chasing the dragon' or chasing. Most opioid drugs can be prepared to be injected, but most pharmaceutical drugs are prepared for oral use.

Quantities used Tolerance develops both to the pleasurable and the hazardous effects of opioids. Experienced users may be outwardly unaffected by a dose that would kill a whole group of first-time users. Some individuals use heroin or other opioids occasionally for recreation, and may use only a small fraction of a gram. A highly tolerant heroin user may consume several grams every day.

Pharmacology Chemical structure: there are a very large number of opioid drugs, which are chemically related but have very different potencies and some variations in effects. Receptor actions: opioids have a number of different specific receptor sites around the body and brain. The effects described below are the result of 'agonist' activity. A smaller number of drugs (e.g. naloxone and naltrexone) block these effects and are therefore known as 'antagonists'. A third group of drugs (e.g. buprenorphine) have mixed actions, and are considered less likely to lead to dependence and safer in the event of overdose.

Main effects Opioids cause people to feel euphoric, dreamy, drowsy and warm. Opioids relieve distress and pain by creating a sense of detachment. Reflexes, including coughing, breathing, pulse and gut movements are reduced. At higher doses sedation may lead to sleep.

Side effects Nausea and vomiting are common early side effects, appetite suppression (for food and sex) and constipation are frequent unwanted effects.

Withdrawal effects Abrupt cessation or reduction in dose leads to symptoms similar to flu: muscular aches and pains, particularly in the joints, hot and cold sweats, shivering, sneezing, goose-flesh, streaming nose and eyes, diarrhoea and vomiting, yawning and muscular spasms. These physical symptoms are rarely objectively severe, disabling or hazardous to health. Dysphoria, depression, insomnia and the loss of a sense of being cocooned against the world, make the experience subjectively highly distressing. Onset of symptoms will depend on the duration of effect of the drug. With heroin the drug needs to be taken around three times per day. Physical withdrawal symptoms are usually substantially reduced within a week and gone within four weeks. Psychological adjustment may take many months or years.

Risks The main health risk from opioids is overdose. Tolerance reduces with abstinence or reduced intake. Overdose is therefore most likely in inexperienced users and in those who have just left detoxification, residential rehabilitation or prison. Most opioid overdoses occur when opiates are taken in combination with other depressant drugs such as alcohol and benzodiazepines. Death usually arises from respiratory depression.

Who uses Heroin has spread across the UK in a number of waves, over the past four decades. From a highly stigmatised, scarce, impure and expensive drug, it is now very much more widely used, and there is probably no longer a 'typical' user. The idea that users of 'dance' drugs would not go on to use heroin is no longer sustainable.

Performance enhancing drugs

Introduction

Drugs have always been used to enhance athletic performance, but until recently most were ineffective. A wide range of drugs are taken for psychological and physiological reasons before, during and after performance. A similar spectrum is now banned by many official sporting bodies who screen athletes for 'doping'. The widespread use of anabolic (muscle building) androgenic (masculinising) steroids (AAS) began in the 1950s. This section will deal only with these drugs.

Classification AAS are a range of synthetic and natural analogues of the male sex hormone testosterone.

What it looks like AAS come in a range of preparations. Injectable liquids usually come in boxes of glass ampoules, oral drugs as tablets. Some are diverted pharmaceutical supplies, but most are manufactured illegally or veterinary products.

Mode of use Drugs are often used in combinations (stacking) using a mixture of oral and injectable drugs. Drug holidays are often included in training regimes, so that drugs are taken in cycles.

Quantities used Legitimate research on doses for different athletic purposes is lacking. Bodybuilders in particular use very high doses compared with the doses used for the rare medical indications.

Preparations Too many to list: sustanon, deca-durabolin and nandrolone are some of the better known names. Some injectable drugs are in gradual release form therefore needing to be taken only weekly or less frequently.

Pharmacology All AAS have similar effects, although the balance between androgenic and anabolic effects, the potency, duration of effect and toxicity all vary. In health, natural testosterone acts directly on a number of organ systems throughout the body. The desired and toxic effects of AAS reflect these systemic effects.

Main effects If used in combination with optimum exercise and diet AAS increase muscle bulk and power. They also give drive and energy during training.

Side effects Irritability and aggressiveness (''roid rage'), depression, mania and paranoia have all been reported. Muscle dysmorphia (reverse anorexia) has been described in some male bodybuilders. Acne, male pattern baldness, changes (increase or decrease) in sex drive, secondary infertility in men and stunted growth (if used before the end of puberty) have also been described. Long-term heavy steroid use may cause damage to the heart (hypertension, ischaemic heart disease and cardiomyopathy), liver (including malignant tumours) and kidneys. In women, irreversible growth of facial and body hair, male pattern baldness, 'breaking' of the voice and enlargement of the clitoris can all be problematic. Disruption of the menstrual cycle is usually reversible.

Withdrawal effects Tolerance and physiological dependence do not occur, and there is no withdrawal syndrome. Bodybuilders sometimes come to greatly fear the physical changes that will occur if they discontinue regular use.

Risks The health risks are the side effects of the drugs as already outlined, the dangers of using counterfeit and veterinary products and the hazards of injecting intramuscularly.

Who uses Over time the use of these drugs has spread from professional athletes and bodybuilders to recreational athletes at all levels. Male bodybuilders and power athletes are most likely to use, but experimental and instrumental use are probably more widespread.

Some other drugs

Ecstacy

Ecstacy (3–4 methylenedioxymetamphetamine) was perhaps *the* drug of the 1990s. Closely related to amphetamine in structure and effects, its unique ability to generate feelings of warmth and empathy (being 'loved up') led to it being christened an 'entactogen'. At its peak perhaps one million ecstacy tablets were being consumed in the UK every weekend. The story of E is a marker of how quickly drug fashions now change: when first available, one (rather expensive) ecstacy tablet would be a typical dose for an evening, and no alcohol or other drugs would be taken. Now ecstacy (perhaps one-fifth the price) is just another drug and is washed down with lager in sometimes very large numbers, alongside whatever else is available. The acute risk of taking ecstacy is of overheating and related problems, which can be fatal. In actuarial terms the risk is equivalent to playing amateur football. There is worrying evidence that ecstacy causes irreversible neurological damage in animals, and some evidence is now accumulating for human users.

GHB

GHB (gamma hydroxybutyrate) is a colourless liquid originally used as an anaesthetic. It causes sedation and euphoria. GHB reactions can include dizziness, vomiting, muscular stiffness, epileptic fits, collapse and coma. Some bodybuilders use GHB because of supposed anabolic effects. Long-term effects and dependence potential are unclear.

Ketamine

Ketamine is another anaesthetic agent in use by veterinarians. It has analgesic and dissociative effects as well as being highly sedating. Derealisation, out-of-body and other bizarre mental states are not uncommon. Raised pulse and blood pressure and impaired coordination may be hazardous.

Poppers

Amyl, butyl and isobutyl nitrate are fruity smelling liquids, usually bought in small bottles and inhaled for their vasodilatory effects. First widely used by gay men, use in clubs is now more widespread. The principle effect is that of a 'head rush', light headedness and dizzyness. Hot flushes (and reddening of the skin) are common, as are headache, nausea, vomiting and coughing. Low blood pressure can lead to collapse.

Over-the-counter drugs

A wide range of drugs with misuse potential are available for sale from pharmacies without prescription. Opioids, antihistamines and ephedrine containing drugs are most widely suspected of misuse by pharmacists. Laxatives are misused to facilitate weight loss, but have no psychoactive effect.

FURTHER READING

Banks, A. and Waller, T.A.N. (1988) *Drug Misuse: A Practical Handbook for GPs*, Oxford: Blackwell Scientific Publications.

Gossop, M. (2000) *Living with Drugs* (5th edn), London: Ashgate Publishers Limited.

Hardman, J. G. and Limbird, L. E. (editors in chief) (2000) *Goodman & Gilman's The Pharmacological Basis of Therapeutics* (9th edn), New York: McGraw-Hill.

Ritson, B. and Thorley, A. (2000) 'Alcohol and its effects', in M. Plant and D. Cameron (eds) *The Alcohol Report*, London: Free Association Books.

Robson, P. (1999) *Forbidden Drugs* (2nd edn), Oxford: Oxford University Press.
Tyler, A. (1995) *Street Drugs* (3rd revision), London: Coronet Books.
Valter, K. and Arrizabalaga, P. (1998) *Designer Drugs Directory*, Amsterdam: Elsevier Science.

CHAPTER 2

EXPLORING SUBSTANCE MISUSE AND DEPENDENCE: EXPLANATIONS, THEORIES AND MODELS

Trudi Petersen

LEARNING OBJECTIVES

By the end of this chapter you will be able to:

1 Identify the factors that relate to substance misuse in Western society.

2 Demonstrate a broad understanding of the concept of dependence and how this might be explored in relation to biological, psychological and societal/environmental theories.

INTRODUCTION

People have used and misused substances since prehistory. Alcohol was used by Neolithic and Stone Age man. Natural psychedelics have become part of our folklore (who could forget Lewis Carroll's hookah smoking caterpillar perched on top of a giant mushroom?). Aboriginals licked hallucinogenic toads whilst Mexicans harvested Peyote cactus to use in rituals. Opium and related substances were used reduce pain and as a tonic. The famous Mariani wine used by Queen Victoria contained both opium and cocaine. Cannabis was used as far back as 2500 BC. Problems derived from substance misuse are not new phenomena either. John Jones, writing about opium and wine in 1700, described the effects of 'a long and lavish use of both' which included:

> Early descriptions, stooping in the back, trembling of the hands, weakness of memory, shortness of life, difficulty and danger in suddenly leaving them off, revive such as sink for want of either, and supply the want of each other.
>
> (John Jones, *The Mysteries of Opium Reveal'd*, 1700)

This chapter looks at some of the reasons why an individual may use or misuse substances and some of the theories which may help to explain why some people continue to misuse substances, or develop problems including that of dependence.

WHY DO SOME PEOPLE USE OR MISUSE SUBSTANCES?

There are a whole raft of reasons why a person may choose to use or misuse a substance for the first time, and a range of influencing factors that may help to explain why they might continue.

Age

One large study of 15–16-year-olds in the UK (Miller and Plant, 1996) identified over 40 per cent reported using an illicit drug. This does not mean that all of these young people will continue to do so. Of the 45 per cent of young people surveyed in the British Crime Survey only 15 per cent reported taking an illicit drug in the previous month (Ramsay and Spiller, 1997) (see Chapter 25).

Historically, males have been more likely to report substance misuse, but recent reports suggest that females may be catching up, certainly in relation to alcohol and tobacco. The ratio of males to females in touch with substance misuse services is usually reported as being approximately 3:1. The Advisory Council on the Misuse of Drugs (ACMD, 1998) suggest that the actual picture is more complicated and that if specific substances are looked at separately this ratio, in some cases, narrows (see Chapter 23).

Ethnicity

Current evidence suggests that drug use is not limited to any one specific group, although some drugs may be widely unacceptable and prohibited or encouraged and abundantly available in different cultures. There is a general lack of research in this area and findings are complicated by the impact of other social factors such as poverty, deprivation and historical issues. There is a need to recognise the impact of different cultures on each other over time, and how these now impact in multicultural societies (see Chapter 26).

Social class

Social class, based on employment classification, has a complex relationship with substance misuse. Factors such as poverty, geography, availability and culture again act as confounders. The unemployed have been reported as being more likely to have used, or to be using illicit drugs, but loss of employment has been shown to reduce alcohol consumption, and higher income is often associated with higher consumption of alcohol and some other drugs.

The impact of peers and family

The impact of peers in substance misuse has been highlighted, especially in relation to prevention and health promotion. The term 'peer pressure' is often used, although this does suggest a somewhat negative, passive, victim like picture. In reality friendships and peer relationships are interactive. Oetting and Beauvois (1988) suggest the term peer 'cluster' instead. Where parental relationships are perceived as inadequate and where substance misuse has commenced, the influence of peers can be stronger. Kandel (1980) suggests that young people choose friends who are like themselves whilst socialisation into friendship groups results in individuals adopting each other's beliefs, attitudes and behaviours. Steinberg *et al.* (1994) found that greater involvement in substance misuse amongst young people predicted that other peer group members would also misuse substances. Young people may develop peer groups as a result of their substance misusing behaviour and may misuse substances as a result of influence from the peer group.

Peer influence is not limited to the young nor is it generally negative. Positive effects of peer relationships include friendship, support and acceptance. These were all aspects identified by McKegany and Barnard (1992) in their study of needle sharing behaviour amongst Scottish injecting drug users. It was recognised that this behaviour was risky but also resulted in positive outcomes of solidarity and trust. Peer influence is used to more positive effect in group treatment, 12 step and other self-help organisations.

The role of the family has come under scrutiny. The idea of the substance misuser coming from a 'broken home' and this being the 'cause' of their problems may be too simplistic. What constitutes a broken home is in itself debatable (Wells and Rankin, 1991). It is suggested that family process in the form of effective parenting and characterised by warmth, affection, consistency and parental supervision is more important than family structure in relation to deviant conduct (ACMD, 1998) (see Chapter 10).

Availability and accessibility

Substance misuse has trends and fashions. This is, in part, to do with individual substance availability. When a substance becomes easily available and cheap it is more likely to be misused. An example of this can be seen in the waves of new heroin misuse to spread across the UK over the past thirty years. Local availability reflects a wider picture. A good crop of coca leaves (the source of cocaine) in South America, combined with better and cheaper transportation, may result in greater quantities of the drug reaching the streets of Europe. With a greater quantity of a drug circulating, market forces will tend to keep, or force the price down.

For a substance to reach the streets it has to pass through many hands. Drug dealing is a business with manufacturers, production operatives, employers and employees and, of course, customers. Like any other business, it is subject to market forces, supply and demand. Such forces can be manipulated. 'Droughts' can occur naturally or deliberately but the effect will be to push up the price and/or reduce the quality and may result in the 'customer' switching to another substance. 'Floods' can also occur, and when this happens after a period of reduced availability the purity of a drug may increase sharply, the price will fall and the risk of overdose will rise rapidly.

Other factors impacting on the availability of a drug include the development of new technology making the production of complex 'designer' drugs within the scope of any jobbing chemist with a basic laboratory and access to the relevant ingredients. The impact of legislation and the success (or failure) of interventions aimed at reducing the supply of drugs will be mediated by the geography of a country's boundaries, the resources available for enforcement and police and customs' priorities (see Chapter 17).

Culture and norms

Accessibility is not just about how easy a substance is to obtain, but is also about the way society views its use or misuse. Cannabis, once demonised as a potentially lethal drug, almost guaranteed to lead to social and moral degradation, is now viewed by many as relatively innocuous, even socially acceptable. Gin, once sold in vast quantities to the poorest people in society and eschewed by the rich, is now a perfectly acceptable aperitif at the poshest dinner parties (though it is rarely served in pint containers these days). The drinking of tea in the eighteenth century was viewed as potentially hazardous, whilst opium and cocaine were available over the counter until the early twentieth century.

Some substances have been specifically linked with cultural fashions, particularly with youth culture and the music scene. One recent example was the explosion of 'dance drugs' during the 1980s and 1990s. Ecstasy became the drug for a generation of rave goers. 'Old' substances such as LSD and amphetamines were 'rediscovered' and given a new cultural identity, alongside music, fashion and literature.

Substances are enjoyable

Although some people do experience outcomes that are negative on first experimenting with a substance (i.e. many new alcohol drinkers are sick) the positive results tend to outweigh the negative. As a practitioner engaged in helping people stop, or control their misuse and seeing at first hand the problems that can be caused by drugs and alcohol, it can sometimes be easy to forget the positive aspects. People don't use substances that make them feel awful unless there is some clear payback. A simple cost–benefit analysis occurs for most people with most substances. If alcohol always makes you ill you probably won't use it regularly or heavily. People misuse substances because they make you feel good, make you feel different, make you more sociable or relaxed, help you perceive things in more depth or in an alternative way, make you accepted by your peers, give you energy, or calm you down. Human beings are curious; we want to experience many things, of which substance use is but one of many. For the majority of people substance use has far more pluses than minuses.

WHY DO SOME PEOPLE EXPERIENCE PROBLEMS WITH SUBSTANCES?

Substance use is different from dependence or addiction. Substance misuse may be:

- experimental – the individual may be trying a substance for the first time, or first few times
- recreational – he or she misuses a substance on an occasional or social basis
- dependent – he or she has developed a dependent pattern of use on the substance and misuses it continuously; in life one should be very judicious in one's choice of addictions, and generally speaking substances are a problematic selection compared to work, exercise, shopping or chocolate.

Problems can occur at any of these stages, not just the dependent stage. For example, volatile substance misuse can result in death even at first experimentation. Recreational misuse of heroin may be intermittent leading to increased risk of overdose as tolerance decreases. Delineating these categories can be difficult. What constitutes 'recreational' use? When is someone 'dependent'? It is possible to be in all of these stages at once; for example someone who is dependent on benzodiazepines may recreationally misuse cannabis and experiment with Magic Mushrooms.

The gateway theory

The idea that misuse of one substance acts as a gateway, leading on to other, more fearful or potentially hazardous substances, is usually referred to as the gateway theory. Caution is necessary in interpreting the evidence. Studies confirm that early uptake of licit substances such as tobacco and alcohol do appear to have predictive value in relation to future misuse of illicit substances (Yamaguchi and Kandel, 1984. Balding, 1995) but there is no evidence to suggest that so-called 'soft' drugs such as cannabis inevitably lead on to 'hard' drugs like heroin. One argument for decriminalising soft drugs is to avoid users having to be in contact with black market sources of a whole range of drugs.

Dependent substance misuse

The World Health Organisation's definition of drug dependence includes recognition that this condition can be psychological and/or physical. It is demonstrated through behaviour and through a compulsion to take the drug either periodically or continuously. This continued use may occur in order to experience the effects of the substance or to avoid withdrawal symptoms. Tolerance need not necessarily be present. This definition also recognises that dependency can occur in relation to more than one substance at a time (WHO, 1969).

Edwards and Gross (1976) proposed a tentative description of an alcohol dependence syndrome, made up of seven elements. The idea of a dependence syndrome has been highly influential on international thinking and research ever since. The individual experiencing dependency syndrome will demonstrate some, or all, of the following;

1 A narrowing of their drinking repertoire. The substance misuse behaviour begins to play a greater part in the person's life, becoming a daily activity regardless of other responsibilities or settings.
2 Salience of behaviour. The substance misuse is prioritised above all else.
3 Increased tolerance. Increasingly larger amounts of the substance are required. This only holds true up to a certain point with some substances. For example, in alcohol misuse tolerance eventually declines to the point where smaller quantities of the substance are needed for intoxication to occur.
4 Repeated withdrawals. On cessation of the substance there are measurable withdrawal symptoms.
5 Relief of withdrawals by further misuse. Withdrawals are avoided by continued or resumption of misuse.
6 Subjective awareness of compulsion. The person may know that their behaviour is causing harm yet will continue to misuse and may find it hard not to think about the substance, experiencing cravings.
7 Rapid reinstatement following abstention. Previous levels of misuse are reached quickly following periods of cessation.

These factors were rapidly seen as relevant to substances other than alcohol and the syndrome idea has been brought in to contemporary definitions of dependence. There are two main tools used to categorise substance misuse disorders in clinical and research settings:

- The International Classification of Diseases (now in its tenth revision: ICD10) which is produced by the World Health Organisation (see Chapter 13), and
- The Diagnostic and Statistical Manual of the Mental Disorders (now in its fourth revision, DSM-IV) produced by the American Psychiatric Association (see Appendix 2.1).

THEORIES RELATING TO SUBSTANCE DEPENDENCE

What use is a theory?

Whilst there are a great many individual factors that may influence substance use and misuse, such factors do not in themselves constitute a theory. The dictionary defines theory as 'a system of ideas or statements explaining something, especially one based on general principles independent of the things to be explained' and 'The formulation of knowledge or speculative thought. The systematic conception of something' (Oxford Shorter Dictionary).

McMurran (1994) highlights that:

- theories work by enabling us to understand the processes which factors influence, and
- theory must fit the observable facts.

> For any theoretic approach to fit the facts [of substance use] it must describe the processes of initiation to, maintenance of and dependence upon the use of any substances and the processes involved in change.
> (McMurran, 1994: 33)

A theory therefore is a dynamic, systematic and explanatory understanding, that can help us direct the most appropriate responses to the issues.

There are many potential theories to underpin substance dependence. These may be broadly divided into (primarily) biological, psychological and sociological models. Some theorists try to insist on 'purity' and exclusivity by dint of professional training, experience, beliefs and values. Perhaps most of us are more closely allied to one particular strand of theory than others. The ability to comprehend the range of potential theoretical explanations enables the practitioner to work from a more considered viewpoint. A broad understanding can help to clarify differences between professional groups and agencies, thereby enhancing multidisciplinary and multiagency working.

Clients themselves are sometimes closely allied to a particular theoretical understanding of their problems. For example, an alcohol misuser who considers 'health' in a broadly physical fashion, who tends to prefer treatment by medication, who has had previous positive experiences of AA, believes that addiction is a disease and who believes strongly that hereditary factors play a major role in his or her condition, will be more comfortable with a counsellor or agency that shares these ideas. As a general rule clients take what they find helpful from any given intervention and care little about the models and beliefs of those trying to help.

The moral model

Early explanations for substance misuse problems focused on moral issues, with dependent individuals being viewed as 'weak willed' or 'sinful'. Such ideas predominated until the nineteenth century, and are by no means unknown now.

The 'treatment' for such a moral failing tends to concentrate on punishment, or on 'saving' the person, often by religious conversion. We may think of the moral model as outdated, but it remains widespread amongst the lay public and a minority of health and social care professionals.

Biological explanations

Within the biological frame there are two broad areas of current interest: those relating to individual biochemical interactions between the person and a substance and those connected with genetic, inherited factors.

Neurones and neurotransmitters

All psychoactive substances work by acting on the nervous system, which is made up of complex networks of neurones. Neurones are individual nerve cells which conduct 'messages' along their length by means of electrical impulses. Connections between neurones occur by means of chemical messengers (neurotransmitters), released when the electrical impulse reaches the synapse (the gap between adjoining neurones). In a connection between two synapses, A and B, an electrical impulse travels along A to the synapse and releases its particular neurotransmitter into the synaptic space. On the other side of the synaptic space, on the surface of the neurone B, lie receptor sites which are specific for different neurotransmitters. On plugging into the receptor, the neurotransmitter may stimulate neurone B to fire off a new wave of electical energy (excitatory), or may dampen it down, making it less likely to fire (inhibitory). Psychoactive drugs often have actions that mimic the effects of neurotransmitters, but may act on the production, metabolism or any other chemical process involved in these fantastically complex electrical and chemical systems. Five neurotransmitters have been particularly studied in connection with addictive behaviour.

The monoamines

Monoamines are a group of neurotransmitters, norepinepherine (noradrenalin), dopamine and serotonin (5-HT). 5-HT deficiency may be associated with risk of alcohol dependence, and dopamine is increasingly being seen as important to reward processing via the so-called dopamine pathway. Research increasingly looks for how pharmacological manipulation of these systems might impact on addictive behaviour.

GABA (gamma aminobutyric acid)

GABA is an inhibitory neurotransmitter in that it slows down or impedes the ability of neurones to fire. Depressant drugs, including benzodiazepines and alcohol, act partly via the GABA system.

Endorphins

Endorphins are the body's naturally occurring opioids, with their own specific receptor sites. They are closely connected with pain recognition and response. Different opioid drugs differ in the strength of their effects at the three main receptor types. Drugs that block the effects of opioids by fitting into receptor sites without effect (opioid antagonists such as naloxone) are already used in the treatment of both opioid and alcohol dependence.

Heredity and genetics

There is evidence that heredity plays a role in the predisposition of a person towards substance dependency. Alcohol studies of families strongly indicate a genetic component. Studies of identical and non-identical twins suggest that the former are very much more likely to be concordant for a substance misuse problem. Studies of adopted children also indicate that despite being brought up in families without alcohol problems, those with alcohol dependent birth parents were more likely to develop alcohol problems (Heath, 1995). It is estimated that 20–25 per cent of those with severe alcohol dependence may have an inherited predisposition (Badawy, 1996).

Biological theories are central to the Western medical approach to addiction. Rapid advances in genetic exploration and neuropsychopharmacology are opening up more possibilities than ever for understanding and for treatment (see Chapters 11 and 12).

Personality

Theories of personality lie somewhere between the biological and the psychological. Personality is a broad term which has no one single definition. Otter and Martin (1996) group explanations of personality into five classes.

- Type theories – the simplest and oldest model based explanations on the main characteristic believed to belong to that person, for example the 'melancholic' type.
- Trait theories – these identify a variable number of traits such as aggression, extroversion, introversion, etc. allowing a matrix to be drawn up to describe the whole personality.
- Social learning theories – focusing on the interplay between the person and their social environment.
- Psychoanalytic approaches – highlighting subconscious drives and defences.
- Phenomenological approaches – the focus here is on the subjective 'lived experience' of the individual and individual meanings.

The term 'addictive personality' is sometimes used, but Nathan (1988) and others have questioned the validity of this construct, concluding that there is no one type of personality more likely to misuse or develop dependence on substances. However, aspects of personality have been linked to substance misuse. Zukerman (1979) identified sensation seeking as a trait that may be common in those who choose to misuse substances, and self-medication for stress-dampening has also been highlighted (Sher, 1987). Other personality factors that are associated with substance misuse include antisocial personality characteristics and personality disorder, risk taking, novelty seeking, reward dependency and lack of harm avoidance (see Otter and Martin, 1996 for an overview of personality and dependency).

Psychological explanations

Psychological theories relate behaviour to processes that take place within the person's mind, as opposed to the physical structure that is the brain. McMurran (1994) highlights six of these as fulfilling the criteria of a 'theory' and having particular relevance to substance misuse and dependency:

- classical conditioning
- operant conditioning
- opponent process theory
- expectancy theory
- social learning theory
- problem behaviour theory

Classical conditioning

Classical conditioning was developed by the Russian physiologist Ivan Pavlov (1849–1936). Pavlov found that dogs produced saliva when they saw a food dish, in expectation of the meal to come. The saliva production was a behaviour which occurred when the animal was able to associate one stimuli (the dish) with another (the food). This association could be learnt. Pavlov went on to test whether dogs could make associations with other stimuli such as a bell rung prior to food delivery. He found they could, eventually the dog would produce saliva in response to the bell even if the food was not forthcoming. The food was the unconditioned stimulus and the initial salivation in response to food is the unconditioned response. The sound of the bell is the conditioned stimulus and the salivation in response to the bell is the conditioned response. Classical conditioning is relevant to cue responsiveness and anticipation in substance misuse.

Operant conditioning

Most of the activities we carry out are learnt. Operant conditioning, derived from the work of Skinner (1904–1990) focuses on how this learning occurs. The likelihood of a behaviour being reinforced depends on the rewards and punishments received in relation to this. Reinforcement may be positive (achieving the sought after intoxicated state) or negative (the avoidance of unpleasant withdrawals). Punishment may decrease behaviour and again may be positive (such as pain) or negative (a desired action is not possible because of intoxication). Reinforcers are subjective – what is pleasurable to one person may be unpleasant for another. The frequency, immediacy and regularity of reinforcement or punishment are mediating factors.

Opponent process theory

Opponent process theory (Solomon, 1980) works on the premise that individuals automatically regulate extremes of pleasure and displeasure. The mind seeks homeostasis (a stable state) by the production of opposing and contrasting affects. Over time the response to a stimuli will decrease and eventually affective withdrawal will occur so that the 'balancing' effect becomes dominant and the person's response is the opposite to that which he or she experienced when they undertook the activity.

Somebody in a bar may initially experience pleasure in response to the alcohol but his brain, in an attempt to balance this out, will produce the opposite affect so that he will cease gaining pleasure and develop a state of displeasure or withdrawal. Over time the individual may come to recognise this and increase his drinking, seeking to re-experience the pleasant reaction, or as a way of avoiding the unpleasant one (returning again to the concept of negative reinforcement). The end result may be a more vehement balancing attempt and greater withdrawal.

Expectancy theory

The ability to predict a potential outcome of a behaviour is addressed by expectancy theory (Tolman, 1932). This is based on the premise that everyone has some knowledge, based on observation and experience, of the probable outcomes of a behaviour. These outcome expectancies may not necessarily relate to the real effects of a substance. For example, the observation of alcohol being used as a relaxant may lead to an outcome expectancy that alcohol induces calm and removes stress. This belief may be tempered according to circumstance, context and internal cues. When tense and tired after a day's work alcohol may be used to relax at home, but if offered a drink at a party when feeling energised and buoyant alcohol will be accompanied by different expectations of increased confidence and liveliness.

Social learning theory

Developed by Bandura (1977) social learning theory has three aspects of particular significance to substance use:

1 Behaviour is shaped by what the person expects to happen as a result of a particular action. The short-term gratifying effects of a substance include feelings of enjoyment or the removal of unpleasant withdrawals. The long-

term benefits of cessation may be less motivating than the short-term rewards of continued misuse.

2 Modelling – the person may learn that certain behaviours have particular outcomes from observing others, either directly or indirectly. This may include, for example, media images and parental behaviour.

3 Self-efficacy – the person's self-perceived ability to change a behaviour is important. Even when the negative effects of a substance are recognised, if a person does not themselves feel capable of change then they are unlikely to try.

Problem behaviour theory

Problem behaviours such as substance misuse are seen clustered in individuals. Three areas, personality, environment and behaviour, are the focus of the theory. Each of these areas has triggers and controls in relation to the different problem behaviours, which combine to produce a level of 'proneness'. This theory argues that it would be unusual to find an individual with substance misuse without this being part of a bigger picture of problematic behaviours.

Other psychological theories may have relevance to initiation and/or continued substance misuse including:

Azjen and Fishbein's (1980) theory of reasoned action

Another integrative theory suggests that action results from a person's attitude towards a behaviour, their belief about a behaviour and the strength of this belief. This is influenced by the person's perception of what other significant people think.

Locus of control

The locus of control (LOC) construct is a single trait theory of personality. It centres around the individual's belief about personal control. The LOC may be perceived as external – the individual perceives their circumstances as hinging on the actions of other people, other factors and fate; or internal – the individual perceives themselves as in control of their situation. Dependent substance misusers may be more likely to have an external LOC, feeling themselves to have less power over their circumstance and less control over change. But the literature on LOC is inconsistent; in some cases substance misusers have been shown to have a higher internal LOC. Martin and Otter (1996) address the implications and potential of the LOC construct in relation to substance misuse.

Stages of change

Prochaska and Di Clemente's transtheoretical model is a multistage cyclical construct centred around motivation and readiness to change (see Chapter 7).

Environmental and social explanations

Though not necessarily constituting a 'theory' in terms of the definitions described above, environmental and social explanations are often drawn upon. The impact of social factors on substance misuse was discussed in the early part of this chapter, and recognition of the role that environmental elements have in relation to sustained substance misuse helps us to see theory within a broader context.

Social deprivation

Social deprivation is a blanket term which includes poverty, poor housing and living conditions, and restricted access to education, transport, work and recreation. Though most often connected with urban decay, deprivation can just as easily be a facet of rural life. The family of four living in a cottage in an isolated part of West Wales may be suffering as much 'deprivation' as a young man on a sink estate in an inner city part of the North of England. The Advisory Council on the Misuse of Drugs points out that deprivation may:

> relate more subtly to age of first use, progression to dependence, intravenous use and risky use, health and social complications of use and to criminal involvement.
>
> (ACMD 1998: 101)

Alternative explanations

Dean (1997) proposes a theory of dependence, centred on the modern science of Chaos Theory, which incorporates the role of chance and uncertainty in relation to Darwinian perspectives on the evolution of the mind and Edleman's theory of natural selection.

Davies (1993) explores issues in relation to attributional theory; the idea that the way 'addicts' describe their behaviour in terms of loss of 'control' or 'addiction' fulfils a social function and expectation. He questions the concept of free will and the idea that non-addicted behaviour is 'free' in a way that 'addicted' behaviour is not. He argues that individuals learn to express themselves using 'addicted' terminology – they 'talk like an addict'. As a result of doing this time and again in social situations the individual's behaviour adapts to fit the stereotype and endorse the social construct that is 'the addict'. Davies (1997) goes on to contest the legitimacy of traditional means of identifying the 'truth' such as psychological tests, questionnaires, etc. and proposes an alternative theory centred around the nature of discourse produced by those who misuse substances.

Conclusion

There are a number of possible reasons why someone may misuse a substance and a range of theories to suggest why this may become a problem for some of them.

Though there are individuals who hold a purist stance, useful contributions to understanding have been derived from biological, psychological and social theorists. No truly integrated theory yet exists and commonly utilised theories are in themselves flawed, obscuring the socially constructed nature of concepts such as 'dependence' and 'addiction'.

One thing is certain, substance misuse is unlikely to disappear. From the time people first discovered that by eating certain plants or animals we are able to experience something 'different' it has been clear that we like artificially altering our mental states. Just as some people will always be in search of the newest 'experience', there will be others who will be in search of 'why' and how best to help those who run into problems. As there is no one substance use experience and no one all encompassing theory, there can be no one specific response.

READER INPUT

Discussion

(a) Look at Table 2.1. Which factors do you think relate most to initial misuse and which to dependency?

(b) Can you suggest how a bumper crop of opium in one part of the world may impact on an individual drug user living in a town in the North of England? How and why could this impact on the many different factors involved in both experimental/ recreational substance misuse and continued misuse?

Groupwork exercise

- Split into two groups.
- Group A takes a strongly biological standpoint whilst group B is aligned with a more psychosocial belief structure.
- Take 10–15 minutes per group to put across the strong points of your particular group using the available evidence.
- As a class, or large group, discuss both the positive and negative aspects of each particular approach.
- This exercise may be done in more depth if you prepare for it in advance, perhaps focusing on one particular substance such as heroin, cocaine, cannabis, etc. Seek out new and contemporary evidence to back up your presentation. Consider a range of substances including licit ones and prescribed medication.

Note – this is not a competition. Neither group will be wholly 'right', rather it is an opportunity to explore the pros and cons of each standpoint.

Table 2.1 An overview of factors impacting on substance misuse and dependency

Biological aspects
- biochemical differences between individuals
- sensitivity to substances, strength and interactions of substances
- genetic predisposition and hereditary factors
- tolerance and withdrawal

Psychological
- personality factors
- experience – of substance, other substances, withdrawal and expectation
- craving
- vicarious observation, social learning and role models
- perceived importance and rationale of use/misuse of substance
- readiness to change – costs and benefits, motivation, self-efficacy in relation to change
- desire for homeostasis
- attribution
- self-image
- beliefs about substance and health messages
- attitudes – own and others
- esteem and assertiveness
- cues
- positive and negative reinforcement
- perception of risk

Socioenvironmental
- impact of peers and family
- availability and accessibility of substance/s – locally and globally
- impact of politics – here and abroad
- culture and norms, including impact of the media
- social and legal sanctions
- trends and fashions
- social factors – age, gender, ethnicity, class
- social costs of use and misuse
- services and help available
- deprivation

Note – these are not in any particular order, nor is the table exhaustive. You may be able to think of other factors which could be included. These factors, although apparently separate, have the potential to work together and affect each other positively or negatively, enhancing risk or protecting against it.

Reflection and self-awareness

- Look at Table 2.1 again and consider the factors in relation to your own substance misuse. Do you ever misuse any substances? Tea, coffee, cigarettes, alcohol, illicit substances? What factors do you consider lead to you initially trying the substance? What impacts on your current behaviour? Perhaps you have ceased misusing a substance – what factors impacted on this? Do you feel you have, or have had, a dependency? What may make you consider this to be the case? Can you relate your experiences to those of other people misusing different substances? Are there similarities or differences? Why might this be the case?

Note – this exercise is designed to be personal, you may not wish to share details with anyone else though you may find it helpful to discuss it with a mentor, tutor or supervisor if you wish.

Case scenario and discussion points

Chris does _______ every weekend. Chris first started doing _______ with a group of like-minded friends. It started off as experimental, they gave it a go to see what it was like. Not all of them continued (some couldn't bring themselves to do it in the first place) but Chris and close friend George carried on. They do it most weekends now. Chris describes how it felt the first time:

'It's brilliant. I get such a kick out of it. Knowing that I'm going to do it gets me really hyped up. I wake up thinking about it and from then until I do it I'm on pins. What's it going to be like this time? I used to get almost sick with anticipation before but now I just look forward to it. Then there's the rush. You get this amazing rush . . . pure adrenaline. If you've never done it you wouldn't believe how intense it can be. After a while it settles down and you get this peaceful feeling. It makes you feel really small in the whole scale of things, sort of in touch with everything, really alive. It really changes your perceptions. Afterwards you feel so good you want to do it again. I don't think anything else really comes close to that first time though and I guess that's what I look for every time I do it. It's fairly risky, I know that. I mean people have died, there was this bloke last year . . . but I know the risks and I'm as careful as possible. If I worried then I wouldn't do it at all, I guess you have to let fate dictate how it turns out to a certain degree. My mother worries herself sick, keeps thinking I'm going to end up in hospital or worse but she doesn't really understand. She's never done it. If I don't get to do it on a weekend now I really miss it.'

Q What is Chris talking about? Heroin? Cocaine? Ecstasy?
A Actually the experience being described is hang-gliding.

- Consider Chris's description of the experience of hang-gliding. How does this relate to concepts such as 'addiction' and 'risk'? How socially constructed do you consider such concepts to be and what might the implications of this be in relation to discourses around substance use and misuse?
- If you discovered Chris was female, divorced and the mother of two children would this impact on your attitude or beliefs.

FURTHER READING

McMurran, M. (1994) *The Psychology of Addiction*, London: Taylor & Francis.

Bonner, A. and Waterhouse, J. (eds) *Addictive Behaviour: Molecules to Mankind. Perspectives on the Nature of Addiction*, Hampshire: Macmillan Press.

Davies, J.B. (1997) *Drugspeak: The Analysis of Drug Discourse*, Amsterdam: Harwood Academic Press.

Dean, A. (1997) *Chaos and Intoxication: Complexity and Adaptation in the Structure of Human Nature*, London: Routledge.

REFERENCES

Advisory Council on the Misuse of Drugs (1998) *Drug Misuse and the Environment*, London: Home Office.

American Psychiatric Association (2000) *Diagnostic and Statistical Manual of Mental Disorders* (4th edn), Text Revision, Washington DC, American Psychiatric Association.

Azjen, I. and Fishbein, M. (1980) *Understanding Attitudes and Predicting Social Behaviour*, Englewood Cliffs, NJ: Prentice-Hall.

Badaway, A.A.B. (1996) 'The neurobiological background to the study of addiction' in A. Bonner and J. Waterhouse (eds) *Addictive Behaviour: Molecules to Mankind. Perspectives on the Nature of Addiction*, Hampshire: Macmillan.

Balding, J. (1995) *Young People in 1994. Social Health Education Report*, University of Exeter.

Bandura, A. (1977) *Social Learning Theory*, New York: Prentice-Hall.

Dean, A. (1997) *Chaos and Intoxication: Complexity and Adaptation in the Structure of Human Nature*, London: Routledge.

Davies, J.B. (1993) *The Myth of Addiction*, London: Harwood Academic Press.

Davies, J.B. (1997) *Drugspeak: The Analysis of Drug Discourse*, Amsterdam: Harwood Academic Press.

Edwards, G. and Gross, M.M. (1976) 'Alcohol dependence: provisional description of a clinical syndrome', *British Medical Journal* 1: 1958–61.

Jones, J. (1700) cited in Porter, R. (ed.) (1991) *The Faber Book of Madness*, London: Faber & Faber, p. 51.

Heath, A.C. (1995) 'Genetic influences on alcoholism risk', *Alcohol Health and Research World* 19 (3): 166–71.

Kandel, D.B. (1980) 'Drug and drinking behaviour among youth', *Annual Review of Sociology* 6: 235–85.

McKeganey, N. and Barnard, M. (1992) *AIDS, Drugs and Sexual Risk*, Buckingham, Open University Press.

Martin, C. and Otter, C. (1996) 'Locus of control and addictive behaviour', in A. Bonner and J. Waterhouse (eds) *Addictive Behaviour: Molecules to Mankind. Perspectives on the Nature of Addiction*, Hampshire: Macmillan.

McMurran, M. (1994) *The Psychology of Addiction*, London: Taylor & Francis.

Miller, P. and Plant, M. (1996) 'Drinking, smoking and illicit drug use among 15 and 16 year olds in the United Kingdom', *British Medical Journal* 313: 394–7.

Nathan, P.E (1988) 'The addictive personality is the behaviour of the addict', *Journal of Consulting and Clinical Psychology* 56: 183–8.

Oetting, E.R. and Beauvois, F. (1988) 'Common elements in youth drug abuse: peer clusters and other psychosocial factors', in S. Peele (ed.) *Visions of Addiction: Major*

Contemporary Perspectives on Addiction and Alcoholism, Lexington, MA: Lexington Books, pp. 141–61.

Otter, C. and Martin, C. (1996) 'Personality and addictive behaviours', in A. Bonner and J. Waterhouse (eds) *Addictive Behaviour: Molecules to Mankind. Perspectives on the Nature of Addiction*, Hampshire: Macmillan.

Ramsay, M. and Spiller, J. (1997) *Drug Misuse Declared: Results of the 1996 British Crime Survey*, London, Home Office.

Sher, K.J. (1987) 'Stress response dampening', in H.T. Blane and K.E. Leonard (eds) *Psychological Theories of Drinking and Alcoholism*, New York: Guilford Press, pp. 227–71.

Solomon, R.L. (1980) 'The opponent process theory of aquired motivation: the affective dynamics of addiction', *American Psychologist* 35: 691–712.

Steinberg, L., Fletcher, A. and Darling, N. (1994) 'Parental monitoring and peer influences on adolescent substance use', *Paediatrics* 93: 1060–4.

Tolman, E.G. (1932) *Purposive Behaviour in Animals and Man*, New York: Appleton Century Crofts.

Wells, L.E. and Rankin, J.H. (1991) 'Families and delinquency: a meta analysis of the impact of broken homes', *Social Problems* 38: 71–93.

World Health Organisation (1969) *Sixteenth Report of WHO Expert Committee on Drug Dependence*, Technical Report Series No. 407, WHO: Geneva.

Yamaguchi, K. and Kandel, D. (1984) 'Patterns of drug use from adolescence to young adulthood. Sequences of progression', *American Journal of Public Health* 74: 668–72.

Zuckerman, M. (1979) *Sensation Seeking: Beyond the Optimal Level of Arousal*, New York: John Wiley and Sons.

APPENDIX 2.1

DSM criteria and definitions

The current edition of the DSM is the DSM-IV. DSM criteria utilises the term substance related disorders as an overall title, but categorises substance use disorders into substance dependence, substance abuse and substance induced disorders which includes substance intoxication and substance withdrawal along with a range of specific substance induced disorders such as substance induced delirium, substance induced persisting amnesia, substance induced psychotic disorder, etc.

Substance dependence

A differentiation is made between dependence and abuse. The former is identified by the presence of three or more criteria in the same 12 month period. Criteria includes:

- Tolerance – defined either by a need for markedly increased amount of the substance to achieve intoxication or desired effect or a markedly diminished effect with continued use of the same amount of the substance.
- Withdrawal – manifested by either characteristic withdrawal syndrome or by the individual taking the substance (or a related substance in order to avoid withdrawals).

- Increases – in amounts of substance taken or in time scale (i.e. the substance is taken for longer than was intended).
- Persistent desire – 'craving' or unsuccessful attempts to cut down or control substance misuse may exist.
- Time spent – much time is spent on activities needed to obtain the substance, use it or recover from it.
- Loss of other activities – this may occur as a result of substance use.
- Continued use despite negative effects – this can occur even where the potential damage is quite clear to the individual.
- Specifiers are added to identify whether the dependency has physiological dependence or not. Further specifiers identifying the course of dependency are added, including remission (full, partial, early or sustained), agonist therapy and the individual being in a controlled environment.

Substance abuse

Substance abuse applies to maladaptive patterns of use which leads to clinically significant impairment or distress, manifested by one or more criteria within a 12 month period. The criteria identified centre on recurrent use that may:

- lead to failure fulfilling major role obligations
- occur in situations which may be physically dangerous
- result in legal problems
- cause or exacerbate social or interpersonal problems.

If the individual fulfils the criteria for substance dependency then a diagnosis of substance abuse does not apply. This category does not apply to nicotine or caffeine.

Intoxication and withdrawal

Substance intoxication criteria highlight three criteria:

- the development of a reversible substance specific syndrome which will vary according to substance
- clinically significant changes due to the substances effect on the central nervous system
- there is no other explanation for symptoms (i.e. another medical or psychiatric condition).

Substance withdrawal also highlights three criteria:

- a substance specific withdrawal syndrome following cessation
- the above withdrawal syndrome results in clinically significant distress or psychosocial impairment
- as with intoxication, there is no other explanation for the symptoms.

Substance induced disorders

A wide range of substance induced disorders are highlighted in the DSM. To reduce the likelihood of differential diagnosis these are included in the manual's sections on those disorders which share similar symptoms. For example, substance induced anxiety disorder is included under the heading of 'Anxiety disorders'. Alcohol is dealt with as a separate diagnostic area and reflects the criteria and definitions set out in the more general substance use and substance induced disorders.

Diagnostic codes

Each diagnosis is given a code number. For example, cocaine dependence (304.20); cocaine abuse (305.60); opiate dependence (304.00); opiod abuse (305.50). Such codes for dependence and abuse are available for most substances. Eleven specific substance classifications are identified (i.e. alcohol, inhalants, nicotine, opiods, sedatives, etc.) alongside polysubstance dependency and other, or unknown substance related disorders. This final classification includes prescribed and over-the-counter medications and toxins, such as heavy metals, antifreeze (ethylene glycol), pesticides and harmful gases. In addition, specific substance induced disorders are listed, for example opiod induced mood disorder (292.84).

CHAPTER 3

WORKING EFFECTIVELY WITH SUBSTANCE MISUSERS

Trudi Petersen

LEARNING OBJECTIVES

By the end of this chapter you should be able to:

1. Identify the skills, knowledge and attitudes involved in effective substance misuse practice, the activities and processes that help to maintain good practice and how these relate to your own practice.
2. Identify your own training needs, the means by which you can attain the relevant skills, knowledge and attitudes and how these might be evaluated.

INTRODUCTION

This chapter looks at the skills, knowledge and attitudes necessary to work effectively with a substance misusing client group and some elements of maintaining good practice. At the end is a short questionnaire – the Competency Assessment Tool (CAT). This has been developed to enable you to identify your own personal learning needs in conjunction with an appropriate supervisor or mentor. It is hoped that this may help you logically to progress in your practice and enable you to identify your current and future training goals.

EXISTING TRAINING AND EDUCATIONAL PROVISION

Self-reported drug use in England and Wales suggests that around 10 per cent of 16–59-year-old adults use an illegal substance annually (Ramsey and Spiller, 1997), and more than 90 per cent drink alcohol. Only a small proportion of these individuals come into contact with specialist substance misuse services. The total number of drug misusers presenting for treatment in the UK, in the six months ending March 1998 was around 30,000 (DoH, 1999b).

Substance misusers come into contact with a wide range of health and social care providers including: emergency health care staff, primary health care teams, social services, acute medical and surgical services, occupational health schemes, criminal justice agencies, child-care workers, community staff, non-statutory sector groups, community pharmacists, housing and benefits agencies – indeed just about everybody. Unsurprisingly, a number of professional groups have identified deficits in the education and training available surrounding substance misuse.

Nursing

A training needs analysis carried out in the mid-1990s (ENB, 1995) suggested that the provision of training and education had not at that time created a workforce considered 'fit for purpose' in relation to substance misuse practice. Disproportionately small amounts of time are spent on nurse education in this regard (Falkowski and Ghodse, 1990). Guidelines developed by the ENB highlight the need for a systematic approach to training and education (ENB, 1996).

Medicine

A training need has also been demonstrated amongst doctors, especially GPs, who, being in the front line are most likely to come into contact with this client group (Glanz, 1986; Bury *et al.*, 1996; Hindler *et al.*, 1996; Martin, 1996). The Department of Health guidelines on the clinical management of drug misusers (DoH, 1999a) defines doctors as:

- Generalists – those not having substance misuse as a main area of work.
- Specialised generalists – those with a special interest in drug misusers but whose work is not primarily centred around this.
- Specialists – those who provide expertise in drug misuse treatment as a main clinical activity.

Training is highlighted specifically for generalists in shared care arrangements. Such training should be locally delivered with the involvement of specialist providers, using national guidelines and material where appropriate and incorporating a list of suggested core topics. The needs of the primary health care team and local circumstance should be taken into account. It is recognised that training has to include the needs of other front line staff such as receptionists, managers and other clinical team members.

The non-statutory sector

Non-statutory sector groups range from large, quasi-professional, organisations capable of developing sophisticated training routes through to two people working part time in shared, rented space. Non-statutory sector training reflects this diversity. Some agencies support employees in gaining accredited, higher level qualifications; for example Alcohol Concern have developed minimum standards for the training of volunteer alcohol counsellors (VACTS) providing the equivalent of Level 3 training for non-professional staff (Alcohol Concern, 1993). In other settings training may be provided in-house with no guarantee of quality.

Other groups listed above will each have their own training needs, influenced by the type of contact they have with substance misusers.

Levels of training and educational need amongst practitioners

Not everyone requires the same level of training. The Advisory Council on the Misuse of Drugs (ACMD 1990) identifies three levels in relation to professional staff.

Level 1 is basic training directed at all staff through pre-qualification courses or via in-service training. This concentrates on basic information about substances, attitudes and knowledge around appropriate referral of clients.

Level 2 is more advanced, aimed at staff who have specific involvement with substance misusers but who would not be classed as 'specialists'. Professional groups could include nursing staff, GPs, the police, etc. Training is provided by in-service training and post-qualification courses. Content is more detailed, looking at a wider range of interventions and specifically at particular professional issues.

Level 3 concentrates on specialist substance misuse practitioners, providing more in-depth theory and practice applications facilitated through accredited courses in substance misuse.

Attitudes

Level 1 of the ACMD professional training levels identifies 'attitude' as central to basic training. Before the early 1980s working with drug users was not considered part of normal practice by health-care workers (Carroll, 1996). It has been argued since that substance misuse is 'everybody's business' (Rassool, 1998). Yet despite increased recognition of professional roles and responsibilities, attitudes often remain poor.

Negative attitudes do not go unnoticed by clients. One small study of twenty illicit drug users in Northern Ireland found that all had experienced 'care' that they felt to be 'filled with judgement, hostility and loathing' (McLaughlin *et al.*, 2000). Research carried out amongst nursing staff has found that attitudes are related to clinical grade; higher status staff having more positive attitudes. It is suggested this may, in part, be to do with peer pressure and autonomy in practice (Carroll, 1996).

Training is linked with improved attitudes (Cartwright, 1980) but content needs to go beyond simple information giving about substances. An examination of exposure of medical students to substance misuse topics found that even those who had a high level of exposure to core topics on substance misuse were unable to demonstrate clinical proficiency in the topic (Wymer *et al.*, 1996). Good working relationships with specialist services have been identified as one potential source of improved confidence (Davies and Huxley, 1997) and better attitudes.

Empathy

Empathy is the ability to understand the meaning of life for another person. Getting 'inside their skin' whilst still maintaining an objective grip on the current clinical situation. It may not always be easy to empathise with someone who misuses substances, especially if this involves lifestyles we could not see ourselves living, as this can make us uncomfortable. Difficulties with empathy are not a problem only for professionals. Ex-misusers often make excellent counsellors and may be able to relate to certain aspects of another person's situation only too well; but having experienced substance misuse is not a 'qualification' for good practice. The experience of substance misuse is always subjective. The ex-misuser/practitioner who is unable to separate their own experiences from those of their client cannot demonstrate accurate empathy.

Reynolds *et al.* (1999) reviewed the literature on empathy, pointing to the difficulties involved in measuring it. They suggested that clients themselves should be consulted to help measure and define empathy. Tschudin (1982) offers a vivid analogy, describing the person in need as having fallen into a ditch. The sympathetic helper is described as lying in the ditch with the person, bewailing the situation. The unsympathetic helper shouts at the victim to get out of the ditch. The empathic helper 'climbs down to the victim but keeps one foot on the bank thus being able to help the victim out of the trouble on to firm ground again'. The skill of empathic working involves keeping a balance between the ditch and the bank.

Exploring your own attitudes and encouraging positive attitudes amongst others

There is a certain amount of truth in the idea that attitudes are 'caught' not 'taught'. Being around people who have negative attitudes can make it difficult to maintain a positive approach. This does not mean that people should not be allowed to express negativity but this should be done in a way that enables the issue to be explored and strategies put in place for managing this. Encouraging a questioning approach to negative attitudes as part of team working is one way of doing this.

Practitioners need to have time for self-awareness, development and reflection. Supervision and support are important components. One of the things that may impact on attitude is the nature of client contact. Many agencies tend to see people only in times of need. It is easy to forget that there are many individuals who do resolve their substance misuse problems, often with no professional input. Possible reasons for change in this population include a general weighing up of the pros and cons of continuing and major events such as alcohol related illness (Sobell *et al.*, 1993). It is important to remember that circumstances and people can and do change.

KNOWLEDGE

The knowledge base of the individual practitioner will vary in relation to role, activities, training, experience and need for specific knowledge. Basic knowledge should be sought in the following areas: substances of misuse, contextual knowledge, basic health knowledge (including mental health issues), treatment options, the law and relevant policy and strategy. Identification of current knowledge and understanding of the means by which knowledge can be enhanced including courses and sources of literature such as books and journals that can help to shape the development of a good knowledge base.

Knowledge of commonly used substances of misuse

- The main effects and side effects.
- An understanding of how the substance is commonly used.
- An awareness of the physical signs of recent or prolonged misuse, i.e. level of consciousness, pupil size, clarity of speech, motor skills, signs of administration such as track marks and withdrawal symptoms.
- The legal status of the substance is useful both for advising clients and to avoid being compromised through ignorance.
- A knowledge of substance combinations is important, especially where this might result in increased risk to the individual.
- An understanding of the concept of tolerance is important, especially in relation to prescribing practices, working with clients in crisis situations and in order to promote health education messages about 'safer' substance misuse (i.e. avoidance of overdose).
- It may be useful to know what the substance looks like though this is not usually essential.
- The background and history of a substance can be interesting but this is rarely essential (see Chapter 2).

Contextual knowledge

- What are the most frequently misused substances? Are there any particular special areas of interest which may not be reflected in other geographic areas? For example, if the area has a lot of gyms and a culture of body-building this may be reflected in the use of needle exchange facilities by anabolic steroid users.

- What are the demographics of the area? Do these reflect the client profile of the available services? What about levels of deprivation and ill health? Economically deprived areas may demonstrate different substance misuse patterns from more affluent areas. How might the socio-economic background influence patterns of use?
- What are local drug prices? What is the drug 'market' like? What is the balance between illicit drugs and diverted pharmaceuticals? How do people generally pay for their illicit drugs? Local agencies and colleagues are good sources of information, but perhaps the best source is the clients themselves.
- What is the make-up and size of agencies and who do they see? What treatment options are available and are there any areas of specialist expertise? What are the links between substance misuse agencies and other agencies such as primary care? Are there gaps in service provision?

Basic health knowledge

- Basic first aid knowledge, including overdose recognition and response.
- Recognition of damage and infection – local and systemic – which may result from injecting substances.
- A basic knowledge of viral diseases – Hepatitis B and C and HIV in particular.
- Recognition of common physical conditions related to substance misuse.
- Recognition of common mental health problems related to substance misuse.
- Knowledge of treatment options including sources of specialist help.
- It is not necessary to be an 'expert' on all forms of therapy but it is useful to have an overall knowledge of the kinds of therapy and treatment that exist, who they may be suitable for, what they consist of, where and how they might be accessed. Again, different practitioners have different requirements. For example medical staff require a good knowledge of prescribing, drug interactions, dose titration, potential side effects, etc. in order to ensure safe practice.

TRAINING

Training is available from many sources. Seminars and short courses are often advertised in journals and in flyers sent to agency managers. Individual agencies may offer their own training packages either alone or in conjunction with other organisations. Accredited substance misuse training up to MSc level is available at several sites in the UK. Many of these are modular or part time, and some are available by distance learning. Trusts, Health Authorities and other local bodies may offer training days.

Funding for training may be possible through your employer or you may find yourself having to pay for it yourself. Are any grants or bursaries available (conferences often offer a number of subsidised places)? Local training departments or research and development (R&D) units should have information on what is available or you can find out through professional bodies such as the RCN. Some training is mandatory for health professionals and should be funded by employing authorities. Where your job necessitates specific training, employers are obliged to ensure that you receive it.

Evidence based practice and clinical effectiveness

Practitioners must ensure that treatments they offer are supported by evidence of effectiveness. In reality this is not always as easy as it sounds. Greenhalgh (1996) points out that there are numerous difficulties involved in establishing how evidence based on any particular practice might be sought, and in substance misuse interventions there are additional methodological and practical complications. Both 'science' and 'art' elements are important components of practice (Sackett *et al.*, 1996), the latter including elements such as interpretation, narrative and intuition.

There is a need to explore what we do in practice. What aspects of our practice are useful? Is our practice safe? Beneficial? What is our rationale for doing what we do? It is simply not enough to say, 'I do this because I've always done it this way', or because 'I have been told to do it like this'. Greenhalgh (1996) provides a medically orientated, context specific, checklist for individual clinical encounters which asks:

'Have you . . .'

- identified and prioritised clinical, psychological, social and other problems, taking into account the patient's perspective?
- performed a sufficiently competent and complete assessment to establish the likelihood of competing diagnosis (or main problem)?
- considered additional problems and risk factors?
- where necessary, sought relevant evidence from systematic reviews, guidelines, clinical trials and other sources?
- assessed and taken into account the completeness, quality and strength of the evidence and its relevance to this patient?
- presented the pros and cons of different helping options to the patient in a way they can understand, and incorporated the patient's views into the final treatment plan?

Being able to identify the relative usefulness of the evidence requires a degree of research awareness and critical reading skill. There are a number of basic textbooks on the subject of research. Most universities offer short modules on research awareness. Is there anyone in your workplace who could help you develop a basic understanding of research issues?

Skills

Interpersonal skills

Substance misuse work is an interactive process. Good communication skills are an essential component. Communication is both verbal and non-verbal. Verbal communication incorporates pitch, speed and tone as well as the vocabulary and grammar used. Communication within a therapeutic relationship differs from that used in everyday conversation. Underlying the therapeutic conversation lies one or more agenda. This may be a requirement to obtain answers to questions, as would be found during an assessment interview, or the need to shape the interaction towards a particular goal such as exploration of feelings or imparting new information to the client. Communication also involves listening. The ability to actively 'listen', and convey empathy and a desire to understand, as opposed to just 'hearing', is a skill in itself. Non-verbal communication includes the use of body language, gesture, eye contact, touch and personal space. The communication skills used in interacting with substance misusers are no different from those used in any other client/practitioner relationship, but there are a few points worth noting.

Effects of substances on body Someone who has recently used a stimulant such as amphetamine will be unable to relax, they may fidget and find it hard to sit still. They may clench their jaw muscles and grind their teeth. Their verbal communication is likely to be rapid and intense. Someone using opiates may come across as drowsy and relaxed. Their speech may be slurred and cognitive functioning appear slow. Withdrawals may make the person uncomfortable. They may be craving and irritable, in a hurry to finish the session and leave.

Interpretation of communication Expressions of bizarre or persecutory ideas or hallucinations may be an indication of underlying mental ill health or may be a result of drug misuse. Poor eye contact may be a sign of shyness and social discomfort or an indication that someone is not telling you the truth and is feeling uncomfortable about it. It may be an indication that they feel their personal space has been invaded, or they may be embarrassed. It may also be a way of the client avoiding your seeing their pupils, which would indicate they have used a particular substance. The client sitting with their arms folded tightly may be feeling anxious, defensive or aggressive, or they may be trying to avoid letting you see trackmarks on the backs of their hands or forearms.

Language Some practitioners express concern over the type of language they feel they should use with substance misusers. The slang of substance misuse can be diverse and confusing, varying according to geography. Having some knowledge of this can aid understanding of what the client (who may never use the technically correct term for a substance) tells you; but beware of the temptation to use slang in an attempt to make the client feel 'at home'. If it is not comfortable for you to use the same language as the client then don't; you will only end up feeling awkward and probably sounding foolish. Inappropriate use of slang may make the client think you are trying to be humorous, sarcastic or perhaps – worst of all – cool.

Good communication skills require practice. One way of doing this is through the use of video recording. Videoing your own interactions, either with a client (ensuring of course that permission is obtained and confidentiality maintained) or via role play can identify strengths and areas for improvement. It can be especially helpful to view and discuss this with a supervisor or mentor.

Boundary setting

Clients need to be made aware of acceptable boundaries of behaviour. Organisations should inform clients of these from the outset. It is useful to have such 'rules' in written form so that the client is able to discuss the rationale with a member of the team and take the material away with them. Whatever service boundaries are agreed, all staff should play a part in their development and must be aware of them. Where a client has transgressed, but the practitioner feels that discharge from the service would be unhelpful, a team agreement should be made as to future actions. An organisation without boundaries is likely to be a chaotic and unsafe place for staff and service users. Over-strict boundaries can make everybody feel too constrained and exclude those most in need from the most appropriate help. When a client is discharged from a service because they have been unable to work within the organisation's ground rules, appropriate alternatives, or future options should be made clear. The Association of Nurses in Substance Abuse use an example of treatment boundaries from a Manchester Drug Service (ANSA, 1997) which prohibits:

- aggressive, offensive or violent behaviour both on the premises and at other sites which may bring the service into disrepute
- bringing illicit drugs or alcohol onto the premises
- theft of property and bringing stolen property onto the premises
- drug dealing on the premises
- prescription loss and altering prescriptions.

Confidentiality

Practitioners should be aware of their own responsibilities within the boundaries of confidentiality and should remember that the information they have about clients is personal and privileged (see Chapter 4).

Working with 'difficult' behaviour

Some individuals can be a challenge to work with. Such clients are sometimes described as 'difficult' or 'problem' clients. This kind of labelling is generally unhelpful. Clients can express challenging behaviours for a variety of reasons, but particularly anxiety and a sense of powerlessness. Sullivan (1995) identifies three common defences employed by substance misusers:

- Denial – the person does not acknowledge the effects of their behaviour. Denial may be demonstrated by lying about, minimising, or blaming others for drug use and other behaviours.
- Projection – the person attributes their own characteristics or behaviour to others.
- Rationalisation – the person may give the impression of having made a considered choice, justifying behaviour and not giving the 'real' reasons for their continued use.

'Manipulation' is another form of 'difficult' behaviour defined by Sullivan as, 'an enduring use of patterns of behaviour aimed at immediately satisfying one's own needs while disregarding the rights and needs of others', Sullivan (1995): 129.

People who are good at manipulating others are rarely caught at it, and are probably running your organisation right now. Those whose social skills point them up as 'manipulative', rarely achieve their goals in relationships and rely on reducing those around them to similarly poor levels of communication and frustration. Such 'manipulative' behaviour triggers emotional reactions, notably anger, in everybody. Expectations and boundaries must be clear to all staff and the client. You must avoid being pulled into the conflict and chaos. Messages need to be simple, clear and consistent and the consequences of boundary breaking need to be realistic, enforceable and followed through. Some clients will inevitably seek to test every boundary raised, and some achieve extraordinarily skill at damaging their own ends in this way. It is important that practitioners involved in dealing with 'difficult' behaviours have access to support through team discussion and clinical supervision.

As Gossop (1993: 181) sagely points out:

> The drug addict is not an evil, vicious and depraved individual; nor is he a perfectly normal person suffering from a metabolic disease. Addicts are individuals. Some are friendly, others are hostile; some are law abiding, many are not. There is no such thing as a single addictive personality nor is there a single addict lifestyle.

Specific task orientated skills

Some areas require specific task orientated skills. If your role requires you to carry out such activities you should ensure that you have appropriate training. Nurses working in substance misuse should have an awareness of the scope of professional practice (UKCC, 1992) and work within the guidelines outlined by this document. Whatever your background you should not participate in any activity that you do not consider yourself adequately trained in or able to carry out. This includes even apparently simple activities such as:

- on site testing of urine samples
- use of a breathalyser
- blood pressure monitoring
- hair test sampling
- methadone dispensing
- giving safer injecting advice
- wound care and dressings
- giving safer sex advice
- pre-test counselling
- writing of records, notes and reports

Stress, burnout and self-management

Cherniss (1995) identifies a variety of potential stresses amongst newly qualified professionals that may ultimately lead to burnout, including:

- Competency crises – the belief that to be 'good' in a particular professional role one always has to be 'on top of things' and not 'failing'.
- Client difficulties. Clients who are unappreciative, dishonest, uncooperative or lacking in basic skills can lead to poor self-esteem amongst staff. Practitioners feel that they are making a commitment and become demoralised and disillusioned when this is not recognised.
- Boredom and routine. The intellectual stimulation of training may not carry over into professional life. Some professionals feel that they do little but meaningless drudgery.
- Lack of collegiality. When feedback and support are not forthcoming from colleagues practitioners can become demotivated, frustrated and unhappy.
- Social factors have an impact including the effect of bureaucracy, society's ambivalence towards helping the needy and an increasingly consumerist/litigious ethos.

For substance misuse practice each of these areas has resonance. Effective self-management is needed to avoid burnout and stress. This can be facilitated in work through supervision and other forms of support. It is also important to realise that work is only a part of life. The healthiest people are those who maintain a balance between work and non-work activities. Johnstone (1999) suggests ways of avoiding and managing burnout including:

- recognising and monitoring stress
- reviewing expectations and obligations
- reviewing support networks
- experiencing success
- the development of a positive 'emotional bank balance'

The reflective substance misuse practitioner

Practice is not static, every action is an opportunity for learning and development. Most people learn from their experiences, often this is not done through a formalised technique but through a more general recognition of what does and doesn't work. We 'muddle through' much of the time, basing some of our actions on research, some on common sense, some on previous experiences and some on intuition. That is the reality of practice. Anyone who claims only ever to carry out actions that are entirely considered and research based can most kindly be considered to lack self-awareness. Sometimes, especially when a situation has been challenging, or the outcome negative, it can be difficult to reflect accurately on what happened. The practitioner may be tempted to see the situation in simplistic terms or resort to the most obvious 'reason'. It is often these situations which are the most potentially fruitful sources of learning. It can be helpful to have a more formalised means of reflecting. There are several reflective tools that can be used. One of the best known is Schon's (1983) cycle of reflection. Schon splits the event being reflected upon into five sections:

1 Description – what was the event, how did you decide to deal with it and why?
2 Reaction – what happened? How did you and other people feel and think about this?
3 Analysis – how do you account for what happened?
4 Evaluation – how can you make sense of this? Could you have done anything else?
5 Synthesis – If this situation arose again what would you do? Would you change anything?

The practitioner is asked to work through each of these in turn, reviewing, learning and finally applying knowledge gained during the reflective process to practice. The use of such a structured model can be helpful as part of clinical supervision.

Clinical supervision

Clinical supervision is described as having three functions (Department of Health, 1994):

- A formative or educational function which aims to develop skills, abilities and understanding.
- A restorative function, which offers support and enables the practitioner to manage the stress and distress that can be generated in clinical practice.
- A normative or management function, which is a form of quality control, enabling standards to be met and maintained.

Supervision is an important aspect of practice. All practitioners should have access to supervision and it should be a management and staff priority. It is tempting, when work pressures are great and time short, to 'put off' supervision, but this is the very time that it is most needed. Clinical supervision is usually carried out by a practitioner or manager of a higher level; but other varieties, including peer supervision and external supervision, can be particularly helpful in some settings.

Lifelong learning

Learning and training should be a central aspect of everybody's professional development. Everybody should have a personal development plan to run alongside appropriate assessment of their work and appraisal of themselves. Such a plan should be reviewed regularly to ensure that old tricks and new knowledge and skills are regularly upgraded. For doctors these processes will soon be central for revalidation, and continued license to practice. The United Kingdom Central Council for Nursing, Midwifery and health visiting point out that:

> Lifelong learning is more than simply keeping up to date. It requires an enquiring approach (to the practice of nursing, midwifery and health visiting), as well as to issues which impact on practice.
>
> (UKCC, 2001)

Professional development and competency require all practitioners to demonstrate responsibility for their own learning and be able to recognise when further learning is required. Some professional groups have a mandatory requirement to demonstrate regular training but the underlying messages of lifelong learning are applicable to any practitioner group.

Reviewing and sharing practice

There are many ways of reviewing practice – individual supervisison and feedback, audit, and performance review amongst them. Good practice can be shared on a local level through team discussion, or on a larger scale through publication, conference presentations or other public fora. Some agencies run 'journal clubs' which are an excellent means of sharing contemporary information with colleagues. Special interest groups exist in some areas for practitioners from a range of backgrounds. Most professional bodies have individual fora for speciality topics and specific associations such as the Association of Nurses in Substance Abuse exist to help practitioners develop a network of colleagues and to promote good practice nation-wide.

Conclusions

Effective substance misuse practice involves knowledge, skills and attitudes. Good practice is dynamic, with a rich mix of theoretical and practical aspects and a range of treatment approaches. Practitioners may be professional or non-professional, rooted in health or social care backgrounds. There are excellent opportunities for career development, specialism, professional growth, lifelong learrning and reflective practice, which offer much for the curious practitioner.

READER INPUT

The reader input for this chapter centres on completion of the Competency Assessment Tool, which is described next.

REFERENCES

Advisory Council on the Misuse of Drugs (1990) *Problem Drug Use: A Review of the Training*, London: HMSO.

Alcohol Concern (1993) *Training Volunteer Alcohol Counsellors: The Minimum Standards*, London: Alcohol Concern.

ANSA (Association of Nurses in Substance Abuse) (1997) *Substance Use: Guidance on Good Clinical Practice for Specialist Nurses Working with Alcohol and Drug Users*, London: ANSA.

Bury, J.K., Ross, A., Van Teijlingen, E., Porter, A.M.D. and Bath, G. (1996) 'Lothian general practitioners, HIV infection and drug misuse: epidemiology, experience and confidence, 1988–1993', *Health Bulletin* 54: 258–69.

Carroll, J. (1996) 'Attitudes to drug users according to staff grade', *Professional Nurse* 11: 718–20.

Cartwright, A. (1980) 'The attitude of helping agents towards the alcoholic client: the influence of experience, support, training and self-esteem', *British Journal of Addiction* 75: 413–31.

Cherniss, G. (1995) *Beyond Burnout*, New York: Routledge.

Davies, A. and Huxley, P. (1997) 'Survey of general practitioners' opinions on treatment of opiate users', *British Medical Journal* 314: 1173–4.

Department of Health (1994) *Working in Partnership: A Collaborative Approach to Care – Report of the Mental Health Nursing Review Team*, London: HMSO.

Department of Health (1999a) *Drug Misuse and Dependence – Guidelines on Clinical Management*, London: HMSO.

Department of Health (1999b) 'Drug misuse statistics for six months ending March 1998', *Statistical Bulletin 1999/7*, London: DoH.

ENB (English National Board for Nursing, Midwifery and Health Visiting) (1995) *Training Needs Analysis: Project on Meeting the Education and Training Needs of Nurses, Midwives and Health Visitors in the Field of Substance Misuse*, London: ENB.

ENB (English National Board for Nursing, Midwifery and Health Visiting) (1996) *Substance Use and Misuse: Guidelines for Good Practice in Education and Training of Nurses, Midwives and Health Visitors*, London: ENB.

Falkowski, J. and Ghodse, A.H. (1990) 'An international survey of the educational activities of schools of nursing on psychoactive drugs', *Bulletin of World Health Organisation* 68(4): 479–82.

Glanz, A. (1986) 'Findings of a national survey of the role of general practitioners in the treatment of opiate misuse: dealing with the opiate misusers', *British Medical Journal* 293: 486–8.

Gossop, M. (1993) *Living with Drugs* (3rd edn) Hants: Ashgate Publishing Ltd.

Greenhalgh, T. (1996) 'Is my practice evidence-based?' Editorial. *British Medical Journal* 313: 957–8.

Hindler, C., King, M., Nazereth, I., Cohen, J., Farmer, R. and Gerada, C. (1996) 'Characteristics of drug misusers and their perceptions of general practitioner care', *British Journal of General Practice* 46: 149.

Johnstone, C. (1999) 'Strategies to prevent burnout', Career focus. *BMJ Classified*, May 1999: 2–3.

Martin, E. (1996) 'Training in substance abuse is lacking for GP's', *British Medical Journal* 312: 186–7.

McLaughlin, D.F., McKenna, H. and Leslie, J.C. (2000) 'The perceptions and aspirations illicit drug users hold toward health care staff and the care they receive', *Journal of Psychiatric and Mental Health Nursing* 7(5): 435–41.

Ramsey, M. and Spiller, J. (1997) *Drug Misuse Declared in 1996: Latest Results from the British Crime Survey*. Home Office Research Study No. 172, London: Home Office.

Rassool, G.H. (ed.) (1998) *Substance Use and Misuse: Nature, Context and Clinical Interventions*. Oxford: Blackwell Science Ltd.

Reynolds, W.J., Scott, B. and Jessiman, W.C. (1999) 'Empathy has not been measured in clients' terms or effectively taught: a review of the literature', *Journal of Advanced Nursing* 30(5): 1177–85.

Sackett, D.L., Rosenburg, W.M.C., Gray, J.A.M., Haynes, R.B. and Richardson, W.S. 'Evidence based medicine: what is it and what isn't it', *British Medical Journal* 312: 71–2.

Schon, D. (1983) *The Reflective Practitioner*, London: Temple Smith.

Sobell, L.C., Sobell, M.B., Toneatto, T. and Leo, G.I. (1993) 'What triggers the resolution of alcohol problems without treatment?' *Alcoholism: Clinical and Experimental Research* 17: 217–24.

Sullivan, E.J. (1995) *Nursing Care of Clients with Substance Abuse*, St Louis: Mosby.

Tschudin, V. (1982) *Counselling Skills for Nurses*, London: Bailliere Tindall.

UKCC (United Kingdom Central Council for Nursing, Midwifery and Health Visiting) (1992) *The Scope of Professional Practice*, London: UKCC.

UKCC (United Kingdom Central Council for Nursing, Midwifery and Health Visiting) (2001) *Suporting Nurses, Midwives and Health Vistors Through Lifelong Learning*, London: UKCC.

Wymer, A., Harrington, M.E., Sundberg, D.K., Cariaga-Lo, L., McGann, K.P., Silvia, L.Y., Camp, L., Dagenhart, M.C., Richards, B.F. and Hoban, J.D. (1996) 'Substance abuse: medical student awareness and clinical skills', *Substance Abuse* 17(3): 159–66.

THE COMPETENCY ASSESSMENT TOOL (CAT):

A personal learning plan for substance misuse practitioners

The competency assessment tool (CAT) has been developed to enable the practitioner to identify their own level of competency in relation to a variety of topics relevant to substance misuse practice. It has been designed specifically for use with a clinical supervisor or mentor.

The CAT is appropriate for new and more experienced practitioners. It is not a validated instrument, but has been piloted and welcomed for its utility and face validity. The author would welcome comments and suggestions. There may be areas which you feel are missing, in which case add them in and let me know.

The CAT consists of a range of competencies grouped under seven broad topic areas:

1 Substances of misuse
2 Service provision
3 Treatment options
4 Specific groups and populations
5 Theory, policy and law
6 Practice issues
7 Professional issues

Filling in the CAT – a summary

- The practitioner is asked to work through each competency identifying their current level of knowledge or skill.
- Each competency is then assigned an importance rating.
- The most important competencies are prioritised.
- The practitioner then works through the list identifying the level of knowledge/skill it is appropriate to attain in each of the prioritised (category C) competencies.
- A timescale for attaining each of these is negotiated.
- A personal development plan is filled in, identifying how this will be attained and how it may be evaluated.
- Finally the whole CAT is reviewed. Whether the competencies have been attained or not is identified.
- A new CAT can be filled in annually.

Identifying your current level of skill/knowledge

Under each of the headings are a series of competencies. You are asked to go through the list identifying what you consider your current level of knowledge/skill for each competency by circling the appropriate score number. Some competencies include both knowledge and skill components. It is possible to score highly on 'knowledge' of a particular practice but to have little experience of delivering it, thus scoring low on the 'skills' score.

Levels are rated from 1 to 5. The scale is subjective and can be agreed by negotiation with your supervisor. What is most important is that you agree. The following guide may be helpful:

5 = Expert level you would expect of a clinical specialist.
4 = A very good level of knowledge – enough to ensure competence as an autonomous practitioner.
3 = Some knowledge but would need to refer to others for help.

2 = Some knowledge but not enough to use it in practice.
1 = Virtually no knowledge.

Note for supervisors/mentors New practitioners in the field may feel overwhelmed by the number of competencies listed and may rate themselves low on a lot of them. It is important that each competency is discussed positively and any existing transferable skill/knowledge is identified as such. Failure to treat this sensitively may leave the practitioner with low esteem, feeling they know 'nothing'.

Identifying the importance of each competency

The importance rating runs from A to C, C being the most important and A the least. You may, for example, have a good knowledge of solvent misuse but you work in an agency which rarely sees solvent misusers, so though your knowledge is good it is not of great importance to your role. Your role may be changing, so that, for example, you may be moving to work with primary health care and would like to develop a knowledge of brief interventions to help train professionals in this setting. This will score highly on the importance rating. (It is perfectly OK to prioritise a competency that is not part of your role if you have ambitions and your manager can see the value of it.)

Prioritising your needs and agreeing a timescale

Go through the CAT and pick out all the C's (most important). These can then be prioritised according to how much knowledge or skill is required for your role. With your mentor/supervisor you will need to discuss a realistic timescale in which you can achieve this. This will depend on your time, the organisations needs and other factors such as existing service provision, support and the kind of work you are doing. For example, some of your clients are at risk of hepatitis, your level of knowledge is low (2) but the service has an infectious diseases nurse who acts as a resource for staff and clients. You feel it is important you can answer some of your clients' questions but you do not particularly want or need to be an 'expert'. You feel that increasing your knowledge by 1 point to a score of 3 over the next four months would be acceptable. The most important thing is ensuring that your intentions and timescales are realistic and achievable. There is no point trying to reach point 5 in a dozen competencies in the next month, you will simply set yourself up for failure. Competencies not prioritised as C are not given an intended knowledge/skill rating, timescale or met/not met indicator – simply do not fill these ones in.

Completing a personal development plan

Once you have negotiated what you need to work on and the timescale in which you will do this, you need to identify how you can do this and how you can demonstrate that you have done this. It is possible that some goals may be combined; for example you may need to increase your knowledge of a specific substance and your contextual knowledge of the local drug scene – cost, availability and so on. There may be a variety of means of achieving goals such as:

- visits to other services
- discussion with colleagues and clients
- reading appropriate literature
- carrying out a search of the literature at the library
- attending training or educational sessions or courses
- observation of colleagues

It is important that this is not a one-sided process. If practitioners are to enhance their knowledge and skills, then the organisation needs to support them in doing this. Again this is dependent on discussion. You may feel that the only way you can achieve a certain competency is to go on a two day a week course for the next six months; but the organisation may be unable to offer this. Negotiation is the key. You might be able to achieve a slightly lower, but acceptable level of competency, by attending a few study days or by some selected reading. Organisational support could include:

- providing some space and time for self-directed learning such as half a day a week or a fortnight to visit the library or study in peace and quiet
- enabling visits to other areas
- providing useful contact details
- supporting requests for external training where appropriate (funding, study days, etc.)
- facilitating management of existing duties, e.g. ensuring that caseloads are not overwhelming
- demonstrating a commitment to staff development as a core aspect of the service

Means of evaluation

The acquisition of new knowledge or skill needs to be demonstrable. With a task such as venepuncture this is relatively simple. The skill may be learnt through attending a recognised training session followed by supervised practice under the guidance of a more experienced practitioner. The evaluation procedure may be a demonstration of venepuncture assessed by an external person such as a phlebotomist and the ability to explain what you are doing, how and why. Other areas offer less scope for visible assessment of competency; but potentially useful evaluation means may include:

- verbal demonstration of understanding
- being able to answer questions
- a short demonstration to colleagues
- written evidence – a short essay or description

- role play
- video performance of role play or actual sessions
- feedback on conferences and study days to colleagues

Has the goal been achieved?

At the end of the agreed time and following evaluation, negotiation of whether you have met your target can be discussed. You may have completely met your target, not met it or it may have been partially met (M, NM or PM) but you feel you still have work to do to achieve your intended skill/knowledge level. It is important that this is discussed from both your point of view and your supervisor/mentor's. Your supervisor may feel you have achieved your target whilst you may feel you still have work to do. Remember that what you are aiming for is your original intended skill/knowledge level. When you have developed a degree of knowledge of a particular area sometimes you come away realising that there is a lot more to this than you originally realised – the more you learn the more you realise you don't know. The aim is not to become an 'expert' (usually), but how much will the skills or knowledge you have developed help you in your job? Do you really need to develop this further? If so then you should identify this in the next review.

Targets may be not met or partially met for several reasons:

- The intended skill/knowledge level was initially too high or unrealistic.
- The timescale may have been inadequate.
- Resources may have been unavailable.
- External factors such as sickness, course cancellations or unavailability of key staff may have impinged.
- Too many competencies were prioritised at any one time.

Reviewing the CAT

Review dates are negotiable. It is not necessary to review at the end of each identified timescale. It is probable that you could have several priorities identified, some may have a one month timescale, some a three month priority, some may be longer still, six months or a year. An annual or biannual review may be most appropriate. This could tie in with other appraisals such as annual performance reviews. During the review a new CAT checklist is completed and the process starts again.

COMPETENCY ASSESSMENT TOOL

COMPETENCY AREA	CURRENT SCORE 1 = least knowledge / skill 5 = most knowledge / skill	IMPORTANCE RATING A = least important C = most important	LEVEL SOUGHT 1 = least knowledge / skill 5 = most knowledge / skill	TIMESCALE Date by which new level is sought	OUTCOME M = met PM = partially met NM = not met
1. SUBSTANCES OF MISUSE **This includes the following** • *Modes of use (IV, Smoked, etc.)* • *Effects and recognition of signs of use* • *Potential side effects and effects of long-term use* • *Potential for dependency* • *Interactions with other substances* • *Cultural aspects*					
heroin	1 2 3 4 5	A B C	1 2 3 4 5		M / PM / NM
other opiates	1 2 3 4 5	A B C	1 2 3 4 5		M / PM / NM
cocaine including crack	1 2 3 4 5	A B C	1 2 3 4 5		M / PM / NM
amphetamine	1 2 3 4 5	A B C	1 2 3 4 5		M / PM / NM
benzodiazepines	1 2 3 4 5	A B C	1 2 3 4 5		M / PM / NM
OTC drugs	1 2 3 4 5	A B C	1 2 3 4 5		M / PM / NM
dance drugs	1 2 3 4 5	A B C	1 2 3 4 5		M / PM / NM
sports drugs	1 2 3 4 5	A B C	1 2 3 4 5		M / PM / NM
alcohol	1 2 3 4 5	A B C	1 2 3 4 5		M / PM / NM
cannabis	1 2 3 4 5	A B C	1 2 3 4 5		M / PM / NM
hallucinogens	1 2 3 4 5	A B C	1 2 3 4 5		M / PM / NM
solvents	1 2 3 4 5	A B C	1 2 3 4 5		M / PM / NM
other (state)	1 2 3 4 5	A B C	1 2 3 4 5		M / PM / NM
	1 2 3 4 5	A B C	1 2 3 4 5		M / PM / NM

COMPETENCY AREA	CURRENT SCORE 1 = least knowledge / skill 5 = most knowledge / skill	IMPORTANCE RATING A = least important C = most important	LEVEL SOUGHT 1 = least knowledge / skill 5 = most knowledge / skill	TIMESCALE Date by which new level is sought	OUTCOME M = met PM = partially met NM = not met
1. SUBSTANCES OF MISUSE					
Understanding of biochemical and neurological processes involved in substance misuse	1 2 3 4 5	A B C	1 2 3 4 5		M / PM / NM
Knowledge of local drug scene – costs, availability, etc.	1 2 3 4 5	A B C	1 2 3 4 5		M / PM / NM
Physical health problems related to misuse	1 2 3 4 5	A B C	1 2 3 4 5		M / PM / NM
Infectious diseases – Hep B, C and HIV	1 2 3 4 5	A B C	1 2 3 4 5		M / PM / NM
2. SERVICE PROVISION					
Knowledge of local services relevant to substance misuse, referral procedures and accessibility. May include non-drug/alcohol services such as HIV support groups.	1 2 3 4 5	A B C	1 2 3 4 5		M / PM / NM

COMPETENCY AREA	CURRENT SCORE 1 = least knowledge / skill 5 = most knowledge / skill	IMPORTANCE RATING A = least important C = most important	LEVEL SOUGHT 1 = least knowledge / skill 5 = most knowledge / skill	TIMESCALE Date by which new level is sought	OUTCOME M = met PM = partially met NM = not met
2. SERVICE PROVISION					
Setting up and managing services					
a) Knowledge of this	1 2 3 4 5	A B C	1 2 3 4 5		M / PM / NM
c) Skills in this	1 2 3 4 5	A B C	1 2 3 4 5		M / PM / NM
Service evaluation					
a) Knowledge of this	1 2 3 4 5	A B C	1 2 3 4 5		M / PM / NM
c) Skills in this	1 2 3 4 5	A B C	1 2 3 4 5		M / PM / NM
3. TREATMENT OPTIONS					
General knowledge of range of potential treatment options	1 2 3 4 5	A B C	1 2 3 4 5		M / PM / NM
Brief interventions					
a) Knowledge of this	1 2 3 4 5	A B C	1 2 3 4 5		M / PM / NM
c) Skills in this	1 2 3 4 5	A B C	1 2 3 4 5		M / PM / NM
Motivational interviewing / approaches					
a) Knowledge of this	1 2 3 4 5	A B C	1 2 3 4 5		M / PM / NM
c) Skills in this	1 2 3 4 5	A B C	1 2 3 4 5		M / PM / NM

COMPETENCY AREA *3. TREATMENT OPTIONS*	CURRENT SCORE 1 = least knowledge / skill 5 = most knowledge / skill	IMPORTANCE RATING A = least important C = most important	LEVEL SOUGHT 1 = least knowledge / skill 5 = most knowledge / skill	TIMESCALE Date by which new level is sought	OUTCOME M = met PM = partially met NM = not met
Behavioural and cognitive behavioural methods					
a) Knowledge of this	1 2 3 4 5	A B C	1 2 3 4 5		M / PM / NM
c) Skills in this	1 2 3 4 5	A B C	1 2 3 4 5		M / PM / NM
Safer injecting and harm reduction					
a) Knowledge of this	1 2 3 4 5	A B C	1 2 3 4 5		M / PM / NM
c) Skills in this	1 2 3 4 5	A B C	1 2 3 4 5		M / PM / NM
Self help and group work including 12 step.					
a) Knowledge of this	1 2 3 4 5	A B C	1 2 3 4 5		M / PM / NM
c) Skills in this	1 2 3 4 5	A B C	1 2 3 4 5		M / PM / NM
Prescribing in relation to alcohol					
a) Knowledge of this	1 2 3 4 5	A B C	1 2 3 4 5		M / PM / NM
c) Skills in this	1 2 3 4 5	A B C	1 2 3 4 5		M / PM / NM
Prescribing in relation to drugs					
a) Knowledge of this	1 2 3 4 5	A B C	1 2 3 4 5		M / PM / NM
c) Skills in this	1 2 3 4 5	A B C	1 2 3 4 5		M / PM / NM

COMPETENCY AREA *3. TREATMENT OPTIONS*	CURRENT SCORE 1 = least knowledge / skill 5 = most knowledge / skill	IMPORTANCE RATING A = least important C = most important	LEVEL SOUGHT 1 = least knowledge / skill 5 = most knowledge / skill	TIMESCALE Date by which new level is sought	OUTCOME M = met PM = partially met NM = not met
Relapse prevention					
a) Knowledge of this	1 2 3 4 5	A B C	1 2 3 4 5		M / PM / NM
c) Skills in this	1 2 3 4 5	A B C	1 2 3 4 5		M / PM / NM
Home detox					
a) Knowledge of this	1 2 3 4 5	A B C	1 2 3 4 5		M / PM / NM
c) Skills in this	1 2 3 4 5	A B C	1 2 3 4 5		M / PM / NM
Alternative therapies					
a) Knowledge of this	1 2 3 4 5	A B C	1 2 3 4 5		M / PM / NM
c) Skills in this	1 2 3 4 5	A B C	1 2 3 4 5		M / PM / NM
Prevention / health promotion					
a) Knowledge of this	1 2 3 4 5	A B C	1 2 3 4 5		M / PM / NM
c) Skills in this	1 2 3 4 5	A B C	1 2 3 4 5		M / PM / NM
Family work					
a) Knowledge of this	1 2 3 4 5	A B C	1 2 3 4 5		M / PM / NM
c) Skills in this	1 2 3 4 5	A B C	1 2 3 4 5		M / PM / NM
Counselling skills					
a) Knowledge of this	1 2 3 4 5	A B C	1 2 3 4 5		M / PM / NM
c) Skills in this	1 2 3 4 5	A B C	1 2 3 4 5		M / PM / NM

COMPETENCY AREA	CURRENT SCORE 1 = least knowledge / skill 5 = most knowledge / skill	IMPORTANCE RATING A = least important C = most important	LEVEL SOUGHT 1 = least knowledge / skill 5 = most knowledge / skill	TIMESCALE Date by which new level is sought	OUTCOME M = met PM = partially met NM = not met
4. SPECIFIC GROUPS AND POPULATIONS / KNOWLEDGE OF . . .					
Dual diagnosis and mental health issues	1 2 3 4 5	A B C	1 2 3 4 5		M / PM / NM
Issues relating to women	1 2 3 4 5	A B C	1 2 3 4 5		M / PM / NM
Young people and substance misuse	1 2 3 4 5	A B C	1 2 3 4 5		M / PM / NM
Older people	1 2 3 4 5	A B C	1 2 3 4 5		M / PM / NM
Drugs in sport /steroids	1 2 3 4 5	A B C	1 2 3 4 5		M / PM / NM
Working with diverse cultures and ethnicities	1 2 3 4 5	A B C	1 2 3 4 5		M / PM / NM
5. THEORY, POLICY AND LAW					
The criminal justice system	1 2 3 4 5	A B C	1 2 3 4 5		M / PM / NM
Knowledge of theories related to substance misuse	1 2 3 4 5	A B C	1 2 3 4 5		M / PM / NM

COMPETENCY AREA	CURRENT SCORE 1 = least knowledge / skill 5 = most knowledge / skill	IMPORTANCE RATING A = least important C = most important	LEVEL SOUGHT 1 = least knowledge / skill 5 = most knowledge / skill	TIMESCALE Date by which new level is sought	OUTCOME M = met PM = partially met NM = not met
5. THEORY, POLICY AND LAW					
National policy and strategy	1 2 3 4 5	A B C	1 2 3 4 5		M / PM / NM
Local policy and strategy	1 2 3 4 5	A B C	1 2 3 4 5		M / PM / NM
Legal issues – substance misuse and the law	1 2 3 4 5	A B C	1 2 3 4 5		M / PM / NM
6. PRACTICE ISSUES					
Screening / brief assessment					
a) Knowledge of this	1 2 3 4 5	A B C	1 2 3 4 5		M / PM / NM
c) Skills in this	1 2 3 4 5	A B C	1 2 3 4 5		M / PM / NM
In-depth assessment					
a) Knowledge of this	1 2 3 4 5	A B C	1 2 3 4 5		M / PM / NM
c) Skills in this	1 2 3 4 5	A B C	1 2 3 4 5		M / PM / NM
Dealing with 'difficult' behaviours					
a) Knowledge of this	1 2 3 4 5	A B C	1 2 3 4 5		M / PM / NM
c) Skills in this	1 2 3 4 5	A B C	1 2 3 4 5		M / PM / NM

COMPETENCY AREA	CURRENT SCORE 1 = least knowledge / skill 5 = most knowledge / skill	IMPORTANCE RATING A = least important C = most important	LEVEL SOUGHT 1 = least knowledge / skill 5 = most knowledge / skill	TIMESCALE Date by which new level is sought	OUTCOME M = met PM = partially met NM = not met
6. PRACTICE ISSUES					
Use of physical screening tools – urinalysis, breathalysers, etc.					
a) Knowledge of this	1 2 3 4 5	A B C	1 2 3 4 5		M / PM / NM
c) Skills in this	1 2 3 4 5	A B C	1 2 3 4 5		M / PM / NM
Safer sex information and advice					
a) Knowledge of this	1 2 3 4 5	A B C	1 2 3 4 5		M / PM / NM
c) Skills in this	1 2 3 4 5	A B C	1 2 3 4 5		M / PM / NM
First aid knowledge	1 2 3 4 5	A B C	1 2 3 4 5		M / PM / NM
Immunisation skills for Hep B vaccination	1 2 3 4 5	A B C	1 2 3 4 5		M / PM / NM
Venepuncture	1 2 3 4 5	A B C	1 2 3 4 5		M / PM / NM
7. PROFESSIONAL SKILLS					
Research awareness (knowledge of types of research, etc.)	1 2 3 4 5	A B C	1 2 3 4 5		M / PM / NM

COMPETENCY AREA *7. PROFESSIONAL SKILLS*	CURRENT SCORE 1 = least knowledge / skill 5 = most knowledge / skill	IMPORTANCE RATING A = least important C = most important	LEVEL SOUGHT 1 = least knowledge / skill 5 = most knowledge / skill	TIMESCALE Date by which new level is sought	OUTCOME M = met PM = partially met NM = not met
Research skills (carrying out research)	1 2 3 4 5	A B C	1 2 3 4 5		M / PM / NM
Knowledge of sources of education and training	1 2 3 4 5	A B C	1 2 3 4 5		M / PM / NM
Sources of information and evidence					
a) Knowledge of this	1 2 3 4 5	A B C	1 2 3 4 5		M / PM / NM
c) Use of these	1 2 3 4 5	A B C	1 2 3 4 5		M / PM / NM
Reflective Practice					
a) Knowledge of this	1 2 3 4 5	A B C	1 2 3 4 5		M / PM / NM
c) Use of these	1 2 3 4 5	A B C	1 2 3 4 5		M / PM / NM

PERSONAL DEVELOPMENT PLAN SUMMARY

Date agreed ______________________________

Review date ______________________________

Mentor ______________________________

Description of competency	Current score	Intended score	How this will be achieved	Timescale	Means of evaluation

PART II

THE CARE AND TREATMENT OF SUBSTANCE MISUSERS

CHAPTER 4

CLIENT ASSESSMENT

Andrew McBride

LEARNING OBJECTIVES

After you have read this chapter you will be able to demonstrate an understanding of:

1 The principles of conducting holistic assessment of alcohol and drug related problems in an individual client.

2 One structured approach to this process.

INTRODUCTION

Assessment is a two-way process. The client will be appraising you and your service from first contact. Who answers the phone and how? How is the appointment letter phrased? How am I greeted when I arrive? In short, is this the sort of agency and person that might help me?

Assessment is a process that does not end until after the client is discharged. Some defined process of early assessment may inform clients about and screen them for the particular helping options available from the professional or the wider agency, but this should not be the only time that the client is appraised for the relevance of what is going on and for evidence of change.

This chapter will mostly be limited to the first few interviews in which basic information is shared. Brief consideration will also be given to the processes of identifying and recording progress towards agreed end points for intervention.

ASSESSMENT IS INTERVENTION

Assessment is the beginning of intervention. In brief interventions 'assessment' and carefully delivered feedback effectively are the intervention. At the end of an initial assessment, 'success' might be chalked up if the client leaves with:

- a clearer common understanding of their difficulties and how these may relate to their use of substances
- confidence in the service and the therapist
- a clear understanding of what is being offered
- achievable targets to begin a change process
- optimism that they can change

At worst the client will leave confused, disempowered, helpless and in need of a cigarette, a drink, a fix and a lie down in a darkened room.

Assessment and philosophy

Assessment cannot be atheoretical. Whether it is knowing the person, or knowing specific facts about them, the information gathered, how it is collected and how it is then recorded, collated and constructed all reflect explicit or assumed theoretical or practical aspects of the assessor's thinking. (In reading my ideas about assessment you must therefore allow for the fact that I am middle aged, British, an atheist with liberal left wing leanings, a doctor, a psychiatrist, a manager, proud of an eclectic theoretical grounding – oh and male. Others might think of other relevant descriptors, but you get the idea.)

Many factors might influence the rate of an individual's progress into and out of a substance misuse problem. To be utterly comprehensive an assessment might cover: macro-economic issues (such as the effects of the collapse of Eastern European chemists' career structures on the quantity, price and purity of designer drugs available in the West), a particular school of psychotherapy might require specific interpersonal and family relationship details and in future some may be primarily interested in the genetic underpinnings of the microscopic structure of the client's synapses. Out here (on planet earth), most assessments are less wide-ranging, and focus on the practicalities of how this person got into this particular set of difficulties, what they are seeking to change, and who and what might help them most effectively.

Purposes of initial assessment

Not all types of help need any formal assessment (and some schools of thought are antipathetic to the very idea). If only one sort of help is available, irrespective of the nature or degree of your problems and if there is no plan to evaluate outcomes, then assessment is unnecessary, beyond determining that the client wants to have that intervention.

There are several good reasons for conducting some sort of early assessment. These include the need to:

- come to a common understanding of the key issues
- develop a shared language for further conversation
- produce a detailed written record of the information collected and the agreements reached
- evaluate risks

The idea that matching individuals with particular characteristics to particular styles of psychological treatment has been undermined to some degree. Background information is therefore of less importance for this purpose than for considering the person's needs holistically. In addition to a substance misuse problem, the client may have physical and mental health difficulties, social problems and practical difficulties in attending for the help you might offer. Deciding on the most appropriate help to offer, in what order and who should be responsible for providing it will often require negotiation with both the client and other agencies. In considering what help may be most appropriate, it is wise to assess the therapy for the client, not the client for the therapy.

Negotiating realistic, short (and sometimes longer) term targets for the client to achieve in terms of altered patterns of substance use is often valuable, although these should always be flexible. For some clients, and in some settings, a written care plan, in the form of a contract, outlining what is to be done and what is expected of the client can be valuable. No one intervention helps all people with all problems all of the time. It is useful to be able to recognise when progress is being made, and when it is time to call a halt and move off in another direction.

Risk assessment

An increasingly important aspect of all areas of the working environment is the assessment of risk. This may cover a number of different areas:

- the client
- the client's family (particularly dependent children)
- you and other professionals
- the wider public

An example of a brief risk assessment is included in Appendix 4.1. Once significant risks are identified, action needs to be taken to reduce the likelihood of harm occurring. Simply recording that somebody is at high risk of suicide, or has threatened to kill another member of staff does nothing to reduce the risk. A discussion, urgently if in any doubt, with your supervisor, manager or the most senior person available, and referral elsewhere to the appropriate professional agency is the minimum acceptable response, and needs to be carefully recorded. Such issues should also be taken to supervision, but action should not be delayed until routine supervision if urgent action is indicated.

PRIORITY SETTING

In services with limited resources, systems may be needed to allow managers and practitioners to prioritise individual clients for available treatments. This often relies on information from the referrer. Any such delays are unsatisfactory because people want help when they ask for it and not some months later. The practical problem with any waiting list system is what criteria are legitimate to make somebody 'urgent': debt, pregnancy, disease, risk of death, divorce, loss of work, offending, age, vulnerability, 'motivation', child-care issues? In the author's experience most people face several of these issues by the time they ask for help. Pragmatically I prioritise pregnancy and identified child-care issues and ignore all the other factors. The alternatives would be too complex and arbitrary to justify. The secret is not to allow waiting lists.

Monitoring

Regular feedback of progress against agreed objectives is valuable for client and therapist alike. During some stages of treatment clients can all too readily doubt that they have made any progress at all, unless reminded of the predicaments they faced when they were first seen. Positive feedback of progress can reinforce changes that have been made, despite setbacks, and encourage self-monitoring.

Record keeping

Without reliable and detailed information about clients at the point they enter the service it is impossible to sensibly evaluate outcome individually, or across the population of people seen by the service. Anybody inheriting a long-standing client, in whose records there is no trace of why they have been on methadone for ten years, or what their pattern of drinking was pre-counselling, will understand the benefits of clear record keeping.

Good notes are also invaluable when passing over continuing clients for a different phase of care, in hospital or rehabilitation, when you leave the agency and if you ever need to write reports for third parties. Records may be demanded by third parties, including courts of law, and all entries need to be written with this in mind. In professional records entries should always be legible, in black ink, signed, dated and timed. All organisations should set standards against which their records can be audited internally, to ensure that basic standards are maintained.

Background

People are generally reluctant to identify themselves as having a substance misuse problem. Once recognised, most will not approach even primary care for assistance. Attending a specialist service is even more potentially anxiety provoking and may require the cooperation of family members and a professional referrer. Making services approachable, geographically, socially, temporally and personally increases the likelihood of attendance and encourages a positive attitude in the client when they first attend.

THE SETTING

The ambience of the room in which assessment takes place can have a marked impact on the experience for all parties. Ideally the setting should be relatively informal, comfortable (furniture, warmth, décor and lighting) quiet and uninterrupted. Such ideals are easily forgotten if you have little choice but to work in a damp, draughty, unsound-proofed, impersonal space. You may get used to it, but for the client it is all new and may reflect too clearly the general sense of unhappiness they are already feeling about being there. If all else fails, check that the chairs are the same height, at an appropriate distance from each other and with you nearer the door in case you need to leave quickly. Is there a 'Do not disturb' sign on the door? Do people know not to put calls through? Are your pager and mobile phone switched off? Are there tissues on the table?

Your behaviour

Whatever the setting, your appearance and behaviour can help to place the client at ease. How informally you dress will determine to some extent what responses you get. Neutral is best because not everybody will warm to your silk Gucci suit or your soiled Anarchist T-shirt, and your appearance probably shouldn't dominate the session. Greet the client, show them where the lavatories are, show them into the room, point them to the chair that you want them to sit in. Explain who you are, how you understand they have reached this point in the proceedings (partner phoned, GP wrote, dropped in). Explain what is going to happen that day, and how long you are going to spend with them. You need to make it clear that you have a limited period of time for each contact, and how long that is. It is not acceptable for the client to begin to disclose sensitive information only to be interrupted because you have run out of time. If you are going to assess them and pass them over to somebody else for help then say so, and introduce them personally.

Confidentiality

It is essential when dealing with sensitive personal information to give unambiguous information about confidentiality and the recording and storage of information. Clients must understand that at the very least they will be discussed with your manager and or supervisor(s) and (if relevant) the referrer. If your model of work includes involvement of the family then explicit consent for disclosure becomes important. If children or young people are involved then your responsibilities under the Children Act also need to be explained. It is increasingly common for courts to obtain and disclose medical information without consent. This can happen if the client is alleged to have committed an offence, but also if they make allegations against a third party. The implications of this have probably not been recognised by the majority of helping agencies. If the client will be notified anonymously to a drugs data-base, this needs to be explained.

Methods of assessment

All information other than that volunteered by the individual should only be obtained with consent. If the client understands the purpose of gathering information from other sources then consent is very rarely refused.

INTERVIEW

The best, most helpful and constructive information will come from talking with the client. This is usually recorded in the form of a history, which records the relevant information, attitudes and expectations. An example of a specialist assessment pro-forma is included in Appendix 4.1. Although daunting at first glance, most people presenting to a specialist substance misuse service will have relevant information under almost every heading. Practice and patience (on both sides) are necessary to fathom the complexities of somebody's life, and it will be the first time for many people that this much interest has been shown in understanding them.

Good interviewers display:

- interest and attention
- empathy
- warmth
- active listening skills
- thoughtfulness (wisdom and knowledge)
- reflectiveness
- an inability to be shocked
- a non-judgemental stance that does not blur into collusion
- a style of questioning that enquires in an open, non-confrontative way about simple, recent stuff

If you have established a good rapport with the individual and they are confident in you, then you will be able to learn more about them than you can possibly need. People sometimes exaggerate or underestimate their substance use, but this is probably no more usual in people with problems than the rest of the population and need not prevent people receiving help and making positive changes.

Important others

Partners or family members may confirm or clarify accounts of substance use and related problem behaviours and are routinely used in research settings to give 'independent' assessment of progress. The importance of appropriate social support in helping the individual is given varying degrees of importance by different forms of intervention (see Chapter 10). People's social networks are likely to have more impact over a longer period than any 'treatment' intervention, however intensive. In gathering information from relatives, scrupulous attention to the confidentiality of the client and continuous attention to the goal of helping the client to change are essential.

Other professionals

It can be very helpful to find out precisely what has already been done, what has proved helpful and what has not. Past records may be helpful, a telephone call may be more so.

Standardised interviews and questionnaires

There are innumerable validated, reliable and sensitive structured interviews and questionnaires covering almost every aspect of substance use and related issues. Use of such tools is probably under-rated by practitioners, despite evidence from research that the very act of systematically reviewing ones own behaviour in such a way can be motivating in itself. Such tools can be used for screening for evidence of problems in at risk populations (e.g. the Alcohol Use Disorders Identification Test), for categorisation/classification/grading of severity in those already identified as having a problem (e.g. the Severity of Dependence Scale), and for monitoring change (e.g. the Opiate Treatment Index).

Appearance and behaviour of the client

Other than what the client says, information can sometimes usefully be obtained from the client's appearance and behaviour, and, if visited at home, their wider environment. As a minimum it is worth considering whether or not there is evidence of intoxication or withdrawal symptoms, neglect, self-injury and track marks. It is not necessary to be trained in psychiatry to be sensitive to evidence of mood disturbance, anxiety, suspiciousness, aggressiveness, confusion or memory impairment. The presence of any of these suggests the need for further skilled professional assessment and intervention.

Medical examination

Physical health problems are common in people who drink heavily and who inject drugs. Relevant physical examination by the client's General Practitioner may be indicated in the event of complaints of physical ill health (see Chapter 13).

Laboratory testing

Screening and diagnostic testing may be undertaken to identify what drugs are being taken and the presence and extent of associated health problems. The results of such tests can be shared with the client to provide objective evidence, for example, that their drinking is having effects on their liver (see Chapter 13) and can be repeated to confirm and reinforce positive changes.

Planning and goal setting

The immediate outcome of an assessment should be the development of a plan of action, drawn up in partnership with the client. Even if no further input is required, the rationale for this and what will happen next should be made clear. For example:

- Your GP, who referred you, will be informed of the outcome of assessment and why, how and when you can come back to see me, if circumstances change in the future.
- Although you do not think that any of the help I can offer is likely to work, you would like to be seen by the agency up the road, and I will pass on all the information I have collected and write to ask them to send you an appointment.

Aims and goals

The overall *aim* of treatment may be broad, for example 'abstinence from opioids', but there are a number of intermediate and component steps that contribute towards the aim. These are *goals*. For example the client may need to stop injecting, stop street drugs, learn to manage anxiety, be able to identify cues to substance misuse and learn how to deal with these, and adapt their social network to their planned new life. A single treatment aim may have several goals. Treatment goals should be SMART:

- Simple – the stated goal should be straightforward and understandable.
- Measurable – the outcome of the goal should be measurable.
- Attainable – the particular change must be possible for the client.
- Realistic – goals need to be practical.
- Time scaled – goals need to have a timescale for review attached to them.

What interventions are going to take place, *How*, *When* and *Who* will be involved all need to be clear.

Conclusion

Assessment is a planned, consistent, repeatable and teachable skill. Talking with people newly presenting for help has great educational value for newcomers to the field. And when you are tired of talking with people about their achievements, potential, vulnerabilities and difficulties, you are tired of life, and certainly shouldn't be working with people.

Note

This chapter talks about 'clients', it could just as easily talk about 'patients'. Most evidence suggests that clients of health services prefer the term 'patient', but I have grown used to 'client' over the years. I ask people what they want to be called, make a note of it, and explain that they may call me Andrew or Dr McBride, whichever they prefer. I am sometimes called worse.

READER INPUT

Questions

(1) How does the agency you work with facilitate the process of assessment?
(2) Could your agency's assessment process be improved upon? How could this happen?

Role play

Take one of the case scenarios found at the rear of this book and take it in turns to practise the roles of assessor and client. Start the process from when 'client' and 'assessor' first meet and consider all the aspects of the assessment including setting the scene and concluding the assessment.

Whilst many clients will take time to tell their story (an initial assessment may last an hour or more) and that assessment may have to take place over a few meetings, you may concentrate on one particular issue in the role play. Oscar winning acting is not necessary to get a feel for the style, approach and questions that feel comfortable from both sides. It can be useful to video such sessions so that you can comment *positively* on how it works out.

(a) What did you find easy, and what more difficult?
(b) What areas of questioning did you find the most challenging (or most uncomfortable) and why?

FURTHER READING

Almost all introductory professional textbooks include a chapter on basic assessment methods relevant to the profession. Try several books, across different disciplines, and also try some of the many introductions to counselling and psychotherapy. These almost always contain sections on establishing a therapeutic relationship.

APPENDIX 4.1

NEW CLIENT ASSESSMENT: Case Number ____________

Key worker (person filling out this form)________________

Date ___/___/______Time______

Client First Name ________________________

Middle Name(s) ________________________

Surname ________________ Known as ________________

Maiden and/or other previous Surnames ________________________

Date of birth ___/___/______ Age ____________

Religion ________________ Ethnicity ________________

First Language ________________________

Address ________________ Home telephone no. __________

________________ Work telephone no. __________

________________ Mobile telephone no. __________

____

Post Code ________________

Telephone no. ________________

Next of Kin (and relationship) ________________________

Address ________________ Telephone no. __________

________________ Aware of appointment Yes/No

Post Code ________________

Source of Referral ________________________

Aware of appointment Yes/No

GP Name ________________ Telephone no. __________

Address ________________ Aware of appointment Yes/No

____

Post Code ________________

Housing Assoc. ________________ Tel No. __________

Pharmacist ________________ Tel No. __________

Probation Officer ________________ Tel No. __________

Social Worker ________________ Tel No __________

Support Worker ________________ Tel No __________

Client's views and expectations

Main problems as identified by the client

1

2

3

4

5

Patterns of drug and alcohol use and injecting: past seven days

	Morning	Afternoon	Evening
Today			
Yesterday			
Day before yesterday			
3 days ago			
4 days ago			
5 days ago			
6 days ago			

Past seven days:	Total number of units of alcohol	________
	Total number of cigarettes	________
	Total amount of main drug (in g)	________
	Total amount of relevant other drug	________
	Total number of injections	________

(For Benzodiazepines convert to mg equivalents of Diazepam. For Opioids convert to mg equivalents of Methadone.)

Appendix 4.1 (cont.)

Patterns of drug and alcohol use and injecting: Lifetime drug
Age of first and last use. Good things about use. Ever dependent. Other less good things about use

Tobacco

Alcohol

Solvents (specify)

Cannabis

Hallucinogens (specify)

Stimulants (specify)

Hypnosedatives (specify)

Opioids (specify)

Anabolic steroids

Injecting drug use

Sharing paraphernalia

Is the past week's pattern fairly typical of:

past month

past six months

past year

If not how has it changed?

Current withdrawal symptoms
(specify nature and degree of symptoms)

Lifetime history of fits (whether or not alcohol or drug related) Yes/No

Lifetime history of Delirium Tremens Yes/No

Current prescribed drugs
(preparation, dose, frequency and duration: check bottles if possible).

Known allergies (especially to medication).

Reasons for use of main drug

Appendix 4.1 (cont.)

Reasons for considering changing pattern of use of main drug

Not so good things about changing *Good things about changing*

Previous attempts at change (who what and when)
Self only, GP, AA/NA, CAT, Residential Rehab (specify), other agency (specify)

What has helped in the past?

Specific/recurrent causes of relapse?

Past psychiatric history and current concerns
Depression, anxiety, panic, phobia, psychosis, deliberate self-harm, deliberate overdose, etc. relevant treatment.

Current sleep pattern
If an issue for past week (work back night by night): Time to bed, time to sleep, quality of sleep, frequency of waking, time finally awake. Time out of bed. Daytime/evening naps?

Past medical history and current concerns
Quality and quantity of recent diet, current bowel habits, current menstrual cycle.

If IV drug use:
Hep. B tested/immunised?
Hep. C tested?
HIV tested?

Past forensic history and current charges
Outstanding charges, past imprisonment, nature of offences. Arson, firearms, offensive weapons, ABH, GBH, wounding, manslaughter, murder, drugs offences, burglary, fraud, take and drive away, shoplifting, sexual offences. Relatedness to alcohol and drug use.

Family history
Genogram with names and ages of parents, sibs, partners and children. Plus relevant alcohol, drug, forensic, medical and psychiatric problems in any known family member.

Appendix 4.1 (cont.)

Relevant personal history
Perinatal problems, pre-school, family stability, nursery, infant and junior education, secondary education, higher education, literacy, numeracy, qualifications and work skills, work experience, sexual and marital history, current partners alcohol and drug use, other close relationships and peer networks, peer groups alcohol and drug use, current life circumstances, accommodation, leisure activities, sources of income (benefits claimed) and expenditure, (specifically, how is substance use paid for) debts. Child-care issues: support and risks. Social services involvement?

Current readiness to change main identified addictive behaviour (tick)

Precontemplation   Contemplation   Action   Maintenance

ICD 10 diagnosis   F __.__/___

History (or risk) of:		Comments/details	Follow-up action
Disturbed behaviour in associationwith mental illness	Yes No		
Disturbed behaviour in association with intoxication or withdrawal	Yes No		
Criminal damage	Yes No		
Arson	Yes No		
Assault, ABH, GBH	Yes No		
Sexual offences	Yes No		
Threats or violence in clinical setting	Yes No		
Carrying a knife	Yes No		

Possessing a firearm	Yes No
Having guard or fighting dogs at home	Yes No
Living with one or more others with such history	Yes No
Suicide	Yes No
Deliberate self-harm	Yes No
Accidental self-harm/ self-neglect	Yes No
Abuse by others	Yes No
Elder abuse	Yes No
Risk to child	Yes No

CHAPTER 5

BEHAVIOURAL AND COGNITIVE BEHAVIOURAL APPROACHES TO SUBSTANCE MISUSE TREATMENT

Paul Bennett

LEARNING OBJECTIVES

After you have studied this chapter you should be able to demonstrate an understanding of:

1 The core theoretical principles underpinning Cognitive Behavioural Therapy (CBT) in relation to misuse/abuse problems.

2 The central elements of CBT used with substance misusers.

3 The effectiveness of CBT in comparison to other therapeutic approaches.

INTRODUCTION

Cognitive behavioural therapy (CBT) is a widely used therapeutic approach that has been applied to the treatment of conditions as varied as depression, anxiety, schizophrenia and non-compliance with medication (Bennett, 2000; Beck, 1976). It is therefore not surprising that it has been adapted for use with people who misuse substances of all kinds. This chapter examines some of the theory underpinning its use, the core techniques that have been applied to its use with people who misuse substances, and considers its effectiveness in relation to other intervention types.

A COGNITIVE MODEL OF SUBSTANCE MISUSE AND ABUSE

The central tenet of cognitive behavioural therapy is that it is not just what happens to us that effects our mood and behaviour but how we interpret such events and our more general beliefs about the world. These each influence our feelings, motivations, and actions. Beliefs that encourage substance misuse may include: 'I cannot cope with going to a party without a hit . . .' or 'Drinking makes me a more sociable person'. Beliefs such as these underlie a vulnerability to substance misuse, and increase the likelihood of use at times of stress or social pressure. These addictive beliefs directly relate to the 'need' to use substances as a means of coping with whatever life throws at the individual.

The nature of addictive beliefs may change over time. At the beginning of a history of substance misuse, positive beliefs such as: 'It will be fun to get high', may predominate. As the individual begins to rely on the substance to counteract feelings of distress, relief-oriented thoughts may predominate: 'I need a shot to get me through the day'.

Not all thoughts or beliefs may support substance misuse. The individual may at times experience a degree of conflict between beliefs that support continued consumption and those that support abstinence. The number and strength of thoughts from each side of the argument will determine the individual's behaviour at any one time. Ironically, these conflicts may, in themselves, make the individual feel uncomfortable and increase the risk of substance misuse.

Substance specific beliefs are frequently accompanied by a wider set of beliefs that may also increase vulnerability. These include a negative view of oneself, one's circumstances, and environment, and may contribute to low self-esteem, depression or anxiety. These emotions, in turn, trigger the addictive beliefs. Such thoughts are typically activated in specific, often predictable, circumstances. Such cues may be both external (e.g. walking past a pub, pressure at work) or internal (e.g. depression, anxiety).

Putting these various elements together, substance misuse is initiated by the presence of either external or internal cues. These trigger both core and addictive beliefs. When the preponderance of thoughts support consumption, these instigate cravings to use a substance. This is then maintained or ceased either by physical incapacity or further cognitive processes.

INTERVENING USING COGNITIVE-BEHAVIOURAL TECHNIQUES

Beliefs as 'facts'

The beliefs we hold about events that have happened or will happen are hypothetical. Some of these guesses may be correct; some may be wrong. The central focus of cognitive behavioural therapy is that people with emotional and/or addiction-based problems not only make inappropriate guesses or assumptions about the world, they also start treating them as facts not hypotheses.

The primary goal of cognitive therapy is to modify maladaptive thoughts that contribute to inappropriate behaviour or emotional states. The nature of the intervention is a collaborative exercise between therapist and client in which the therapist acts as an 'educator', teaching new skills to help people cope with their problems. Treatment assumes an appropriate relationship between therapist and client. At its most basic, this involves the therapist showing warmth towards the client, being able to understand the difficulties the client is facing from their perspective and reflecting this back to them (empathy), and being honest in their relationship (Rogers, 1967).

The first phase of any intervention is to ensure that both client and therapist share the same point of reference and that the client can identify the relationship between cognitions, emotions and behaviour.

The education phase

The education phase involves both direct and indirect elements. The former may involve didactic information provision. However, making CBT relevant to the client involves their active participation. One way of making clients aware of the relationship between thoughts and feelings is to ask them to think about the feelings and thoughts they have had in the recent past: even while waiting for the interview. These are then identified as 'automatic thoughts' and the relationship between them and their mood at the time is discussed. The relationship between thoughts and substance misuse should then be assessed in some detail.

A second way that clients can learn the association between thoughts, feelings and behaviour, is through the use of 'homework' assignments. Clients may be asked to record their thoughts at the time they are feeling depressed, angry, or prior to use of a substance. These records can be brought to subsequent sessions and used as a basis for discussion.

Beliefs as hypotheses

Once clients are able to catch their thoughts and identify the association between thoughts, emotions and behaviour, a variety of strategies can be developed to help them identify errors of thinking they may be having.

The Socratic method

An important therapeutic strategy within CBT is known as the Socratic method or 'guided discovery' (Beck, 1976). This is used to help clients identify distorted patterns of thinking that are contributing to their problems. It encourages them to consider and evaluate different sources of information that provide evidence of the reality or unreality of the beliefs they hold. One technique that has been developed specifically to help identify and challenge core beliefs is known as the downward arrow technique (Beck *et al.*, 1979). When clients express what seems to be inappropriate thoughts or reactions to events, the downward arrow technique can be used to identify distortions in core beliefs that are contributing to their problems. Key questions include:

- What is your concern about . . .?
- What would the implications be . . .?
- What would the consequences be . . .?
- What would the ultimate consequences be . . .?

An example of the use of the downward arrow technique is provided by this extract from a session with a problem drinker adapted from Beck *et al.* (1993):

Therapist: You feel quite strongly that you need to be 'relaxed' by alcohol when you go to a party. What is your concern about being sober?
↓
Client: I wouldn't enjoy myself and I wouldn't be much fun to be with.
↓
T: What would be the implications of that?
↓
C: Well, people wouldn't talk to me.
↓
T: And what would be the consequence of that?
↓
C: I need to have people like me. My job depends on it. If I can't entertain people at a party, then I'm no good at my job.
↓
T: So, what happens if that is the case?
↓
C: Well, I guess I lose my job!
↓
T: So, you lose your job because you didn't get drunk at a party?
↓
C: Well, put like that, I think I may have not had it in the right perspective.

Here, the technique has been used both to identify some of the client's core beliefs and to get them to reconsider the accuracy of those beliefs.

Homework assignments

Homework assignments can also be used to identify and challenge thoughts underlying substance misuse. The most commonly used strategies are monitoring and challenging distorted thinking, and behavioural assignments that challenge distorted thinking.

Keeping a cognitive diary

Thoughts and thought challenges between sessions can be monitored through the use of a diary in which the client records any thoughts and challenges they may have in relation to their substance misuse or other relevant issues. These should be reviewed in the session following the period of diary keeping. Questions the client may use to challenge assumptions include:

- What evidence is there that supports or denies my assumption?
- Are there any other ways I can think about this situation?
- Will getting drunk now do any good?
- Has it helped before?
- Could I be making a mistake in the way I am thinking?

Behavioural challenge

A second strategy is to set up homework tasks that directly test the cognitive beliefs that clients may hold. For example, if a client believes that they cannot go to a party without drinking, they may be set the homework task of trying to do so. Clearly such challenges should be realistic or they simply serve to maintain the pre-existing beliefs. However, they are an important part of any intervention. Success in these tasks brings about long-term cognitive, behavioural and emotional changes. They should therefore be chosen with considerable care and with the collaboration of the client. Clients should have a high degree of confidence that they will be able to complete the challenge successfully.

OTHER STRATEGIES

Although identifying and challenging cognitive distortions is central to the cognitive-behavioural approach, these are not the only strategies CBT employs. A useful precursor to therapy follows the principles of motivational interviewing (see Chapter 6), and is known as the Advantages–Disadvantages Analysis. Because of its similarity to motivational interviewing this will not be described further here (but see Beck *et al.* 1993).

Activity monitoring and scheduling

A frequently employed strategy involves planning things that interfere with substance misuse. Initially, a diary may be used to identify which behaviours the person engages in that are associated with substance misuse. Once these have been identified, alternative behaviours that interfere with the risk of this occurring may be scheduled at critical times. A problem drinker who finds it difficult not to drink in the evening and night, for example, may plan to go to places, such as the cinema or non-drinking friends, which prevent drinking at such times.

Behavioural rehearsal and role play

The therapy session permits a number of skill deficits to be identified and rehearsed prior to their use in the 'real world', often through the use of role-play. The skills taught will depend on the needs of the individual, but may include social and assertion skills, refusal, or conflict resolution skills among others. Behavioural rehearsal frequently involves a staged approach, in which complex skills are broken down into smaller components which are practised alone, before being integrated into a larger set of skills.

The emphasis is on ensuring success in the acquisition of skills to improve self-confidence and their continued use (Bandura, 1986). Skills may be rehearsed within sessions and practised in the 'real world' between sessions. Role-play in which the client acts as someone who is affected by another's substance misuse may also be used to help gain insight into the problems other people experience as a consequence of their behaviour.

Coping with cravings

Clients often experience powerful urges to take their substance of choice. Learning to cope with these cravings is a central element within the cognitive-behavioural approach. A number of strategies have been developed within this framework, including:

Distraction techniques

These involve clients changing the focus of their attention from their cravings to some other aspect of their environment. These may include concentrating on events or things within the environment: counting people, looking for car number plates that begin with a 'T', etc. The focus can be on anything that results in some form of attentional change (Blagden and Craske, 1996).

Flashcards

Flashcards can be particularly useful when clients are in high stress situations. Their content can be generated within therapy sessions, and should be short ('Think how well things have gone until now – don't let things slide'), and sufficiently general to be relevant under most conditions in which they may be necessary.

Imagery techniques

A number of imagery techniques can be used. One simply involves distraction, with the focus of the distraction being on an internally generated image rather than an external event. This can be enhanced by preceding such images with a technique known as thought stopping (Burk *et al.*, 1985). This involves saying to oneself

'Stop!' at the same time as generating an image that reflects the same sense such as a Stop sign or a road that goes over a cliff. A second strategy involves replacing positive thoughts about the value of substance misuse with a more negative outcome, such as having an argument with a partner.

Relaxation skills

Because many individuals use substances to help them cope with stress, it can be useful to teach some stress management skills. The simplest of these is relaxation training, the goal of which is to enable the individual to relax as much as is both possible and appropriate throughout the day and at times of particular stress. Learning relaxation may also lead to an increase in actual or perceived control over the stress response, a valuable outcome in itself.

The first stage of learning relaxation skills is to practise them under optimal conditions, augmented by continued practice at home, typically using taped instructions. The relaxation process most commonly used is a derivative of Jacobson's deep muscle relaxation technique (see Stetter, 1998). This involves alternately tensing and relaxing muscle groups throughout the body in an ordered sequence. As the individual becomes more skilled, the emphasis of practise shifts towards relaxation without prior tension, or relaxing specific muscle groups whilst using others in order to mimic the circumstances in which relaxation will be used in 'real life'.

At the same time as practising relaxation skills, individuals can begin to monitor their levels of physical tension throughout the day. Initially, this provides an educative effect. After a period of monitoring tension and learning relaxation techniques, individuals can begin to integrate them into their daily lives. Relaxation is best used, initially, at times of relatively low levels of excess tension. The consistent use of relaxation techniques at these times can prepare the person to cope with times of greater tension.

Rehearse, cope, reflect

Meichenbaum (1985) suggested that when an individual is trying to change their behaviour, the opportunity should be taken to rehearse new coping strategies before they are implemented. This can be done within therapy sessions, via role play, or by the client on their own. Once in the situation planned strategies should be enacted. Finally, after the situation has occurred, time should be given to review what occurred and the successes or failures that can be learned from. This process, in itself, can be as powerful a process of achieving change as any of the strategies previously described.

How effective is CBT in the context of substance misuse?

Cognitive behavioural interventions have achieved substantial success with other disorders. There is no reason to assume that they will not repeat this success in the treatment of substance-related problems. CBT is relatively simple to implement, will meet with good success rates, and has high face validity. However, success rates do not appear to be significantly greater than for other individual treatment approaches.

Reflecting the findings of studies in other populations, Project MATCH (Matching Alcoholism Treatments to Client Heterogeneity, 1998), for example, found no advantage in the use of CBT in comparison to other recognised treatments. They compared three treatment approaches in over 1,500 American problem drinkers: twelve-step facilitation, CBT, and Motivational Enhancement Therapy. By the end of treatment, 41 per cent of the CBT and twelve-step clients were abstinent or drank moderately: 28 per cent of the Motivational Enhancement group achieved the same criteria. However, by one- and three-year follow-ups, there were few differences between the three groups. Disappointingly, the researchers were unable to identify any client characteristics that predicted success or failure in any intervention. How culturally bound these results were, and whether they would translate to a UK population is unclear. What is clear is that CBT should not necessarily always be used on its own.

Couples therapy is a highly effective intervention in the treatment of substance misuse problems (Stanton and Shadish, 1997), and may usefully be combined with individually based CBT. Any combination of therapies need not necessarily just involve psychological therapy. Anton *et al.* (1999) reported a combination of Naltrexone and weekly CBT to be a more effective treatment than CBT alone.

Summary and conclusion

Interventions based on cognitive behavioural principles have a number of common elements and strengths. They are based in the present, focus on coping with specific problems, assume that cognitions guide our behaviour and that maladaptive cognitions drive maladaptive behaviour. The focus of any intervention is therefore both on the behaviour itself and the cognitions that are assumed to underpin that behaviour. Both need to be the focus of interventions, as the reciprocity between the two means that cognitive change will facilitate behavioural change, and behavioural change will facilitate cognitive change. Successful completion of homework tasks will result in increased confidence in the ability to achieve change: perhaps more so than any indirect cognitive procedure (Teasdale, 1985).

The focus on techniques provides a clear set of principles for therapists to use. However, it is important that those who use these techniques gain adequate supervision in their use from an experienced and competent supervisor. The results of Shaw *et al.* (1999) clearly indicate that therapist competence is an important determinant of the outcome of CBT.

Finally, despite its strengths, it should be remembered that CBT is not the only effective intervention that can be used to help people with substance abuse problems. The key to its successful use is the ability of the therapist to determine whether this approach is best for the individual they are working with. It may also be usefully employed in combination with other methods. Although it is a promising single approach, people with substance and alcohol problems typically face a multiplicity of problems in a variety of domains. No one type of intervention is likely to be totally effective in all cases and with all problems. Integration of cognitive-behavioural principles into a wider set of interventions may prove more effective than the 'purist' use of CBT techniques alone.

READER INPUT

Questions

(1) Briefly describe the central focus and primary goal of CBT.
(2) How might a client be encouraged to make associations between their thoughts, emotions and behaviours?
(3) List five strategies which may be employed to help the client identify errors of thinking and associated behaviours?
(4) How might a client be taught to manage cravings?
(5) Read Chapter 2 on theories relevant to substance misuse again. Which theoretical standpoints relate best to the principles of CBT?
(6) Read Chapter 10 on family interventions – can you identify how CBT might be used in a family/significant others setting to enable the client to reduce or cease their substance misuse and/or to provide help for the people who have to cope with the clients problem drinking or substance misuse?

FURTHER READING

Beck, A.T., Wight, F.D., Newman, C.F. and Liese, B.S. (1993) *Cognitive Therapy for Substance Abuse*, New York: Guilford.

Meichenbaum, D. (1985) *Stress Inoculation Training*, New York: Pergamon.

REFERENCES

Anton, R.F., Moak, D.H., Waid, R., Malcolm, R.J., Dias J.K. and Roberts, J.S. (1999) 'Naltrexone and cognitive behavioral therapy for the treatment of outpatient alcoholics: Results of a placebo-controlled trial', *American Journal of Psychiatry* 156: 1758–64.

Bandura, A. (1986) *Social Foundations of Thoughts and Actions: A Social Cognitive Theory*, Englewood Cliffs, NJ: Prentice-Hall.

Beck, A.T. (1976) *Cognitive Therapy and the Emotional Disorders*, New York: International Universities Press.

Beck, A.T., Rush, A.J., Shaw, B.F. and Emery, G. (1979) *Cognitive Therapy for Depression*, New York: Guilford.

Beck, A.T., Wight, F.D., Newman, C.F. and Liese, B.S. (1993) *Cognitive Therapy for Substance Abuse*, New York: Guilford.

Bennett, P. (2000) *An Introduction to Clinical Health Psychology*, Buckingham: Open University Press.

Blagden, J.C. and Craske, M.G. (1996) 'Effects of active and passive rumination and distraction: a pilot replication with anxious mood', *Journal of Anxiety Disorders* 10: 243–52.

Burk, E.M., Randolph, D.L. and Probst, C. (1985) 'Effects of several thought stopping treatments on worry cognition', *Psychology* 22: 31–41.

Meichenbaum, D. (1985) 'Stress inoculation training', New York: Pergamon.

Project MATCH Research Group (1998) 'Matching alcoholism treatments to client heterogeneity: Project MATCH three-year drinking outcomes', *Alcoholism: Clinical and Experimental Research* 22: 1300–11.

Rogers, C.R. (1967) *The Therapeutic Relationship and its Impact*, Madison: University of Wisconsin Press.

Shaw, B.F., Elkin, I., Yamaguchi, J., Olmstead, M., Vallis, T.M., Dobson, K.S., Lowery, A., Sotsky, S.M., Watkins, J.T. and Imber, S.D. (1999) 'Therapist competence ratings in relation to clinical outcome in cognitive therapy of depression', *Journal of Consulting and Clinical Psychology* 67: 837–46.

Stanton, M.D. and Shadish, W.R. (1997) 'Outcome, attrition, and family couples treatment for substance abuse: a meta-analysis and review of the controlled, comparative studies', *Psychological Bulletin* 122: 170–91.

Stetter, F. (1998) 'Relaxation techniques in psychotherapy', *Psychotherapeutics* 43: 209–20.

Teasdale, J.D. (1985) 'Psychological treatments for depression – how do they work?', *Behavioural Research and Therapy* 23: 157–65.

CHAPTER 6

MOTIVATIONALLY BASED INTERVENTIONS FOR BEHAVIOUR CHANGE

Meurig Davies and Trudi Petersen

LEARNING OBJECTIVES

After you have studied this chapter you will be able to:

1 Identify some of the factors that influence motivation and behaviour change.

2 Demonstrate an understanding of how a motivational approach can be utilised in practice.

INTRODUCTION

Most practitioners working within the fields of health and social care come into contact with clients experiencing substance misuse problems and will be aware of the importance of the individual's 'motivation' if they are to change their behaviour. Traditionally, motivation was seen as an innate characteristic of the individual. The client was either motivated to change, or not. If the client was not motivated they would 'fail' regardless of the intervention. Interventions were based on confrontation and advice, and inability or unwillingness to change or maintain change, was rationalised as the client having inadequate motivation.

In the past twenty years thinking in most UK settings has moved on influenced, among other things, by Prochaska and DiClemente's (1983) model of behaviour change, which recognises motivation to be a shifting phenomenon (see Chapter 7).

THE DEVELOPMENT OF MOTIVATIONAL INTERVIEWING

Motivational interviewing was developed by the American psychologist William Miller. In 1982 whilst supervising a group of psychologists working with substance misusers he found himself questioned about his methods. He began to explore his particular approach and wrote a concept paper which led on to further theory and empirical research (Miller, 1983, 1996).

It became clear to Miller that motivation is central to change processes. Ambivalence, a desire to carry out one action tempered by the desire to carry out an opposing action, is a potent influence on motivation. Also important is the way that practitioners interact with clients. Practitioners demonstrating greater empathy and possessing the ability to practise reflective listening have a significant positive effect on behaviour change (Miller and Baca, 1983).

Rollnick and Miller (1995) describe motivational interviewing as being 'directive' and 'client centred'. It is defined as a way of working, a 'counselling style', which aims to 'elicit behaviour change'. This is done by 'helping clients to explore and resolve ambivalence'.

Miller and Rollnick make a distinction between 'spirit' and technique. Becoming immersed in technique may risk loss of the overall spirit of what is being attempted. It is recommended that only interventions aimed at increasing readiness to change and embodying the spirit of Motivational Interviewing should be actually termed 'Motivational Interviewing' (Rollnick and Miller, 1995). Miller's original ideas have been developed and adpated by a variety of theorists and practitioners.

Utility of the motivational interviewing model

The principles of motivational interviewing can be used in any health care setting in which a behaviour change is sought in order to achieve health gains. It has been shown to be of use in interventions with both alcohol using and drug using clients. Noonan and Moyers (1997) reviewed eleven clinical trials of motivational interviewing, nine supported it as a useful intervention.

Motivational interviewing (including brief interventions) has been adapted and developed to address other client groups, resulting in motivationally based approaches to a variety of behaviours, including diabetes care (Stott *et al.*, 1995), risk reduction in HIV (Baker and Dixon, 1991) and the treatment of sex offenders (Garland and Dougher, 1991). Noonan and Moyers (1997) also cite its potential in pain management, coronary heart disease rehabilitation and eating disorders. The common features of these applications are behaviour change, the limitations of direct persuasion and working with ambivalence. Miller (1983) described four key aspects of motivational interviewing:

A de-emphasis on labelling

Negative labelling can serve to rationalise failure and inability to change. This may occur in either client or practitioner, e.g. 'I am a drug addict therefore I am bound to be addicted to some drug'. 'Substance misuse clients lie and shouldn't be trusted.' Labelling is discouraged.

Individual responsibility

Responsibility for issue identification and change rests with the client. A decision to maintain the *status quo* and resist change may be a viable position, despite the possibility that it may be seen by others as an 'unwise' decision. The client is treated as an adult, capable of making responsible decisions about their behaviour and finding an appropriate course of action to follow. This approach is consistent with humanistic psychology. The principles of motivational interviewing have been identified as congruent with the empowerment focus of social work (Hohman, 1998).

Internal attribution

When the individual identifies the potential for change as residing inside themselves rather than the result of external factors, change is generally greater. Positive internal attribution is consistent with developing feelings of self-esteem and self-efficacy.

Ambivalence

Where an individual recognises that their behaviour is inconsistent with their beliefs, attitudes or feelings, discrepancy or ambivalence, develops. In order to restore a balance, change is necessary.

Miller outlined several conditions required in order for motivation to be directed towards behaviour change:

- Self-esteem is increased.
- Self-efficacy (confidence) is increased.
- Discrepancy is initially increased.
- A reduction in discrepancy is sought through behaviour change.

The practitioner's role centres around identifying and increasing ambivalence whilst increasing the client's belief that they can generate change. It is important to note that increasing ambivalence without having the resources to reduce or restore internal inconsistencies can lead to stress. Stress has been described as a global precursor of relapse (Wanigaratne *et al.*, 1990).

A motivational process

Initially a process of engagement and affirmation is undertaken using a client centred approach as outlined by Rogers (1951). The practitioner attempts to build a rapport with the client. Practitioner skills of empathy and reflection focus the process on the client and enable the development of feelings of self-worth.

This early stage also involves agenda setting. When a client presents with a variety of issues, or a generalised desire to 'change things', identifying a realistic agenda concentrating on one particular aspect at a time will focus sessions and make them manageable. Rollnick *et al.* (1999) describe a collaborative agenda setting chart which may be adopted in such circumstances.

Readiness for change

The client's readiness to change can be assessed using Prochaska and DiClemente's model. Readiness to change can be established by simply asking the question: 'How ready to change are you?' Or it can be explored using a numerical rating scale (as described in 5. Support self-sufficiency). (See Chapter 7.)

Basic principles

Miller and Rollnick (1991) identify five basic motivational principles. We will now look at these in relation to specific practitioner activity.

1. Express empathy

Empathy can be expressed in a number of ways. Think of situations when you have felt that another person really understands what you are saying. They may nod, showing they are listening, make you feel comfortable, have open body language, congruent facial expressions and good eye contact. They may demonstrate an understanding of your feelings, i.e. 'I see how that could have been difficult for you'. One specific way of doing this is by reflection, feeding back what the client says. Miller (1983) asserts that reflection should not be a passive process but should be selective.

Reflection as reinforcement The intended effect is to increase the client's awareness of an important point or points and to facilitate further exploration and consolidation.

Reflection as restructuring Content may be slightly restructured, placing this in a different light or perspective such as in positive reframing. For example, a slip at a social event may be reflected as a relapse avoided, rather than a catastrophic indication of vulnerability.

2. *Develop discrepancy*

Awareness building is directed towards increasing cognitive discrepancy. The object of this process is to elicit from the client how their behaviour differs from their preferred lifestyle, aims and objectives. The client is encouraged to consider the benefits of continuing their behaviour, the benefits of changing or seeking out alternatives to that behaviour and the consequences of changing, or not changing, the behaviour.

Client preconceptions about what is expected of them may make it difficult for them to identify positive aspects of substance misuse for fear of professional judgement. The wording of questions needs careful consideration. For example, terms such as 'problem' are value laden. Asking the client to identify the 'useful' or 'beneficial' things alongside the 'not so useful' or 'not helpful' aspects of their substance use is better than asking them to list the 'bad things'.

The aim is to create a situation where the client considers behavioural change necessary in order to restore internal consistency. This can only be effective if the client is actively engaged in increasing awareness and identifies the problems and consequences of continuing or changing their behaviour themselves.

Miller (1983) outlined two means of achieving this.

- *Eliciting Self-Motivating Statements*. Self-motivating statements are positive statements, generated by the client in order to recognise problems related to substance misuse, develop concern regarding these and identify a need to change behaviour.
- *Integrating Objective Assessment*. Objective measures such as alcohol dependency scores and blood test results are fed back to the client. The way that this is done is important. (A challenging approach may result in resistance.) The aim is not to frighten the client but to elicit their interpretation of the data.

3. *Avoid argument*

Argument is avoided. This does not, however, mean that resistance is ignored. Resistance should be looked for and, once identified, attempts made to reduce it.

4. *Roll with resistance*

Resistance may take a variety of forms: argument, denial, excuses, blaming, interrupting and ignoring. The passive individual may be expressing as much resistance as the red-faced, angry person.

Overt persuasion of someone experiencing ambivalence is likely to lead to resistance. Miller and Rollnick (1991) refer to this as the 'confrontation-denial trap'. The more reasons the practitioner gives for stopping a behaviour the more the client reasserts their reasons to continue. Miller and Rollnick (1991) identify three 'traps' where resistance may develop and suggest strategies for dealing with these.

1 Control is taken from the client. If the client feels they are losing their autonomy resistance may occur. A re-emphasis on personal choice and control can help alleviate this.
2 The client's readiness to change or confidence levels are misjudged. A reassessment of these issues may be needed.
3 Meeting force with force. When confrontation is met with resistive force by the practitioner even deeper resistance may develop. Backing off and coming alongside the client through the use of reflective listening skills can help avoid this.

5. Support self-efficacy

The client's perceived importance of change and their confidence that they can change are key aspects. Rollnick *et al.* (1999) suggest the use of a rating scale to ascertain these. (Asking the client to rate how important change is to them and how confident they are about change on a scale where 1 = 'not at all' and 10 = 'extremely'.) Such scales can be used to elicit self-motivational statements. At first glance a logical approach would seem to be to ask the person why they didn't go for a higher number, but this is likely to elicit negative statements such as, 'I didn't go for a 4 because I can't . . .' This can quickly revert to a situation where they exhaust themselves by trying to persuade the client that they can do something, providing further material for resistance. Eventually the practitioner runs out of ideas and the client has confirmed to themselves their inability to carry out an action. What the practitioner is aiming for is positive statements. If the client is asked why a 3 not a 2 they are more likely to give positive statements, e.g. 'I chose a 3 because I have managed to stop using for short periods in the past'. The practitioner then uses their skills to build on these. Positive factors and successes, both past and current, are reinforced by the practitioner and a sense of optimism is encouraged. A realistic approach is necessary; forced over-confidence and idealistic goal setting will be counter-productive.

Moving towards change

Summarising

The client's expressed needs, feelings, ambivalent statements, decisional balances and self-motivational statements are brought together and fed back to the client in a selective, reflective way. The client is asked to comment on this summary in order to ensure that the feedback is complete and accurate.

Alternatives for behaviour change

The client may already be aware of appropriate strategies for change and has made attempts to change. The practitioner should help to explore these further. The directive nature of a motivational approach enables the practitioner to have a role in presenting alternative strategies for change. This is not done prescriptively, 'You should do this', but for example, 'This has been found to work with people in your situation, do you think this might be helpful?' Alternatives can then be practised by role play and evaluated in future sessions.

The scaling process can be used to help the client identify ways to change. Asking the client how they can move up the 1–10 scale may elicit specific actions, which can be worked towards, or particular ways that the practitioner can help. Brainstorming all potential strategies is one way of doing this.

Skill

The practitioner should be consistently non-judgemental, accepting and client centred. Necessary skills include the ability to reflect, participate in active listening, summarise, ask open-ended questions, clarify and affirm, demonstrating congruent non-verbal communication, sensitivity and empathy. Alongside this the practitioner needs to be able to direct the interaction in a positive fashion. The practitioner's role is not one of professional 'expert' with 'all the answers'; rather it is that of a 'partner'.

Conclusion

Motivational approaches offer a positive option for both practitioner and client but it is important that those using this approach are comfortable with it. Discomfort may lead to a loss of its 'spirit'. Role play can be very useful, especially if this is videoed. It is important that the practitioner has adequate support and good clinical supervision. Whether utilised in a brief intervention or as part of a more comprehensive treatment package motivationally centred approaches have potential in a wide variety of settings for a range of issues.

READER INPUT

Questions

(1) Developing a rapport, setting an agenda and identifying the client's readiness to change are early stages. How might you go about achieving these goals with a client and how might these influence follow-up interaction?

(2) What is ambivalence and what is the rationale for increasing ambivalence?

(3) How could you identify and increase ambivalence and direct the client in resolving this positively.

(4) What are self-motivational statements?

(5) How could you explore the client's belief in the importance of changing their behaviour and their confidence that they might be able to change? How might you use these to increase motivation?

Discussion

How might the practitioner:

(a) Give information whilst ensuring the client retains responsibility?
(b) Deal with negative statements or resistance whilst avoiding argument?
(c) Facilitate the client in developing and evaluating change strategies?
(d) Ensure client's goals and strategies are realistic and achievable?

Activity

Consider role-playing your own scenarios using characters who range in age and substances misused and who may vary in their stage of change, ambivalence and resistance. This can be done in pairs, one person playing the client, the other the practitioner. It can be helpful to video this, critically appraising it afterwards. Look especially at the use of open-ended questions, evidence of reflective listening, indications of a non-judgemental approach, recognition of ambivalence and management of this, argument avoidance and resistance management strategies.

REFERENCES

Baker, A. and Dixon, J. (1991) 'Motivational interviewing for HIV risk reduction', in W.R. Miller and S. Rollnick (1991) *Motivational Interviewing: Preparing People to Change Addictive Behaviour*, New York: Guildford.

Garland, R.J. and Dougher, M.J. (1991) 'Motivational Intervention in the treatment of sex offenders', in W.R. Miller and S. Rollnick (1991) *Motivational Interviewing: Preparing People to Change Addictive Behaviour*, New York: Guildford.

Hohman, M. (1998) 'Motivational interviewing: an intervention tool for case workers working with substance abusing parents', *Child Welfare*, LXXVII 3: 275–89.

Miller, W.R. (1983) 'Motivational interviewing with problem drinkers', *Behavioural Psychotherapy* 11: 147–72.

Miller, W.R. (1996) 'Motivational interviewing: research, practice and puzzles', *Addictive Behaviours* 21(6): 835–42.

Miller, W.R. and Baca, L.M. (1983) 'Two year follow up of bibliotherapy and directed controlled drinking training for problem drinkers', *Behaviour Therapy* 14: 441–8.

Miller, W.R. and Rollnick, S. (1991) *Motivational Interviewing: Preparing People to Change Addictive Behaviour*, New York: Guildford.

Noonan, W.C. and Moyers, T.B. (1997) 'Motivational interviewing', *Journal of Substance Misuse* 2: 8–16.

Prochaska, J., DiClemente, C. (1983) 'Stages and process of self-change of smoking: towards an integrative model of change', *Journal of Consulting and Clinical Psychology* 51: 390–5.

Rogers, C.R. (1951) *Client Centred Therapy*, London: Constable.

Rollnick, S., Heather, N., Bell, S. (1992) 'Negotiating behaviour change in medical settings: the development of brief motivational interviewing', *Journal of Mental Health* 1: 25–37.

Rollnick, S., Mason, P. and Butler, C. (1999) *Health Behaviour Change, A Guide For Practitioners*, London: Churchill Livingstone.

Rollnick, S. and Miller, W.R. (1995) 'What is motivational interviewing?' *Cognitive Behavioural Psychotherapy* 23: 325–34.

Saunders, B., Wilkinson, C., Phillips, M. (1995) 'The impact of a brief motivational intervention with opiate users attending a methadone programme', *Addiction* 90: 415–24.

Stott, N.C.H., Rollnick, S., Pill, P. and Rees, M. (1995) 'Innovation in clinical method: diabetes care and negotiation skills', *Family Practice*.

Wanigaratne, S., Wallace, W., Pullin, J., Keaney, F., Farmer, R. (1990) *Relapse Prevention For Addictive Behaviours*, London: Blackwell Scientific Publications.

FURTHER READING

Bien, T., Miller, W., Boroughs, J. (1993) 'Motivational interviewing with alcohol outpatients', *Behavioural and Cognitive Psychotherapy* 21: 347–56.

Miller, W.R., (1985) 'Motivation for treatment: a review with special emphasis on alcoholism', *Psychological Bulletin* 98(1): 84–107.

Rollnick, S., Heather, N., Gold, R. and Hall, W. (1992) 'Development of a short "Readiness to Change" questionnaire for use in brief, opportunistic interventions among excessive drinkers', *British Journal of Addiction* 87: 743–54.

Rollnick, S., Mason, P. and Butler, C. (1999) *Health Behaviour Change, A Guide For Practitioners*. London: Churchill Livingstone.

CHAPTER 7

BRIEF INTERVENTIONS, BRIEF INTERACTIONS

Ray Hodgson

LEARNING OBJECTIVES

By the end of this chapter you will be able to:

1. Describe the stages of change and be able to identify how these relate to brief interventions.
2. Demonstrate an understanding of how a brief intervention may be carried out in practice.

INTRODUCTION

We know from our own life experiences that even a few words can influence our future behaviour. The Chinese saying, 'If you can't make time for exercise then you will have to make time for illness', has nudged at least one person into taking regular exercise. A distinction is sometimes made between minimal interventions (less than 30 minutes) and brief interventions (up to three or four one-hour-sessions). Both types will be considered in this chapter.

Rollnick *et al.* (1999) point out that practitioners in health care are under pressure from the public health lobby to view every contact as a potential for brief intervention. They suggest this may not necessarily be helpful to practitioners or clients, with concerns including time problems, relationship damage, privacy issues and clients' perceptions of feeling overwhelmed with 'good' advice. So, are brief interventions helpful or merely a vehicle for raising client's guilt? One of the major criticisms of traditional 'advice giving' interventions is that they do not take into account the client's perceptions about what is important and why, or how ready the person is to address their 'non-healthy' behaviour. This chapter has an emphasis on one particular source of short-term communication, that which centres on motivation. Chapter 6 explores the idea of motivational approaches in detail, concentrating on longer-term and more specialist input. It is recommended that these two chapters are read in conjunction with each other.

INTERVENTION OR INTERACTION?

The dictionary definition of 'intervention' is:

> The action, or an act, of coming between, or interfering, especially so as to modify or prevent a result.
>
> (Brown, L. (ed.) *The New Shorter Oxford English Dictionary*, Vol. 1: 1401)

The dictionary definition of 'interaction' runs thus:

> Reciprocal action; action or influence of persons or things on each other.
>
> (Brown, L. (ed.) *The New Shorter Oxford English Dictionary*, Vol. 1: 1391)

This chapter concentrates on client centred approaches to short-term inputs, highlighting the need for recognition of the client's understanding and position in relation to change. The concept of reciprocation seems more apt than that of interference. Although the term 'brief interventions' is used throughout, the reader is encouraged to read 'intervention' but think 'interaction'.

STAGES OF CHANGE

First it is necessary to consider the ways in which people change. Readiness to change is sometimes strong, sometimes weak, but more often fluctuating. According to Prochaska and Di Clemente (1983) there are at least five stages of change:

1 Precontemplation.
2 Contemplation.
3 Readiness for action.
4 Action (behaviour change).
5 Maintenance.

An additional aspect is relapse.

In the precontemplation stage the individual does not intend to change in the near future. The perceived benefits of substance misuse may outweigh the perceived costs. Costs may be played down because of ignorance or denial. The contemplation stage covers that period when costs and benefits are being reappraised and ability to cope with change is assessed. This stage can last a few minutes or a few years. Contemplation becomes determination when a commitment is made. In the action stage positive steps are being taken. Finally, the maintenance stage begins a few months after successful change. In this stage vigilance is still relatively high, in an attempt to prevent relapse. Prochaska and Di Clemente describe the stages of change as a cyclical process rather than a linear progression. A person may swing backwards and forwards between stages. For example, thinking about changing, gearing up toward change then choosing not to follow this through and returning to the contemplation stage is common.

One mistake often made is to assume a readiness for action. Ambivalence is frequently experienced and motivation can vary daily. Furthermore a person in the contemplation stage needs a different approach from a person who is ready for action. So the first basic principle that applies to brief interventions is to take into account their stage of change, i.e. has the person considered changing their behaviour or have they made any plans to do this? Do they even consider their behaviour to be a cause for concern? A non-contemplative substance misuser might be encouraged to see connections between substance misuse and personal problems. On the other hand, someone in the action stage could be encouraged to consider various change strategies or ways of coping with temptation.

The second basic principle is to focus upon natural processes of change (Table 7.1). Prochaska and Di Clemente (1986) present evidence that these processes are differentially linked to particular stages of change. Raising awareness and self-re-evaluation are dominant during a move into the contemplation stage. Self-liberation is a key process in moving from contemplation to action, whereas counter-conditioning, stimulus control and contingency management are crucial during the action and maintenance stages.

So one of the aims of brief interventions is to identify an area associated with substance misuse that could possibly be changed. This may not necessarily be specifically related to the substance itself. In the following example an isolated client achieved abstinence by transforming his social environment after a brief intervention (personal communication – Karen Hicks).

Example 1

The client had retreated into himself after an accident that left him with some disability. He was asked by the practitioner to bring a friend with him to the counselling session. He brought along a close female friend who was happy to give support but, she pointed out, the communication between them had deteriorated. Just two sessions were sufficient to improve communication and facilitate the development of positive activities together. The aim was to 'have fun'. Within weeks the client had changed from a silent, solitary drinker to a talkative, social abstainer as a result of this 'nudge in the right direction'.

Table 7.1 Processes of change

Raising awareness	This can be the result of a therapeutic intervention or alternatively a life event.
Self re-evaluation	Taking stock of one's current situation often precedes cognitive and behavioural changes. 'What are my talents and skills?' 'What do I want to achieve?'
Social-environmental re-evaluation	A substance misuser might consider that they are locked into a social network of other substance users and decide that a change of environment is called for.
Self-liberation	At some stage during change a feeling of freedom and confidence is experienced. Perceived self-efficacy or ability to cope is an important milestone and a predictor of future success.
Social liberation	This occurs when the person becomes more confident in social situations and is less likely to experience social pressure to use substances.
Counter conditioning	This process involves replacing substance use with other activities. At another level it is the process of counteracting craving by replacing substance use thoughts with other thoughts.
Stimulus control	Avoiding substance misuse cues or desensitising them is one component of more behavioural approaches to treatment.
Contingency management	If abstaining leads to immediate benefits then the new lifestyle will be reinforced.
Dramatic relief	Catharsis and conversion sometimes occur during psychological treatment or after a substance misuse related catastrophe. Sometimes dramatic attitudinal change occurs after less obvious trauma, i.e. an experience of impotence.
Helping relationships	Self-help groups, befriending schemes and professional counselling are based upon the belief that it is easier to change with the help of empathetic help.

The Prochaska and DiClemente model puts the substance misuse issue in perspective, enabling the practitioner to ask a number of relevant questions, the main ones being

1 What stage of change has this person reached?
2 What change processes should now be the focus of attention?

EVIDENCE OF EFFECTIVENESS

There is good evidence that minimal and brief interventions can be effective, at least for alcohol related problems, in both primary care and hospital situations (Heather, 1998; Raistrick *et al.*, 2000). Wallace *et al.* (1998) used an intervention that involved the assessment of alcohol problems, followed by information about how to cut down on drinking and using a drinking diary. Control group patients received the usual care. One year on, the proportion of men drinking excessively had fallen by 44 per cent in the treatment group, compared to 26 per cent in the control group. A World Health Organisation study involving 1,655 heavy drinkers in 10 countries achieved similar results with a 5 minute intervention following on from a 15 minute assessment (Babor and Grant, 1992). These studies demonstrate effectiveness in primary care settings but it is suggested that brief interventions can also be effective in hospital settings. One of the first investigations to focus on brief interventions involved patients on a general medical ward (Chick *et al*., 1985).

There are still unanswered questions. Are brief interventions effective within a social work or probation setting? Do the effects last longer than one year? What kind of person responds to which kind of intervention? Most importantly, we need to know much more than we do about the change processes that are involved.

BRIEF MOTIVATIONAL COUNSELLING

One approach that performed well in a randomised controlled trial is Motivational Enhancement Therapy (MET) (Project MATCH, 1997). It was found that four sessions of MET were as effective as twelve sessions of other treatment approaches, even with people more severely alcohol dependent. At the heart of this approach is the view that motivation to change can be enhanced by a practitioner and, once enhanced, the client has available the skills to implement change. Miller and Sanchez (1994) describe six 'active ingredients' of brief interventions. They are summarised by the acronym FRAMES.

Feedback of personal risk or impairment.
Responsibility for change.
Advice to change.
Menu of alternative change options.
Empathy on behalf of the practitioner.
Self-efficacy or optimism in the client is facilitated by the practitioner.

Crucially important is the therapeutic style central to the MET approach. It has been demonstrated that an empathetic therapeutic style is a powerful predictor of success.

Basic principles of MET

The approach begins with the assumption that the responsibility and capacity for change lie within the client. The practitioner's task is to create a set of conditions that will enhance the client's own motivation for and commitment to change. The practitioner seeks to mobilise the client's inner resources and those inherent in the client's natural helping relationships in order to help the client initiate, persist in and comply with behaviour change efforts. Miller and Rollnick (1991) describe five basic motivational principles underlying such an approach.

1 Express empathy.
2 Develop discrepancy.
3 Avoid argumentation.
4 Roll with resistance.
5 Support self-efficacy.

This approach can be divided into two major stages: building motivation for change and strengthening commitment. To use MET as a brief intervention needs training and supervised practise. A useful MET manual is available from the National Institute on Alcohol Abuse and Alcoholism (see website address in Further Reading at end of chapter).

A menu of options

The MET approach outlined underpins both brief and minimal interventions. A menu of items is considered by the practitioner then selected. Items include:

- Establishing rapport.
- Raising the topic of alcohol or drug misuse.
- Exploring concerns.
- Assessing motivation and confidence.
- The pros and cons of substance misuse.
- Change strategies.
- Reviewing and summarising.

Raising the issue of substance misuse must be accomplished sensitively. One sure way of turning the client off is to demand, 'What are you going to do about your alcohol (or drug) problem?' A direct approach may be occasionally appropriate but generally the topic needs to be addressed more carefully, for example by a general discussion on health, stress at work or home, or accidents and injuries. This offers the opportunity to ask the client how their substance use fits in. There are many ways of exploring concerns in a non-threatening way, for example:

1 'What effect does alcohol have on you?' This can provoke discussion on good and bad effects.
2 'Tell me about a typical day when you are drinking or using drugs.' This elicits specific situations and events such as 'I've been stopped twice by the police whilst walking home from the Dog and Gun'.

Perceptions of positive effects from substances predict onset of use, problematic use and relapse after treatment. One of the goals of a brief intervention is to identify positive effects and emphasise the positive effects of moderation or abstinence to keep the balance of pros and cons tipped in one direction.

The focus is on motivation to change rather than techniques for producing change, nevertheless the client's confidence in their ability to change and their motivation as a result of this can sometimes be influenced by a brief discussion of potential change strategies. The following simple approaches may be slipped into a brief session or if the client requests advice.

- **Goal setting.** Change requires the setting of reasonable short-term goals such as drinking only on Wednesday, Friday and Saturday for two weeks.
- **Frequent recall of the benefits of change.** General intentions usually lead to naught. One strategy is for the client to imagine the positive benefits of change every time they carry out a regular activity such as when they have a sip of tea or coffee.
- **Develop other pleasant activities** and enlist the support of a friend or relative.
- **Reviewing.** People can often forget information communicated by health professionals. It is essential to review key points that emerge.

A five minute intervention

Minimal interventions have been seen to impact on behaviour. Smith *et al.* (2000) found a single 15 minute intervention was effective in reducing alcohol consumption in young men with alcohol related injury. However, in some busy settings it is not possible to incorporate even a 15 minute intervention into routine service provision. The WHO study mentioned earlier demonstrated that change could be facilitated by an intervention as brief as 5 minutes. Example 2 (below) outlines a 5 minute intervention focusing on alcohol misuse in an accident and emergency setting.

Example 2

This scenario concentrates on alcohol misuse in an accident and emergency setting but could be relevant for other settings/substances where time is pressured.

- **Empathise and develop a non-confrontational style**
  'What happened? How did you get this injury?' 'We ask quite a few questions about the causes of accidents because we want to work out how to prevent them. Could you tell me about your injury?'
- **Initiating discussion about excessive alcohol use as a risk factor**
  'For many A&E patients alcohol was one of the reasons they were injured. Do you think alcohol could have played a part in your injury?'
- **Give feedback about their level of consumption**
  'Some of your friends probably do drink as much as you but you do drink more than is recommended and more than average.'
- **Discuss the benefits of reduced consumption**
  'Do you think your life would improve in any way if you cut down on your drinking?' 'Would you be in more control?' 'Would you be healthier?'
- **Discuss intentions and commitment**
  'Do you plan to drink less in the future?' We are giving out booklets which give information about alcohol, would you like one? Do you think you might read it?'

The above steps and suggested questions can be summarised by another acronym, BRIEF:

> Benefits – the client should be informed of the benefits of sensible drinking.
> Risk factor – investigation into the substance (i.e. alcohol) as a risk factor in the client's current situation can raise awareness.
> Intentions – clarify the client's future intentions.
> Empathise – the practitioner should retain a non-judgemental attitude.
> Feedback – the practitioner should give the client feedback on their levels of consumption.

Right time, right place, right person

A brief intervention such as this can be given at the same time as other medical procedures, adding little to the time involved. The aim of the intervention is to raise awareness and motivation to change whilst facilitating decision making. Lengthy discussion would be discouraged though specialist referral may be one possible future option. A few words given at the right time by the right person can have a significant influence. Health professionals have status and credibility. A nurse or doctor may be the right person to carry out this activity and immediately after an event may well be the right time.

Conclusion

The evidence supports the case for routine implementation of brief interventions. Some of the time such an approach will be all that is needed, but for some individuals a brief intervention may be the first step in a process of stepped care. For many prolonged psychotherapeutic approaches it is the early sessions that are associated with greatest change. The first few sessions prime a number of key change processes, including awareness and motivation, planning, understanding the nature of the 'problem' and the sharing of this with a practitioner.

Primary care and medical settings are suitable for the development of brief interventions; however, for this to be facilitated a number of beliefs commonly held by health professionals may need challenging. Practitioners need to be made aware of the evidence relating to effectiveness. They also need to believe that it is their job to intervene (role legitimacy) and have to learn the relevant skills in order to carry out such an approach effectively (role adequacy). Finally the health care system will have to provide better support with both training and shared care for 'difficult' cases (role support). Just as smoking and exercise are targets when considering the prevention of heart disease so should substance misuse be seen as a target when considering accidents, injury and a wide range of diseases as well as family and social problems. Brief interventions can help shift our perspective and see the potential benefit of early interventions.

READER INPUT

Questions

(1) What do the acronyms FRAMES and BRIEF stand for?
(2) How many settings can you think of that may offer an opportunity for brief interventions?

Role play

Imagine the following scenario: Steve has come to the outpatients' clinic for a follow-up appointment after treatment for a facial injury he received during a fight at a night club. How might the practitioner at the clinic:

(a) Raise the issue of alcohol with Steve?
(b) Identify his readiness to change?
(c) Carry out a brief intervention around Steve's alcohol use?

Consider role playing this scenario in each of three ways:

(a) Steve is a little concerned about his alcohol use but is ambivalent about whether he wishes to change his behaviour.
(b) Steve does not consider his alcohol use an issue.
(c) Steve has been concerned about his alcohol intake and has made some steps towards cutting down but he is still ambivalent about this and unsure of exactly how to go about doing so effectively.

Post-role play discussion

How did the person role playing the practitioner come across during the activity? What kind of questions did they ask? What was their use of language and non-verbal communication? What kind of attitude did they convey and how? How did the person role playing Steve feel during the interaction? What was the pattern of communication between them?

FURTHER READING

National Institute on Alcohol Abuse and Alcoholism http://www.niaaa.nih.gov.

REFERENCES

Babor, T.F. and Grant, M. (1992) *Programme on Substance Abuse: Project on Identification and Management of Alcohol-related Problems. Report on Phase 11. A Randomised Clinical Trial of Brief Interventions in Primary Health Care*, New York: World Health Organisation.

Brown, L. (ed.) (1993) *The New Shorter Oxford English Dictionary*, Oxford: Oxford University Press.

Chick, J., Lloyd, G. and Crombie, E. (1985) 'Counselling problem drinkers in medical wards. A controlled study', *British Medical Journal* 290: 965–7.

Heather, N. (1998) 'Using brief opportunities for change', in W.R. Miller and N. Heather, (eds) (1998) *Treating Addictive Behaviours* (2nd edn) New York: Plenum.

Miller, W.R. and Rollnick, S. (1991) *Motivational Interviewing: Preparing People to Change Addictive Behaviour*, New York: Guilford Press.

Miller, W.R. and Sanchez, V.C. (1994) 'Motivating young adults for treatment and lifestyle change', in G.S. Howard and P.E. Nathan (eds) (1994) *Alcohol Use and Misuse by Young Adults*, Notre Dame, IN: University of Notre Dame Press.

Prochaska, J. and DiClemente, C. (1983) 'Stages and processes of self-change of smoking: towards an integrated model of change', *Journal of Consulting and Clinical Psychology* 51: 390–5.

Prochaska, J.O. and DiClemente, C.C. (1986) 'Toward a comprehensive model of change', in W.R. Miller and N. Heather (eds) *Treating Addictive Behaviours* (2nd edn) New York: Plenum.

Project MATCH research group (1997) 'Matching alcoholism treatments to client heterogeneity: Project MATCH post treatment drinking outcomes', *Journal of Studies on Alcohol* 58(1): 7–29.

Raistrick, D., Hodgson, R.J. and Ritson, B. (2000) *Tackling Alcohol Together*, London: Free Association Books.

Rollnick, S., Mason, P. and Butler, C. (1999) *Health Behaviour Change, A Guide For Practitioners*, London: Churchill Livingstone.

Smith, A., Hodgson, R.J. and Shepherd, J. (2000) *Reducing Alcohol Consumption in Young Men with Alcohol Related Facial Injuries*. London: Alcohol Education and Research Council.

Wallace, P., Cutler, S., Haines, A. *et al.* (1988) 'Randomised control trial of General Practitioner intervention in patients with excessive alcohol consumption', *British Medical Journal* 297: 663–8.

CHAPTER 8

HARM MINIMISATION

Richard Pates

LEARNING OBJECTIVES

After reading this chapter you will be able to:

1 Understand the concept of harm minimisation.
2 Show how this can be put into practice.

INTRODUCTION

> Harm reduction is the intersection between public health and human rights.
>
> (Nadelmann, 2001)

Harm minimisation (also known as harm reduction) is a model of working that has been associated with drug use since the mid-1980s. This was a response to the need to try to minimise the harm caused by injecting drug use at the beginning of the HIV epidemic. The model acknowledges that people will continue to use drugs despite the risks and sometime prohibition, and works on the principle that some of the risks of drug use can be reduced and minimised. Prevention measures and education are important but if they are unsuccessful we must work with the consequences of drug use.

Drug use can be harmful because of the effects of the drug itself, contaminants mixed with the drug, the method of delivery and the effects on others. The effects of injecting drugs include not only the actions of the drug but also possible infection and damage caused by the process of injecting.

Harm minimisation is about educating drug users to the risks of drug taking and helping them take responsibility for themselves. Harm minimisation is a process and not a treatment and should be integrated with other forms of intervention.

People who use drugs (including alcohol) are part of the wider community. It is in the public interest that those members of the community who use drugs do so with the minimum of damage to themselves and others and that the means to minimise harm are available.

THEORY

Newcombe (1992) suggested a theoretical framework for harm minimisation. He proposed a classification using a two-dimensional model, one dimension classifying the type of consequence of drug use (health, social or economic), and the other dimension the *level* of consequence (individual, community or societal). For example:

- Cirrhosis of the liver caused by excessive alcohol consumption would be seen as an individual health harm.
- Stigmatisation of the relatives of drug users as a community social harm.
- The cost of drug law enforcement as a societal economic harm.

Psychoactive drugs bring about benefits as well as causing harm, and Newcombe points out that we need to consider the balance between the two. For example:

- The use of cannabis is illegal and has social consequences for the user but is used widely for symptom control in some diseases such as multiple sclerosis and AIDS.
- Drinking small amounts of alcohol on a regular basis may have benefits to the cardiovascular system whereas large quantities of alcohol consumed on a daily basis will have damaging health effects.
- High levels of alcohol consumption have harmful effects on health but produce large amounts of money in taxes.

Newcombe suggests that a more accurate classification of the harm and benefits of drug use should include a time dimension (e.g. short, medium and long-term effects), a duration dimension (temporary or permanent) and a scale dimension (minor, moderate or major effects). Using such a model, an organisation, be it the government or a local non-statutory agency, can decide on its strategic priorities and what it can afford to do.

The Advisory Council on the Misuse of Drugs, which advises the British government, recognised in a report on AIDS and Drug Misuse (ACMD, 1988) that individuals who use drugs may not wish, or be able to become abstinent at the point of first contact with services. ACMD suggested a hierarchy of harm reduction measures, from stopping people sharing injecting equipment, through persuading them to cease injecting to becoming abstinent. This model allows the process of change to start from where the drug user is, and for the helping agency to remain in contact to facilitate further change while maintaining credibility with the individual.

Assessment

It is inadvisable to accept that a user of substances knows, for example, the difference between a vein and an artery, why they should not inject into an artery and how to avoid this risk. Some drinkers are likewise unaware that four cans of 9 per cent ABV lager contain the equivalent of two-thirds of a bottle of spirits (18 British units). By finding out what people are doing, it becomes possible to educate them into safer practices. This means that individuals working with people with substance problems must have full knowledge of their subject in order to give relevant and accurate information to help clients make informed choices.

Clients should also be provided with information about themselves via objective testing. This may be a blood test to determine the state of the liver in heavy drinkers, testing for the presence of antibodies for hepatitis B and C or HIV so that immunisation or treatment can be offered, or cognitive testing to determine whether impairment has resulted from heavy substance use. All these again provide the client with objective information so that they can make informed choices.

METHODS

Alcohol

Attempts to limit the harm caused by alcohol have been attempted through legislation and education. The 1751 Gin Act introduced legislation to limit the issuing of licences to sell gin and stiff penalties for the unlicensed selling of gin. This reduced the consumption of gin, which had been having a devastating effect on the urban population of England, from 11 million to 2 million gallons per year. Prohibition under the Volstead Act in the USA tried to halt the selling of alcohol from 1920 onwards. This is a good example of a policy that was misguided and driven mainly by crusading moralists (Behr, 1997). It was misguided in that it led to the involvement of organised crime in the alcohol trade, comparable perhaps with the heroin and cocaine trades today. Prohibition did reduce the incidence of cirrhosis of the liver in the USA during this period, but at a high price. The law is also used to minimise alcohol related harm by restricting the age of permitted alcohol purchase and licensing restrictions including the times and places from which alcohol may be sold. Economic measures have also been used, increasing taxes on alcohol to reduce overall consumption. It has been suggested that a substantial increase in alcohol taxation would lead to an overall reduction in alcohol related harm (Kenkel and Manning, 1996).

Harm reduction for alcohol may include not only approaches aimed at the individual drinker but also at a policy or environmental level (Larimer *et al.*, 1998). The individual may be 'taught' to drink in a controlled way (Sobell and Sobell, 1995) and educated on the dangers of alcohol and certain styles of drinking, e.g. binge drinking.

Other approaches include public education and advertising campaigns, and greater information about the products themselves, such as the amount of alcohol by volume, being printed on packaging. These approaches must be seen against the background of powerful alcohol producers who market their products to increase the amounts sold and introduce people at a young age to alcohol use as an acceptable, desirable part of life.

Graham and Homel (1997) have reviewed the effects of the environment on alcohol related aggression. The design of the bar, level of cleanliness and décor, quality of the air within the bar (i.e. effects of tobacco smoke) and provision of food can all affect the expectations of clients and reduce levels of alcohol related aggression. The use of glasses and bottles that shatter rather than splinter is also useful, as it limits the injuries that can be caused by using glasses as weapons. Staff training has been shown to reduce levels of alcohol consumption, levels of drink driving and alcohol related injuries (Saltz, 1997).

Illicit drugs

Harm minimisation processes surrounding the use of illicit drugs have attracted the most publicity. The harm that drugs may cause has been recognised for most of the last century, but it is only since the beginnings of the HIV epidemic in the 1980s, that concerted attempts have been made to minimise related harm.

The harm that may be caused by drug use will depend upon the drug, the method of administration and the characteristics of the taker. Harm minimisation advice about the drugs themselves can be divided into advice about the drug (dosing), about the effects of mixing drugs, and about the short- and long-term effects. With this information, people are able to make choices about the level of risk to which they will expose themselves. For example, users of stimulants need to know that these drugs will raise blood pressure and heart rate, to dangerous levels in some individuals. They may also be more disinhibited and take more sexual risks under the influence of the drug and that they may experience a 'come down' after use. They also need to know about the long-term effects of appetite suppression and psychosis that can all follow long-term stimulant use. The way in which drugs are taken can also be important; injection of drugs being perhaps the most hazardous (see Chapter 14).

In addition to advice, important interventions can be made which have been shown to be effective in limiting the spread of disease caused through drug injecting. Needle and syringe exchanges provide injecting drug users with free sterile needles, syringes, in some cases sterile water and other paraphernalia, and condoms. Exchanges also provide a means of safer disposal of used equipment. Needle exchange users are far less likely to share other people's used equipment. Attendance at a needle exchange also gives the opportunity to ask advice about injecting and health issues and to obtain referral to treatment services if requested (see Appendix 8.1).

The provision of substitute prescribing programmes is another important harm minimisation intervention (see Chapter 11).

The availability of testing for infections also provides harm minimising opportunities. Immunisation, e.g. for hepatitis B or tetanus, may be offered as protection against these diseases. These are not 'cures' for drug use but recognise that if the spread of diseases is to be curtailed then pragmatic responses are needed.

Dance drugs

Harm minimisation principles have been deployed innovatively with 'dance drugs' which are used by many thousands of young people at clubs and dance events (Tyler, 1995). Ecstasy increases body temperature and the venues will themselves be hot, so that there are risks of overheating and exhaustion. Measures have evolved including the provision of 'chill out' rooms where dancers can sit and cool down and the availability of free water to help dancers avoid dehydration. Another example of harm minimisation on the dance scene has been seen in Holland, where drug testing has been introduced so that users can have a sample of their pill tested to ascertain the content. Again the intention is to provide information so that the user can make a more informed choice about the risks they are willing to take.

Other interventions that are used with drug users include outreach and detached services to make contact with users who will not normally come into contact with services and to provide them with clean injecting equipment, advice and condoms. Provision of condoms is particularly important for commercial sex workers, many of whom also use drugs and are therefore doubly at risk in terms of HIV and other infections.

DOES HARM MINIMISATION WORK?

Many varieties of harm minimisation have been evaluated and found to be effective. For example, Robertson *et al.* (1986) estimated an alarming 85 per cent prevalence rate for HIV amongst intravenous drug users in an area of Edinburgh in Scotland. In neighbouring Glasgow the rate was less than 4 per cent. One major difference between the two cities was the availability of needles and syringes. In Edinburgh there was a strict policy of confiscation of injecting equipment by the police and this meant higher rates of sharing. There was also poor access to treatment. With improved availability of treatment and access to clean injecting equipment the prevalence of HIV in Edinburgh has dropped dramatically.

Stimson (1996) reviewed the strong evidence that harm minimisation approaches averted an HIV epidemic among drug users in the United Kingdom. Others have made the comparison with other countries, without harm minimisation strategies, that have experienced catastrophic rates of HIV among their drug using populations. Bastos *et al.* (1998) have noted that across the world, cities where harm reduction policies were adopted at the beginning of the HIV epidemic have much lower prevalence rates than those which did not implement these policies for either political or economic reasons. They also point out that the speed at which the epidemic grew in those countries was extremely rapid, with prevalence in at risk groups increasing from zero to more than 50 per cent in a very few years. Stimson warns that, 'The message to the UK government is *not* that the epidemic never happened and that resources may be directed elsewhere; rather, that evidence to date suggests that prevention investment has paid off, that public health prevention works with this population, and that this needs to be sustained in order to preserve the beneficial situation in which we find ourselves.' One has also to remember that this real public health achievement has been made against a background of increasing illicit drug use.

Burrows and Urban (2001) in reviewing the effectiveness over time of harm reduction programmes have said that a period of at least six years is needed to develop an adequate response in a large country with widespread injecting drug use, and at least three to four years in a smaller country. Where policies are not harm reduction oriented and where HIV already exists, the implementation of harm reduction initiatives will show a progressive and real impact.

Hawks and Lenton (1995), reviewing harm reduction in Australia, stated: 'Overall conclusions from randomised controlled trials and observational studies are that methadone treatment reduces heroin use, crime, injection related risks and premature mortality among people on opioids.'

From a public health perspective harm minimisation works and has cost benefits because the cost of such interventions are much cheaper than the cost of treating people with HIV. Wiebel (2001) has stated that the costs associated with not attending to public health threats such as HIV/AIDS, hepatitis C, bacterial endocarditis, overdose death, chemical dependence and the like are real and large. Ultimately, no society can afford to let these problems escalate unabated.

In the UK the battle to prevent the spread of HIV is being won, but the war is not over. The rates of hepatitis C in the UK among drug users is very high and there may be people becoming users now who were not exposed to the measures developed in the 1980s and 1990s. Harm minimisation policies and practices need to remain in place, evolve to meet new challenges and receive adequate funding.

Questions about the efficacy of harm minimisation measures for alcohol problems remain. Aspects of alcohol harm reduction have clearly had an effect, for example in terms of drink driving. Not only are rates now much lower but there is a general public acceptance that driving after drinking is unacceptable. This is a direct result of the introduction of the breathalyser thirty years ago.

Despite harm minimisation measures for alcohol and other drugs, unacceptably high levels of harm are caused to individuals, communities and society. We know that we cannot eliminate the use of drugs, nor perhaps would we wish to when there are benefits when used in moderation. Measures that effectively reduce the harm caused must continue to be pursued.

READER INPUT

(1) Using the framework proposed by Newcombe classify:
  (a) An agency that you are familiar with and which has some degree of involvement with substance misuse problems. Does the agency see any of its function as being within a harm reduction framework?
  (b) Your own pattern of drug use.
  (c) The pattern of drug use of somebody you have met who has a problem.

(2) What aspects of needle exchange cause you most anxiety? How might needle exchange be made more accessible in your area? How can needle exchange be modified to combat the spread of hepatitis C more effectively?

(3) Drug and alcohol use are legally constrained, and in some instances prohibited. Consider both sides of the arguments that:
  (a) Alcohol related violence should be tackled by stricter enforcement of licensing laws.
  (b) Drug users should be told about the risks of injecting and then left to their own devices.

FURTHER READING

Derricott, J., Preston, A. and Hunt, N. (1999) *The Safer Injecting Briefing: An easy to use comprehensive reference guide to promoting safer injecting*, Liverpoool: HIT Publications.

Marlatt, A. (1998) *Harm Reduction. Pragmatic Strategies for Managing High-Risk Behaviours*, New York: The Guilford Press.

O'Hare, P.A., Newcombe, R., Matthews, A., Buning, E.C. and Drucker, E. (eds) (1992) *The Reduction of Drug Related Harm*, London: Routledge.

Stimson, G. (1996) 'Has the United Kingdom averted a major epidemic of HIV-1 infection among drug injectors?' *Addiction* 91(8): 1085–8 (plus commentaries on pp 1089–99).

Whitfield, J. (1996) 'A scientific perspective on harm reduction', *Drug and Alcohol Review* 15(2): 117–19.

REFERENCES

Advisory Council on the Misuse of Drugs (1988) *AIDS and Drug Misuse Part 1*, London: HMSO.

Bastos, F., Stimson, G.V., Telles, P. and Barcellos, C. (1998) 'Cities responding to HIV-1 epidemics among injecting drug users', in G.V. Stimson, D.C. Des Jarlais, and A. Ball (eds), *Drug Injecting and HIV Infection*, London: University College London Press.

Burrows, D. and Urban, W. (2001) 'The time it takes: When to start harm reduction programmes for HIV prevention among IDUs', paper presented at the 12th International Conference on the Reduction of Drug Related Harm, New Delhi, India.

Behr, E. (1997) *Prohibition*, London: Penguin Books.

Graham K. and Homel, R. (1997) 'Creating safer bars', in M. Plant, E. Single and T. Stockwell (eds) *Alcohol: Minimising the Harm – What Works?* London: Free Association Books.

Hawks, D. and Lenton, S. (1995) 'Harm reduction in Australia: has it worked? A review', *Drug and Alcohol Review* 14: 291–304.
Kenkel, D. and Manning, W. (1996) 'Perspectives on alcohol taxation', *Alcohol Health and Research World* 20(4): 230–8, cited in Marlatt, A. (ed.) (1998) *Harm Reduction. Pragmatic Strategies for Managing High-Risk Behaviours*, New York: The Guilford Press.
Larimer, M.E., Marlatt, G.A., Baer, J.S., Quigley, L.A., Blume, A.W. and Hawkins, E.H. (1998) 'Harm reduction for alcohol problems. Expanding access to and acceptability of prevention and treatment services', in A. Marlatt (ed.) (1998) *Harm Reduction. Pragmatic Strategies for Managing High-Risk Behaviours*, New York: The Guilford Press.
Nadelmann, E. (2001) 'Globalization of harm reduction: practice, politics, principles', The Rolleston Oration, 12th International Conference on the Reduction of Drug Related Harm, New Delhi, India.
Newcombe, R. (1992) 'The reduction of drug related harm. A conceptual framework for theory, practice and research', in P.A. O'Hare, R. Newcombe, A. Matthews, E.C. Buning and E. Drucker, (eds) *The Reduction of Drug Related Harm*, London: Routledge.
Robertson, J.R., Bucknall, A.B.V., Welsby, P.D. *et al.* (1986) 'An epidemic of AIDS-related virus (HTLVIII/LAV) infection among intravenous drug abusers in a Scottish general practice', *British Medical Journal* 292: 527–30.
Saltz, R.F. (1997) 'Prevention where alcohol is sold and consumed: server intervention and responsible beverage service', in M. Plant, E. Single and T. Stockwell, (eds) *Alcohol: Minimising the harm – what works?* London: Free Association Books.
Sobell, M.B. and Sobell, L.C. (1995) 'Controlled drinking after 25 years: How important was the great debate?' Editorial in *Addiction* 90: 1149–54.
Stimson, G. (1996) 'Has the United Kingdom averted a major epidemic of HIV-1 infection among drug injectors?' *Addiction* 91(8): 1085–8.
Tyler, A. (1995) *Street Drugs*, London: Hodder & Stoughton.
Wiebel, W. (2001) 'Harm reduction – a historical view from the trenches', *International Journal of Drug Policy* 12(1): 41–3.

APPENDIX 8.1

AN OVERVIEW OF SAFER INJECTING ADVICE AND INFORMATION

Trudi Petersen

NEEDLE EXCHANGE ASSESSMENT

The following areas should be explored in relation to the client's knowledge, skills and attitudes, as well as the client's previous experiences.

What substance is the client injecting?

What is the person using? Are they using an appropriate means of administering the substance. Anabolic steroids should not be injected in any way other than intramuscularly (IM). Crack cocaine is often injected but this should be avoided as this can cause vein damage (and loss of good sites) very quickly. Tablets are sometimes crushed and injected but clients should be advised against this as particles and chalk can enter the blood stream causing local and distant problems.

PREPARATION OF THE SUBSTANCE

How are they preparing the injection? Heroin is usually mixed with an acid (usually citric acid) to allow it to dissolve. Citric acid should be bought in powdered form from a chemist. Lemon juice and vinegar should not be used because they contain toxins that can cause tissue damage.

How is the client injecting?

How are they injecting? Intravenously (into a vein)? Skin popping (subcutaneously)? Intramuscularly (into muscle)? Is the client using the most appropriate way of injecting? What is their technique? For IV injection the needle should be inserted at a 45 degree angle smoothly into the vein, the plunger should be drawn back and the blood observed. If the blood re-entering the syringe is bright red and frothy the client may have hit an artery. If no blood enters the barrel then the needle is not in a vein. The substance should be injected slowly, fast injection may cause the vein to 'blow'. If a tourniquet is used it should be removed before the needle is withdrawn.

A note on anabolic steroid injectors

IM injection of anabolic steroids is not possible with a 1 ml integrated syringe and needles. The client should be advised to use larger gauge needles and 2 or 5 ml syringes. Injection should be into the upper outer quadrant of the buttock. It is important that injection takes place here to avoid hitting the sciatic nerve, damage to which can cause paralysis. Most steroid users who inject into the buttock are injected by a friend. If possible the injector should be spoken to. An alternative site is the outer part of the upper thigh. The solution should be checked for air bubbles prior to administering and bubbles removed by flicking the syringe, withdrawing and pushing back the plunger. The needle should not be pushed in right up to the hilt. IM injections should be given slowly.

Steroid injectors should be encouraged to take some time 'off cycle'. Where health checks such as LFT's and blood pressure monitoring are possible these should be offered.

Where are they injecting?

The 'safest' IV sites are found in the superficial veins on the arms, in the crook of the elbow (the ante-cubital fossa). The legs may be used but the further sites get from the heart the slower the blood supply and the greater the risk of problems. Injecting should always take place with the flow, i.e. towards the heart. Small veins on the hands and feet should be avoided because they have thin walls and will be more easily damaged.

Does the client know how to avoid hitting an artery or major nerve? They should not inject anywhere that there is a pulse. Does the client know how to feel for a pulse? Groin injecting should be discouraged as it is dangerous – the main artery, nerve and vein all lie in close proximity to one other. Advice on safer groin injection should only be given by an experienced substance misuse worker. 'No go' areas include the neck, breasts, armpits and genitals.

Does the client know how to feel for a vein. Having a sensitive feeling technique is more helpful than simply looking. Not everyone has highly visible veins. The client may be advised on how to raise a vein – warming the area with hot water, exercising/pumping by squeezing the hand into a fist repeatedly. If it is possible to avoid using a tourniquet this is preferable. Does the client know that resting sites will reduce the risk of damage and help keep the vein healthy and the site available? Can they learn to be ambidextrous? Rotating sites should be encouraged.

KNOWLEDGE OF SAFER INJECTING AND SHARING PRACTICES

What is their knowledge of safer injecting practices? For many people 'sharing' means using someone else's needle and syringe after they have used it. The practitioner should make it clear that 'sharing' involves both passing on works and using other people's. It also involves 'sharing' with sexual partners and old friends. Knowing someone a long time is no guarantee of safety. Believing that someone has undergone testing for blood-borne viruses is no guarantee either – false negatives can occur, most viruses have a window period where antibodies are not detectable, they may have contracted a virus since the test and they may not have understood or correctly disclosed their results.

It is possible to pass on disease via any form of shared equipment. This includes spoons, filters, water for flushing or mixing and swabs. The client may attempt to reduce harm by cleaning equipment, sometimes simply by washing out, sometimes by washing through with bleach and cold water. This may be relatively effective in relation to HIV but has been shown to have little impact on hepatitis B or C. It is not possible to remove every trace of blood from a needle and the amount needed for transmission is very small. The client should be strongly advised not to share at all. This can be difficult in 'real life'. Cleaning is probably better than not cleaning but should not be encouraged as a first line measure. Instead it is worth exploring contingency measures that the client may have in place to help avoid sharing, such as keeping an 'emergency' injecting pack somewhere accessible but not too accessible. Would the client be prepared to try an alternative means of administering a drug on the occasions they have no clean equipment, such as smoking instead of injecting? What other ideas do they have to plan for this situation in advance?

Environmental preparation and cleanliness

Injecting through dirty skin can cause bacteria to enter the blood stream resulting in cardiac damage. Does the client clean their injection area beforehand? Swabs are no longer given out by needle exchanges as their efficacy is debatable – most injecting drug users do not leave the solution to dry on the skin before injecting. Plain washing can remove a lot of surface dirt. Hand washing can also help prevent hepatitis A.

What about the 'cooking up' area? A clean piece of paper can help keep new works away from dirty surfaces (which may have traces of old blood on them).

Risky practices, such as frontloading and backloading where the contents of a syringe are shared out between two people, should be discouraged.

Particular care should be taken if injecting another person. The client may use different 'works', spoon and water, but may still transmit viruses by, for example, needle stick injury, or simply pressing the site with their thumb to stem bleeding and then using that same thumb to feel for their own vein.

Overdose risk and misuse of other substances

How often are they using? Is there a risk from accidental overdose due to reduced tolerance? If so the client may be advised to try smaller amounts first by splitting the dosage? There is no guarantee of quality for street drugs; even substances from the same supplier may vary in strength and purity. Is the client using any other substances which may enhance risk? For example, alcohol, benzodiazepines and opioids can all cause respiratory depression.

FIRST AID KNOWLEDGE

What is the client's knowledge of first aid? Would they know what to do in the following situations?

- Hitting an artery: apply pressure, raise area and seek medical help immediately.
- Local infection (the area may be red, swollen and hot); the client should seek medical help quickly.
- Systemic infection: the client should seek medical help immediately.
- Arterial obstruction (the skin becomes pale and then blackens with severe

pain or loss of feeling): the client should seek medical treatment immediately, as treatment can prevent death or loss of the limb.

- Deep vein thrombosis (the first sign of this is usually a hot sore area – often at the back of the calf. Blood clots arising from DVT's can travel to the lungs (pulmonary embolus) with frequently fatal results: the client should seek medical help immediately.
- Overdose: the client should be informed of basic first aid in the event of overdose and advised on ringing an ambulance for help. Some drug users fail to stay with the person until an ambulance arrives, fearing police intervention. It must be stressed that staying with the person may keep them alive.

Services and environmental safety

What is the client's knowledge of how and where to obtain clean injecting equipment? The client should be informed of all sources including needle exchanges and community pharmacies. It should be explained that the latter will involve some cost if the pharmacy is not part of an exchange scheme.

Where is the client injecting? Do they inject alone? Is their locality safe? For example: injecting alone in a derelict building late at night during a cold winter spell and not telling anyone where you are carries particular risks. If a group of people inject is it possible for one to remain less intoxicated as a source of help for potential overdose, etc.? Has the client received basic resuscitation training (Airway, Breathing, Cardiac Output, and Cardiopulmonary resuscitation)? Do they know how to put somebody in the recovery position? Does the client have a mobile phone? (Does it have credits and is the battery working?)

How does the client keep their equipment and drugs? Are they out of the reach of children, other people and animals? How do they dispose of used equipment? Clients should be provided with 'burn bins' for safe disposal and advised on how to use these, i.e. not overfilling them, how to close them properly, not reaching into them to dispose of works.

Is the client aware of hepatitis and HIV issues? Have they been tested or do they wish to be tested? Can appropriate arrangements be made for clients to take up hepatitis B vaccination?

GIVING SAFER INJECTING ADVICE AND INFORMATION

- Always check out what people know before you offer advice. If they can tell you what you were going to tell them, you can save time, reinforce positive messages and avoid alienating the client.
- Information should be given slowly and backed up with written information. (Bear in mind that some clients may be illiterate.)
- As with any demonstration of a practical skill, 'telling' should be backed up by 'showing'. Pointing to injection sites can help the client to identify them.

The client can be shown how to feel for a vein. Do not ask to see the client inject themselves as you may find yourself in the position of having encouraged and witnessed an illegal act and having allowed this to happen on your work premises, which could place you and your employer at risk of prosecution. (Some agencies have legitimate, sterile, equipped injecting rooms, but this is now rare in the UK.)

- Not all information will be taken in at any one visit. Information should be provided in small, easily understood chunks and should be repeated at later visits.
- Be specific – asking to look at someone's arms is of no use if they inject into their groin or legs. Ask to look at their injection sites instead. Ask if they inject anywhere else.
- Ask open-ended questions and concentrate on how? why? where? when? and what?
- Check understanding by using open-ended questions. Asking 'Do you understand?' will simply elicit a yes/no answer. Asking 'Can you tell me how you would. . . .?' offers an opportunity to identify deficits in knowledge.
- Don't assume – just because someone has been injecting for a while does not mean that they are doing so in the safest way possible.
- Avoid jargon – the client may not understand terms like 'frontloading' or 'backloading'. Explain what you mean to avoid ambiguity.
- A positive, non-judgmental approach will help develop rapport.
- A contextual awareness of specific risk taking behaviour may enable client and practitioner to work together to develop innovative ways of injecting more safely. Simply stating that injecting/sharing is dangerous is of little help if the client feels coerced by another person for example. In a situation like this it may be helpful to work on the client's assertiveness and self-efficacy.
- Along with safer injecting, clients should be provided with information about safer sex. Condoms should be provided.
- Needle exchange offers an opportunity for awareness raising about other forms of help and may enable the client to move towards reducing their substance use or seeking treatment.
- Needle exchange is skilled work and practitioners should endeavour to keep up to date by reading appropriate literature. There are a number of needle exchange and harm reduction forums and groups which offer the opportunity to network and share best practice.
- Finally, remember – there is no such thing as 'safe' injecting; the best that can be aimed for is 'safer' injecting.

FURTHER READING

Derricot, J., Preston, A. and Hunt, N. (1999) *The Safer Injecting Briefing*, Liverpool: HIT Publications.

Petersen, T. and Llewellyn, J. (2002) *Safer Injecting Booklet*, available from the British Specialist Drug Service, Blackberry Hill Hospital, Bristol.

CHAPTER 9

TWELVE STEP APPROACHES

Caroline Williams

LEARNING OBJECTIVES

Once you have studied this chapter you should be able to demonstrate an understanding of:

1 The core principles of the 12 step model and the 'tools' used to achieve recovery.

2 The potential usefulness of 12 step in substance misuse treatment.

INTRODUCTION

The 12 step programme consists of a range of self-help groups which have their origins in the recovery philosophy of the first 12 step programme – Alcoholics Anonymous. The Minnesota Model is an adaptation of the 12 step programme used in some specialist treatment settings.

HISTORY

The 12 step movement developed out of Alcoholics Anonymous (AA), a self-help organisation founded in the 1930s by Bill Wilson and Bob Smith. They formulated

Table 9.1 The 12 steps of Alcoholics Anonymous

1	We admitted we were powerless over alcohol – that our lives had become unmanageable.
2	Came to believe that a power greater than ourselves could restore us to sanity.
3	Made a decision to turn our will and our lives over to the care of God as we understood Him.
4	Made a searching and fearless moral inventory of ourselves.
5	Admitted to God, to ourselves, and to another human being the exact nature of our wrongs.
6	Were entirely ready to have God remove all the defects of character.
7	Humbly asked Him to remove our shortcomings.
8	Made a list of all persons we had harmed and became willing to make amends to them all.
9	Made direct amends to such people wherever possible, except when to do so would injure them or others.
10	Continued to take personal inventory and when we were wrong promptly admitted it.
11	Sought through prayer and meditation to improve our conscious contact with God as we understood Him, praying only for knowledge of His will for us and the power to carry that out.
12	Having had a spiritual awakening as the result of these steps, we tried to carry this message to alcoholics, and to practice these principles in all our affairs.

Note: The 12 Steps are reprinted with the permission of Alcoholics Anonymous (Great Britain). Permission to reprint this material does not indicate that AA has approved or reviewed the contents of this publication nor that AA agrees with the views expressed in this publication. AA is a programme of recovery from alcoholism only. Other self-help organisations address other addictions.

the 12 steps and principles of AA from their own experiences of maintaining sobriety (Table 9.1) by sharing with others, when they had not managed to do this alone. The book describing all this, *Alcoholics Anonymous*, published in 1939 is the core text of AA, affectionately known by members as 'the Big Book'.

In the 1940s and 1950s three centres in Minnesota were established that incorporated the AA philosophy: Pioneer House, Hazelden and the Wilmer State Hospital. These centres developed an integrated treatment programme generically known as the 'Minnesota Model'. The Wilmer State Hospital programme particularly influenced the present Minnesota structure, combining medical treatment, multidisciplinary team work, individual counselling, groupwork and a therapeutic community environment. Medical staff and psychologists worked alongside clergy and lay counsellors who were themselves recovering alcoholics.

From its initial focus on alcohol, the 12 step model broadened to incorporate other chemical dependency with Narcotics Anonymous, and later the treatment of behavioural addictions such as gambling and eating disorders. Family support groups – Al Anon (for the families of problem drinkers) and Families Anonymous (for families of drug misusers) – have evolved in parallel with the treatment groups.

The movement has spread internationally to 134 countries. A recent survey carried out by the organisation (Alcoholics Anonymous, 2000) found there are 3,300 meetings weekly in the UK, and 97,000 meetings world-wide. Membership in the UK stands at 40–50,000, and world-wide the figure is over two million. Literature is available in many languages as well as Braille, sign language, audio and other formats.

HOW DOES THE 12 STEP MOVEMENT VIEW ADDICTION?

Addiction as a loss of control

Addiction is seen as the inability to control one's use of any mood altering substance or behaviour despite awareness of its damaging consequences. It is seen as arising from attributes of the person as well as the substance. This concept of addiction, encapsulating behaviours (i.e. gambling, etc.), is not dependent on evidence of physical dependence such as tolerance and withdrawal effects as outlined in diagnostic criteria.

In the past much store was placed in accepting the label of 'addict' or 'alcoholic'. Some early treatment facilities were quite confrontative over this issue. It has since been recognised that aggressive confrontation can be detrimental. Though it is still important to accept the concept of being 'addicted', this is a self-defined, arbitrary concept.

Addiction as a long-term condition

It is believed that this population who have 'lost control' remain vulnerable to future loss of control. Addiction is viewed as a lifelong condition which, unchecked, would be progressive and potentially fatal and which can be arrested by intervention but not 'cured'. Controlled drinking is not seen as a realistic aim, complete abstinence being the only safe option.

Addiction as an illness

The controversial 'disease' concept need not be confused with a biological model. Addiction can be seen as an illness in a similar way as certain psychological conditions such as obsessive compulsive disorder. There may well be a genetic or physiological component but it is not necessary for the condition to have a wholly biological basis in order to be termed an 'illness'.

The use of the word 'illness' is largely pragmatic. It releases the person from guilt and shame, which only serves to worsen addictive behaviour. The person is then free to forgive themselves and focus their energy on recovery. It may be argued that the use of an illness model may lead to development of the 'sick' role. This is not the message. The person is seen as responsible, not for the 'illness' itself but for the consequences of their behaviour and for the decision to change.

Apart from the use of the term 'illness' the 12 step philosophy does not espouse any specific cause for addiction, although there are some members who hold the belief that they are literally 'intolerant to' or 'allergic to' a substance.

The model is in fact compatible with a multifactoral model of causation and is opposed to a 'moral model'. Within Minnesota treatment centres there is widespread belief in a multifactoral model with people being genetically predisposed to increased risk, some being more predisposed by aspects such as personality, development, environment, social circumstance, learning and conditioning.

Addiction as a primary condition

Although a multifactoral model may be accepted in relation to causation, 12 step beliefs claim that once developed, addiction can be regarded as a primary condition with characteristic symptoms or patterns of thinking and behaviour.

The addictive personality; shame and co-dependence

The term 'addictive personality' is often used to describe this characteristic pattern of thinking and behaviour and in this sense could describe an effect of the illness in progress rather than just a pre-existing personality predisposing to addiction (Nakken, 1998). The 12 step approach suggests that it is not necessary to understand cause in order change thinking and behaviour. Bradshaw (1988) suggests that the common core underlying addictive traits is a sense of shame causing an emotional dis-ease, akin to low grade chronic depression, which predisposes the individual to seek mood altering substances or behaviours. Also predisposing to other patterns of relating, often termed 'co-dependence', e.g. problems with self-esteem, boundary setting, impulse control and the management of feelings.

HOW DOES THE 12 STEP MOVEMENT VIEW RECOVERY?

The movement is abstinence based but because addiction is viewed as a pattern of thinking and behaviour, recovery is not only about abstinence from a substance. 'Sobriety' is seen as the development of a healthier attitude to oneself and others. In AA the state of 'abstinence' without 'sobriety' is often called being 'dry drunk'. As relapse commonly occurs as a response to painful emotions (fear, anger, guilt, etc.) emphasis is placed on learning to cope with these feelings and on lessening these by changing thinking in ways that enhance feelings of acceptance and well-being or 'serenity'.

Recovery is achieved by attendance at meetings and 'working the programme' with the mutual support of others who are trying to do the same: 12 step organisations do not provide counselling, medical advice or treatment, housing or financial support.

Minnesota Model treatment uses the principles and tools of the 12 step movement in a professional treatment context, alongside other treatment methods. Most treatment centres are residential. They have some overlap with broader therapeutic community approaches in that everyone is encouraged to be part of the practical running of the house and decision making. Members are encouraged to use the support of others in the community to seek feedback and challenge unhealthy attitudes and behaviours, with staff help as necessary. Programmes typically involve a combination of group therapy, counselling, lectures and video-audio material. There may be 'share' sessions from recovering ex-residents and participants are encouraged to attend relevant local 12 step meetings.

The 'tools' of the recovery programme

There are a number of elements to the programme. The tools of recovery may be divided into:

- those which promote fellowship
- those for changing thinking and behaviour
- those which promote the development of spirituality

Tools which promote fellowship

'Fellowship' is central to the movement. It is achieved by the giving and receiving of support through attendance at meetings, telephone contact, sponsorship and through 'service roles'.

Meetings

Meetings are usually around one to one-and-a-half hours long. Some are 'closed' for members only, others are open to interested people such as health professionals. There are no restrictions on membership, the only requirement being a desire to stop using a substance (or behaviour). There is no formal commitment to attend. Members may attend as many (or few) meetings as they wish at any of the group's locations. The format of meetings varies. The most common is the 'discussion meeting' where everyone is encouraged to share their views and experiences around a topic such as a specific step or a more general theme, such as anger. In 'speaker meetings' an in-depth share from a member or guest takes place. Groups may vary in structure but there is considerable consistency because of the standardised guidelines and literature.

Sharing

Sharing is central to the 12 step philosophy. Members discuss their own experiences and feelings in an accepting environment. Others are asked to refrain from interruption, advice and criticism. This aims to dispel feelings of isolation whilst aiding self-acceptance and instilling hope.

Support

Members are encouraged to stay in touch between meetings and advised to attend regularly. Whilst attendance anywhere is possible, the maintenance of a 'home' group enables the member to become part of a community support network. In areas where there are no meetings postal contact is possible. More recently support has become available via the Internet.

Sponsorship

This is a one-to-one mentor relationship with another person further along the road of recovery. As recovery develops, sponsoring others provides another opportunity for personal development as well as a continuing support system for new members.

Service roles

The rotation of service roles (i.e. chair, treasurer, tea maker, etc.) gives everyone a chance to take responsibility and work as part of a team.

Much of the benefit of the 12 step movement may derive from the group experience itself. Yalom (1985) described eleven factors contributing to the beneficial effect of therapeutic groups. These factors can all be applied to 12 step methods.

1. The instillation of hope.
2. Universality.
3. Imparting information.
4. Altruism.
5. Corrective recapitulation of the primary family group.
6. The development of socialising techniques.
7. Imitative behaviour.
8. Interpersonal learning.
9. Group cohesiveness.
10. Catharsis.
11. Existential factors.

Tools which summarise the programme's philosophy for changing thinking and behaviour

Adherence to the philosophy of the approach

A range of aids exist to remind the individual of the core concepts of the movement and facilitate behaviour and attitude change. These include reading the 'approved' literature and the use of 'slogans' along with the 'serenity prayer'.

The core of the programme involves working through the 12 steps in an attempt to change thinking and behaviour (see Table 9.1).

Step 1
This encourages letting go of self-blame over loss of control whilst encouraging an honest acceptance about the extent and consequences of this. Accepting 'powerlessness' encourages acceptance of help from others.

Steps 2–3
The programme makes clear that a 'higher power' may be anything the person chooses, including the programme itself.

Steps 4–7
These promote self-awareness and development; a realistic appraisal of individual assets and shortcomings. Self-blame is not encouraged though accuracy in identifying destructive traits is.

Steps 8–10
These aim to alleviate the burden of guilt by attempting to repair harm done. This is done to obtain release from negative emotions and does not depend on a particular response from others.

Step 11
Regular periods of reflection are encouraged to actively maintain the process of recovery.

Step 12
Individuals are encouraged to give, as well as receive support, creating a continuing resource for all members.

The serenity prayer and slogans

The serenity prayer is a short prayer encouraging the individual to focus on those aspects which can be changed, whilst accepting that there are some things which it must be accepted cannot be changed. Slogans are used as reminders of the key elements of the programme, e.g. 'one day at a time'.

The 12 traditions

The 12 traditions are not the same as the 12 steps. The traditions outline the principles by which the 12 step movement runs. They aim to safeguard the group against unhealthy dynamics and keep the focus on recovery. For example, 12 step groups are self-supporting, have no political or financial affiliation, no leaders and strict personal anonymity.

Tools for developing spirituality and alternatives

Although the steps identify a need to enlist a 'higher power' in seeking help and the term 'God' is used in the literature, the idea of a greater power need not necessarily refer to a traditional deity. For some a higher power may be a more abstract concept. Prayer or meditation can be seen as tools used to enhance spirituality. For those who feel they that cannot align themselves with this, alternative organisations exist – the Secular Organisations for Sobriety (SOS) and Rational Recovery (RR).

THEORETICAL ASPECTS

The 12 step approach has elements common to other approaches. The belief that changed attitudes aid recovery may be seen as analogous with the principles of cognitive behavioural therapy. Similarly the use of slogans, short soundbites which aim to provide the individual with reassurance and a reminder of their goals, is similar to some techniques used in CBT. The non-judgemental philosophy is akin to the person centred approach of Carl Rogers (1951). Social learning theory (Bandura, 1977) suggests that behaviour is guided by expected consequences. Vicarious learning can influence the individual. The use of a sponsor as role model is a form of positive learning. Efficacy expectations are as important as outcome expectations. The structured building of esteem in the 12 steps includes the regular contact with others who are also 'succeeding' and may generate a belief that success is possible. Azjen and Fishbein (1980) claim that behaviour is influenced by the belief a person has about that behaviour and how strongly they feel that belief to be true, as well as the individual's perceptions of what other people (that they value) will think of their behaviour. Where the individual values the members of the group he or she will want to behave in ways that make them accepted. The use of social networks as a form of support has been a feature of recent family and social based interventions.

The evidence base

Does 12 step work?

Research data in relation to AA has historically been notoriously difficult to obtain (Bebbington, 1976). Although 12 step is appearing more often in contemporary literature, methodological challenges still remain, the main difficulties being the anonymity of group members and self-selecting nature of the organisation. Cook (1988) reviewed a number of studies showing the Minnesota Model to be effective in drug and alcohol dependence but points out that many studies have weaknesses particularly in regard to a lack of control groups for comparison. Chappel and DuPont (1999) reviewed recent studies, suggesting evidence of effectiveness of 12 step. This included one eight-year follow-up study of 628 previously untreated alcoholics (Humphreys *et al.*, 1997). The number of AA meetings attended in the first three years predicted remission, lower depression and higher quality relationships. The 12 step facilitation was found to be equal in effectiveness to CBT and MET in the Project MATCH study of drinking outcomes (Project MATCH research group, 1997). Miller (1995) suggests that although all methods seem equally effective in the short term, 12 step groups appear to be more effective long term.

Who might it be suitable for?

The notion of who 12 step may be most appropriate for has been highlighted. Janowsky *et al.* (1999) suggest that particular personality variables may predict abstinence and self-help group attendance, notably high levels of persistence and low levels of shyness and fear of uncertainty. This study concentrated on abstinent individuals at one month post-detox only. Sample size was small but the authors point out that most relapses occur within the first one to two months and it is suggested that this study has potential relevance for future replication. Indicators of AA affiliation have included female gender, older age, more authoritarian and extroverted. Adolescents were likely to have had less parental involvement in treatment, more feelings of hopelessness, a history of prior treatment and non-drug using friends (Hohman and LeCroy, 1996). However, earlier work by Emrick (1989) suggested it was not possible to predict who would affiliate. Christo (1999) studied attendees and non-attendees of Narcotics Anonymous (NA). NA attendance was related to less drug use amongst those who had left residential care whilst a wish not to abstain from alcohol was seen as the main reason why drug users failed to engage with NA. Christo suggests that improvements in psychological health may take up to five years after abstinence and long-term support is therefore advantageous. This is usually not available in most treatment settings but is easily accessible through self-help.

The future?

Though the positive effects of 12 step are recognised by many researchers, the general consensus across the literature is that more rigorous research is needed, especially over the long term and amongst larger groups. Some 12 step non-alcohol groups such as NA have even less evidence base and may be a focus for research. How researchers will deal with the challenges involved in regard to this remains to be seen.

Conclusion

There is a lack of knowledge and training regarding 12 step methods amongst professional groups. Misunderstandings are common. However, 12 step approaches offer another useful resource which is widely available, free, open to anyone, flexible in terms of commitment and provides support at times when other agencies are unavailable. It is not exclusive and can be used alongside many other forms of therapy.

The evidence base is scanty in comparison to other approaches but continued uptake and growth of the movement provides support for its use. The positive effects of 12 step have been identified by some researchers but more rigorous research is required.

It will not be suitable for everyone but this approach can be a useful alternative or adjunct to other treatments for some clients. Professionals would benefit from a knowledge of this which may encourage greater openness and understanding of its use.

READER INPUT

(1) Find out where your nearest AA or NA group meets. (AA and NA can both be found in the phone book – regional offices will be able to tell you where your nearest group is based.) If it is possible for you to attend an open session, go along. Explain why you are attending. Please ring beforehand to let them know you are coming and so you do not clash with a 'closed' session. You are asked to retain sensitivity and respect for the organisation and the people who are there when you attend.

FURTHER READING

Bradshaw, J. (1988) 'Healing the shame that binds you', Audiotape, Health Communications Inc.

Nawinski, J. (1999) 'Self help groups for addictions', in B.S. McCrady and E.E. Epstein (1999) (eds) *Addictions: A Comprehensive Guidebook*, NewYork: Oxford University Press.

Parker, J. and Guest, D.L. (1999) *The Clinicians' Guide to 12 Step Programs: How, When and Why to Refer the Client*, Minnesota: Auburn House.

The practitioner is also encouraged to obtain and read the material or view/listen to audio/visual material, produced by the AA and other 12 step groups.

REFERENCES

AA members survey 2000. *Alcoholics Anonymous*.

Azjen, I. and Fishbein, M. (1980) *Understanding Attitudes and Predicting Social Behaviour*, Englewood Cliffs, NJ: Prentice-Hall.

Bandura, A. (1977) *Social Learning Theory*, New York: Prentice-Hall.

Bebbington, P.E. (1976) 'The efficacy of Alcoholics Anonymous: the elusiveness of hard data', *British Journal of Psychiatry* 128(6): 572–80.

Bradshaw, J. (1988) 'Healing the shame that binds you', Audiotape, Health Communications Inc.

Chappel, J.N. and DuPont, R.L. (1999) 'Twelve step and mutual help programs for addictive disorders', *The Psychiatric Clinics of North America* 22(2): 425–46.

Christo, G. (1999) *Narcotics Anonymous as Aftercare. Executive Summary* No. 62, London: The Centre for Research on Drugs and Health Behaviour.

Cook C.H. (1988) 'The Minnesota Model in the management of drug and alcohol dependency: miracle, method or myth?' *British Journal of Addiction* 83: 625–34 (Part 1), 735–48 (Part 2).

Emrick C.D. (1989) 'Alcoholics Anonymous: Membership characteristics and effectiveness as treatment', in M. Galanter (ed.) *Recent Developments in Alcoholism* Vol. 7: 37–53. New York: Plenum Press.

Hohman, M. and LeCroy, C.W. (1996) 'Predictors of adolescent AA affiliation', *Adolescence* 31: 340–52.

Humphreys, K., Moos, R.H. and Cohen, C. (1997) in J.N. Chappel and R.L. DuPont (1999) 'Twelve step and mutual help programs for addictive disorders', *The Psychiatric Clinics of North America* 22(2): 425–46.

Janowsky, D.S., Boone, A., Morter, S. and Howe, L. (1999) 'Personality and alcohol/substance use disorder, patient relapse and attendance at self help group meetings' *Alcohol and Alcoholism* 34(3): 359–69.

Miller, N.S. (ed.) (1995) *Treatment of the Addictions: Applications of Outcome Research*, New York: Haworth Press.

Nakken, C. (1998) *The Addictive Personality* (2nd edn), Minnesota: Hazeldon.

Project MATCH Research Group (1997) 'Matching alcoholism treatments to client heterogeneity: Project MATCH post treatment drinking outcomes', *Journal of Studies on Alcohol* 58(1): 7–29.

Rogers, C.R. (1951) *Client Centred Therapy*, London: Constable.

Yalom, I.D. (1985) *The Theory and Practice of Group Psychotherapy* (3rd edn), New York: Basic Books.

Websites

Alcoholics Anonymous: www.alcoholics-anonymous.org.uk

Narcotics Anonymous: for the UK the website is www.ukna.org A global site is also available at www.na.org

CHAPTER 10

FAMILY INTERVENTIONS IN SUBSTANCE MISUSE

Richard Velleman and Lorna Templeton

LEARNING OBJECTIVES

Once you have studied this chapter you will be able to:

1. Demonstrate a basic understanding of the impact of substance misuse on the family, and the importance of the family in interventions in this area.
2. Identify the types of interventions that are available to families and an overview of the theories that underpin these interventions.

INTRODUCTION

There are almost two million adults in the UK drinking at 'harmful' levels (i.e. more than 50 units per week for men or more than 35 units per week for women) (ONS, 1997). The numbers of problem drug users in the UK are harder to estimate, but figures suggest that there are in excess of 200,000 (ISDD, 1997). Conservatively assuming that every substance misuser will negatively affect at least two close family members, this suggests about five million family members in this country are living with the negative consequences of drug and alcohol misuse.

Relatives suffer bio-psycho-social stresses as a result of living in this environment, which may impact on physical and mental well-being and lead to the development of problems both for themselves and other family members (Velleman, 2000; Velleman *et al*., 1993). This is a world-wide phenomenon

(Orford, 1990). These relatives need help, both for themselves and in order to deal constructively with their substance misusing relation. Between a third and a half of calls to alcohol advice centres come from partners, families and friends (Brisby *et al.*, 1997). Similar percentages apply in the area of drug misuse. A particularly important area is the impact of drug and alcohol problems on children and the realisation that their needs are not adequately met within current service provision (Velleman, 2000; Velleman and Orford, 1999).

It makes sense to utilise family members as participants in interventions aimed at the substance misuser. Systemic thinking implies that an intervention will be more likely to succeed if there is wider family involvement.

Poor service provision

Services which involve relatives – either as service users in their own right, addressing their own problems, or as part of a wider family intervention – are minimal. A recent report by the National Society for the Prevention of Cruelty to Children (NSPCC) and the Alcohol Recovery Project (ARP) (Robinson and Hassall, 2000) described the results of a brief national survey within the UK of services for family members. Only a small number of such services were identified: two child-focused services, five family-focused services (which tended to be residential), and seven adult-focused services.

Theory suggests that family members should be involved in order to draw substance misusers into treatment and to ensure that changes which are made impact on the whole system. In British practice, however, such interventions are not mainstream although Vetere (1998: 127) has argued for 'a systemic couples and family service as part of every community alcohol service'.

INTERVENTIONS

Historical development

The majority of early research focused on the female spouses of 'alcoholics' (as people with drinking problems were known then). This work was dominated by a 'blame' approach that sought to understand men's alcohol misuse with reference to women's negative characteristics. Much of this research focused on signs of 'psychopathology' or the 'personality traits' that spouses purportedly had, which 'promoted' their husband's alcoholism (Orford, 1994). Recent research has approached this issue in a less accusatory fashion. There are now a range of theories around the impact of substance misuse on the family, and a range of interventions and therapies designed to help these families.

A systemic approach

Many of these more recent approaches adopt behavioural or systemic standpoints (Collins, 1990), suggesting that the family 'learns' how to deal with substance misuse, or operates as a system where the actions of each person impact on everybody else, so that particular acts function to control, encourage, or prevent substance misuse behaviour. Even negative behaviours can serve to maintain balance in such a family system.

Working with relatives in this vein can build on family interactions, and change behaviour to bring a different, more 'normal' balance to that system, to break the habits of learnt behaviours, or change reinforcement patterns so that more positive and less negative behaviours are reinforced.

An extreme version of this systemic view is the co-dependency theory, which states that spouses and partners (typically female) become 'addicted' to the relationship they are in, the drinking behaviour, and its (usually negative) consequences. This theory suggests that if the co-dependency cycle is not broken, the partner may remain in the relationship or enter another relationship with the same consequences. Many of the family or couple interventions which stem from systemic or behavioural theories suggest that the family member(s) should receive help alongside the misuser, or join concurrently running group sessions for family members and misusers.

Unilateral family therapy

Unilateral family therapy is a more contemporary advance in the development of family interventions. This approach also utilises the systemic model, but suggests that it is possible to alter the ways that a family works without all members of the family system being present in therapy sessions. It is possible to alter someone's substance misuse even if they never present for treatment. Working with other members of the system and helping them to change their behaviour will, it is argued, automatically impact on the user's behaviour as well. This approach was designed to be most suitable for attracting the most 'unmotivated, treatment-resistant [drinkers]' (Meyers *et al.*, 1996).

Co-operative counselling

Yates (1988) found that problems with someone else's drinking were more likely to be reported than were problems related to personal drinking. On this basis, a 'co-operative' counselling service was established and evaluated, which worked with 'affected others' to encourage problem drinkers into treatment. Results indicated that relatives valued the help that was offered to them, in particular the relief felt by the relative, confirmation that the drinking was a serious issue and the advice on how to develop effective strategies to use with the drinker to help the situation. Working with 'affected others' brought several problem drinkers into treatment. Although seen as relatively successful, Yates' study has been little replicated in the UK. In the USA, however, such approaches are more widely available (Edwards and Steinglass, 1995; O'Farrell, 1993).

Community reinforcement training and social networks

Community reinforcement training (Meyers *et al.*, 1996), first developed in the 1970s, is another example of an approach that aims to work with 'concerned others' to reinforce non-drinking behaviour through a positive reinforcement process. A related way of working is the ARISE intervention (Garrett *et al.*, 1998), which utilises family and other network links to encourage substance misusers into treatment, whilst also trying to help the family in its own right. Galanter's (1993a,b) cognitive behavioural network therapy also involves the engagement of social networks to help the substance misuser and the wider family. Here, the misuser, a key significant other (usually, but not necessarily, a relative) and other relatives, friends and significant others (for example, a work colleague or other professional) are all engaged in work on someone's substance misuse. The family is seen as central to co-attend therapy sessions with the misuser, to introduce and maintain the misuser into treatment, and then to prevent relapse.

The stress-coping-support model

The primary focus of the interventions outlined so far is to use the family member to engage and maintain the user in treatment, and to work on using their positive family functioning to stop the substance misuse. Outcome measures are primarily related to the abstinence or reduced substance use of the misuser, as opposed to measures of couple or family functioning, or individual symptomatology of the other family members. Little or no attention is paid to working with relatives as people with problems in their own right as a result of living with an active substance misuser.

A different theoretical approach underpins the 'stress-coping-support' model developed by Orford and colleagues (Orford, 1998). This suggests that substance misuse is usefully conceptualised as a 'chronic stress' (in a similar way to Alzheimer's disease, dealing with serious conduct problems in adolescence, or dealing with severe psychological distress), where family members have to deal or cope with the often distressing behaviour of one of their relatives, and where the availability of outside social support can be a crucial determinate of how well they succeed at this coping. Therapeutic interventions emerging from this perspective focus on affected relatives receiving help in their own right. An early version of this approach is the Al-Anon movement which is discussed later in this chapter.

Intervention approaches utilising this stress-coping-support model, aim to develop interventions and services which focus on the help that family members need in their own right to deal with the high levels of problems they experience. Although not the primary aim of these interventions, these forms of working with the relative sometimes also do have a positive impact on the problem drinking of the misuser. Such approaches have been developed in both primary (Copello *et al.*, 2000a,b) and secondary care (Howells, 1997).

Copello and colleagues successfully developed and evaluated a brief intervention in the primary care setting, aimed at affected family members, which required facilitated input from a primary care professional (Copello *et al.*, 2000b). This is now being further evaluated alongside a self-help version of the same intervention, with the aim of exploring the effectiveness of individual self-help compared to a facilitated intervention. Self-help groups and books (Meyer, 1982) are important examples of the effectiveness of this way of working with family members. A self-help manual, based on the Pressures to Change model, and developed for female partners of heavy drinkers, was found to be no less effective than counselling (Barber and Gilbertson, 1998). Bower *et al.*'s (2001) systematic review has promoted the effectiveness of self-help manuals and interventions in the field of anxiety and depression.

In the secondary care setting, Howells (1997) developed and evaluated a counselling intervention for the partners of problem drinkers. This intervention was aimed both at those partners who wanted to stop or control the problem drinking of their relative, and at those who wanted to help themselves without helping the drinker. The intervention was found to be effective in terms of decreasing the overall stress and psychological symptoms of the spouses, and in the reduction of the amount of 'self-sacrificing' coping of the partner (thought to be the least beneficial).

Al-Anon

Al-Anon is probably the most famous example of an approach aimed at relatives in their own right. A huge international self-help movement, based on the '12-step' approach developed by Alcoholics Anonymous, it focuses exclusively on the needs of the (mainly) spouses and partners of alcohol misusers. Al-Anon has been joined more recently by Al-Ateen, a 12-step approach to helping young children exposed to drinking problems. Families Anonymous is a similar self-help movement for families and children of drug misusers (see Chapter 9).

THE EVIDENCE BASE

There is a growing evidence base for behavioural, community reinforcement and family approaches (O'Farrell, 1993). Meyers *et al.*'s (1998) study involving community reinforcement and family training (CRAFT) recruited sixty-two concerned significant others, 74 per cent of whom managed successfully to engage their previously treatment-resistant drug misusing relative into treatment. This also led to a reduction in physical and psychological symptoms for the non-misusing family member. Sisson and Azrin's (1986) behavioural approach gave community reinforcement counselling to twelve relatives, with positive results on the alcohol misuser seeking treatment and reducing their drinking. McCrady's evaluation of three types of behavioural based intervention found that it was an effective way of working with couples, but that no one of the three treatments was any better than the other two (Collins, 1990). Edwards and Steinglass's (1995) review of twenty-one studies of interventions which involved family participation concluded that these interventions were both helpful and cost-effective.

There is a similar growing evidence base for ways of working which involve the engagement of social networks. Liepman *et al.* (1989) recruited and evaluated twenty-four of these types of social networks, finding that the alcohol misusers were more likely to enter treatment and remain abstinent.

Evidence for the effectiveness of interventions aimed at relatives in their own right is emerging. Copello *et al.* (2000b) demonstrated that, when engaged, relatives of substance misusers reported a significant reduction in both physical and psychological symptoms, a reduction in forms of coping believed to be least beneficial to relatives and that attitudes and motivation towards working with relatives of substance misuers of primary health care professionals improved. Howells (1997) has shown positive results of good practice through anecdotal evidence.

Al-Anon/Al-Ateen

Although there is a dearth of 'scientific' evidence in relation to 12 step approaches such as Al-Anon, anecdotal reports are plentiful and the numbers of groups (about 28,000 groups world-wide), its breadth of coverage (including via the Internet) and continued uptake of the service, suggests good practice.

Other treatment services have adopted the 12 step approach. In the UK, the Family Service offered at Clouds Residential Service, a residential programme comprising group therapy, lectures and practical advice, has been successfully developed. Evaluation concluded that:

> The family programme [makes] a clinically significant contribution to the psychological well-being of this often neglected group.
>
> (Georgakis & Shepherd, 1998: 19)

Primary care

The primary care environment has been identified as an appropriate one to work in, given that over 98 per cent of the British population are registered with a GP and there are millions of consultations with primary health care professionals every day. GPs and primary care teams are trusted and appointments are valuable opportunities for health promotion and prevention. The results of the feasibility study reported earlier (Copello *et al.*, 2000b) found training and supporting primary health care professionals to use an intervention, based on the stress-coping-support model, in their work with relatives of substance misusers to be an effective way of improving the relatives' situation.

Despite its evidence of minimal service provision, the aforementioned NSPCC and ARC report (Robinson and Hassall, 2000) provides a model of good practice for the development of more family focused work within the UK. The report stresses that new funding for this work is crucial if it is to develop.

Strengths and weaknesses of family/social network centred approaches

The future in this area is that interventions involving (or aimed specifically at) family members are becoming more widespread, and developing a better evidence base. The USA influence, the recent shift to a more community/primary care approach, and a realisation that other family members (not just spouses) can be affected have all aided this gradual move. A further strength is the fact that interventions which utilise relatives in the treatment of people who misuse substances make good common sense: people can easily understand why involving relatives is more likely to lead to a more beneficial outcome. One major weakness, however, is that these interventions are not mainstream, and that it is still rare to find couple or family work being utilised as a matter of course within substance misuse services.

A second major weakness is that, even where a family perspective is utilised, the focus is still usually on the 'relative as adjunct' as opposed to being entitled to services in their own right, due to their high morbidity and high distress. Future service development needs to ensure that a focus remains on helping relatives with their own problems, whilst allowing for the potential that the misuser may also be helped.

There is a growing evidence base for behavioural, community reinforcement, family, and social network approaches to involving relatives as adjuncts to substance misuse interventions; and for the effectiveness of interventions for relatives in their own right.

READER INPUT

Questions

(1) In which ways might family members or significant others such as friends, neighbours, employers be helped to:
- (a) Improve their knowledge base about the substance and its effects and side effects?
- (b) Be encouraged to put strategies into practice?
- (c) Access suitable peer or social support?

Discussion point

(2) What challenges might the practitioner face in working with family members and how could these be addressed?

REFERENCES

Barber, J. and Gilbertson, R. (1998) 'Evaluation of a self-help manual for the female partners of heavy drinkers', *Research on Social Work Practice* 8: 141–51.

Bower, P., Richards, D. and Lovell, K. (2001) 'The clinical and cost-effectiveness of self-help treatments for anxiety and depressive orders in primary care: a systematic review', *British Journal of General Practice* 51: 838–45.

Brisby, T., Baker, S. and Hedderwick, T. (1997) *Under the Influence: Coping With Parents who Drink too much – a Report on the Needs of the Children of Problem Drinking Parents*, London: Alcohol Concern.

Collins, R. (1990) 'Family treatment of alcohol abuse: behavioural and systems perspectives', in R. Collins, K. Leonard and J. Searles (1990) (eds) *Alcohol and the Family: Research and Clinical Perspectives*, New York: Guildford Press.

Copello, A., Orford, J., Velleman, R., Templeton, L. and Krishnan, M. (2000a) 'Methods for reducing alcohol and drug related family harm in non-specialist settings', *Journal of Mental Health* 9: 319–33.

Copello, A., Templeton, L., Krishnan, M., Orford, J. and Velleman, R. (2000b) 'A treatment package to improve primary care services for relatives of people with alcohol and drug problems', *Addiction Research* 8, 471–84.

Edwards, M. and Steinglass, P. (1995) 'Family therapy treatment outcomes for alcoholism', *Journal of Marital and Family Therapy* 21: 475–509.

Galanter, M. (1993a) 'Network therapy for addiction – a model for office practice', *American Journal of Psychiatry* 150: 28–36.

Galanter, M. (1993b) 'Network therapy for substance misuse – a clinical trial', *Psychotherapy* 30: 251–8.

Garrett, J., Landau, J., Shea R., Stanton, M.D., Baciewicz, G. and Brinkmansull, D. (1998) 'The ARISE intervention – using family and network links to engage addicted persons in treatment', *Journal of Substance Abuse Treatment* 15: 333–43.

Georgakis, A. and Shepherd, S. (1998) 'Forgotten families', *Addiction Counselling World* (Spring), 17–20.

Howells, E. (1997) 'Coping with a problem drinker: the development and evaluation of a therapeutic intervention for the partners of problem drinkers in their own right', Unpublished PhD thesis, University of Exeter.

ISDD (1997) *Drug Misuse in Britain, 1996*, London: Institute for the Study of Drug Dependence.

Liepman, M., Nirenberg, T. and Begin, A. (1989) 'Evaluation of a program designed to help family and significant others to motivate resistant alcoholics into recovery', *American Journal of Drug and Alcohol Abuse* 15: 209–21.

Meyer, M. (1982) *Drinking Problems = Family Problems: Practical Guidelines for the Problem Drinker, the Partner, and all those involved*, Lancaster: Momenta.

Meyers, R., Dominguez, T. and Smith, J. (1996) 'Community reinforcement training with concerned others', in V. Van Hasselt and M. Hersen (eds) *Sourcebook of Psychological Treatment Manuals for Adult Disorders*, New York: Plenum Press.

Meyers, R., Miller, W., Hill, D. and Tonigan, J. (1998) 'Community reinforcement and family training (CRAFT): engaging unmotivated drug users in treatment', *Journal of Substance Abuse* 10: 291–308.

O'Farrell, T. (1993) (ed.) *Treating Alcohol Problems: Marital and Family Interventions*, New York: Guilford Press.

ONS (1997) *Living in Britain – Preliminary Results from the 1996 General Household Survey*, London: Office for National Statistics.

Orford, J. (1998) 'The coping perspective', in R. Velleman, A. Copello and J. Maslin (eds) *Living with Drink: Women who Live with Problem Drinkers*, London: Longmans.

Orford, J. (1990) 'Alcohol and the family: an international review of the literature with implications for research and practice', in L. Kozlowski, H. Annis, H. Cappell *et al.* (eds) *Research Advances in Alcohol and Drug Problems*, Vol. 10, New York: Plenum.

Orford, J. (1994) 'Empowering family and friends: a new approach to the secondary prevention of addiction', *Drug and Alcohol Review* 13: 417–29.

Robinson, W. and Hassall, J. (2000) *Feasibility Study Report on a Specialist Family Alcohol Service*, London: NSPCC & ARP.

Sisson, R. and Azrin, N. (1986) 'Family-member involvement to initiate and promote treatment of problem drinkers', *Journal of Behavioural Therapeutic Experimental Psychiatry* 17: 15–21.

Velleman, R. (2000) 'The importance of the family', in D. Cooper (ed.) *Alcohol Use*, Edinburgh: Radcliffe Medical Press.

Velleman, R., Bennett, G., Miller, T., Orford, J., Rigby, K. and Tod, A. (1993) 'The families of problem drug users: a study of 50 close relatives', *Addiction* 88: 1281–9.

Velleman, R. and Orford, J. (1999) *Risk and Resilience – Adults who were the Children of Problem Drinkers*, Reading: Harwood Academic Publishers.

Vetere, A. (1998) 'A family systems perspective', in R. Velleman, A. Copello and J. Maslin (eds) *Living with Drink: Women who Live with Problem Drinkers*, London: Longmans.

Yates, F.E. (1988) 'The evaluation of a "Co-operative Counselling" alcohol service which uses family and affected others to reach and influence problem drinker', *British Journal of Addiction* 83: 1309–19.

CHAPTER 11

MEDICAL APPROACHES AND PRESCRIBING: DRUGS

John Merrill

LEARNING OBJECTIVES

After you have studied this chapter you will be able to:

1. Describe the theoretical basis for treating drug dependence in terms of maintenance and abstinence-orientated treatments, substitution and symptomatic therapy.
2. Understand how medical treatments for dependence on the main groups of drugs are implemented.
3. Be aware of good practice issues and the legal framework for prescribing.
4. Know the sorts of treatment that are currently being developed and are likely to become available in the near future.

INTRODUCTION

Although the management of substance misuse demands diverse skills of professionals and non-professionals from multiple backgrounds, medical interventions are crucial and becoming increasingly important. Several reasons explain the increased medicalisation of substance misuse. These include:

- an increased understanding of the way substances act on the brain and the chemical changes that underlie psychological processes
- advances in pharmacology and the development of new drug therapies
- the relative ease by which pharmacological treatments lend themselves to evaluation in clinical trials
- increased demands from drug users, the general community and political leaders for effective treatments for drug problems and the resulting harms to individuals and society.

Some individuals with drug problems may require only medical interventions, but these are the minority. Common sense tells us that unemployed homeless drug users will do better in treatment if they can be found stable accommodation and a job. For some the requirement for non-medical aspects of treatment may be less obvious, but most drug users will benefit from interventions aimed at increasing or sustaining motivation to change, boosting self-esteem and developing networks of friends who do not use drugs. There is much research evidence to show that outcomes from medical treatment programmes are largely determined by the range and quality of psychosocial interventions that are provided.

This chapter will address solely the medical aspects of treatment, and only the treatment of drug dependence. Other interventions, for example the treatment of acute intoxication and overdose, co-morbid physical and psychological disorders, are addressed in other chapters.

TREATMENT AIMS

The aim of treatment is to stop or reduce the use of drugs and to prevent or reduce the harms resulting from drug use. Treatment can be viewed as addressing three specific, though overlapping areas: detoxification, relapse prevention and maintenance.

Detoxification

Once dependence upon a drug has developed, stopping using the drug will cause unpleasant withdrawal symptoms. The nature, severity and duration of withdrawal depend on the type of drug, the extent and duration of dependence and from one individual to the other. Detoxification is the process of easing the transition through withdrawal to asymptomatic abstinence.

Relapse prevention

There is a high risk of relapse following detoxification. This is because yearning to experience the effects of drugs (craving) persists well beyond the end of detoxification. Much of relapse prevention is psychological rather than medical but drug treatments are becoming increasingly valuable adjuncts in relapse prevention.

Maintenance

Many individuals are unwilling or unable to undergo abstinence-orientated treatment. This introduces the option of prescribing a substitute drug in non-reducing doses. The substitute may be the actual drug to which dependence has developed but, more often, a better and safer alternative is available. Maintenance treatment with a substitute drug eliminates withdrawal symptoms and allows individuals to address concurrent issues. Thus, an individual on maintenance may be able to stop injecting, stop illicit drug use, reintegrate with their family and non-drug using friends, obtain stable accommodation and resume education or employment. For some, the period of maintenance may be short and precede detoxification – sometimes known as 'maintenance to abstinence' treatment. For others, maintenance may be indefinite or even life-long.

MEDICAL MANAGEMENT OF OPIOID DEPENDENCE

Principles of treating opioid dependence are similar no matter which opioid drug an individual is dependent upon. Heroin dependence is by far the most common drug problem presenting to services and principles of managing heroin dependence form the basis for treating dependence upon other drugs.

Treatment with methadone

Methadone is a synthetic opioid, which has been used as a substitute treatment for over thirty years. It has several properties that make it an excellent substitute for other opioids and heroin in particular. These include:

- a long duration of action so it can be taken once daily
- being available in liquid form which deters injecting
- having relatively little euphoriant effect, thus eliminating withdrawal symptoms without reinforcing continued use

Methadone can be used in reducing doses for detoxification or in non-reducing doses for maintenance.

Initiating treatment with methadone

Starting treatment with methadone is not easy. Caution is necessary because a therapeutic dose to those who are dependent on opioids can be fatal to those who are not. Although in theory it may be possible to calculate the equivalent dose of methadone to street heroin, heroin users may exaggerate how much heroin they take, their daily heroin intake may vary considerably depending upon the funds they have available, and the purity of street heroin may fluctuate. The need to obtain a thorough history supplemented by urine tests to confirm dependence before starting treatment with a substitute cannot be overemphasised.

An initial daily dose of methadone will usually be between 10 and 40 mg. This should be in the form of methadone mixture 1 mg per 1 ml. The patient should be seen each day with dose increases limited to 10 mg daily unless there are obvious signs of severe withdrawal. Stable blood levels of a drug are only established after a period equivalent to five or six half-lives of the drug, i.e. five or six days after the last increase in methadone dose. If methadone is being prescribed for detoxification, the starting dose for detoxification will be the minimal dose required to prevent withdrawal symptoms.

Methadone reduction

Methadone reduction in the community is most likely to succeed if the patient has managed to stabilise on methadone without using any street heroin. The rate at which the dose of methadone is reduced should be between 5 mg and 10 mg every week or fortnight. Dose reduction can be quicker if slowed towards the end of the reduction. An element of flexibility should be allowed, with dose reductions temporarily stopped if the patient feels the need to take things more slowly. Enforced dose reductions are unlikely to succeed.

For those who are motivated to detoxify but have difficulty doing so whilst in the community, admission to an inpatient unit may be required. Dose reduction can then proceed more quickly: typically over ten days. It is important to inform patients that such rapid reductions will result in peak withdrawal symptoms at about the time of their final dose of methadone, with a further ten days required before withdrawal symptoms become minimal.

Methadone maintenance

The dose of methadone required for maintenance treatment is usually more than the minimal dose that relieves withdrawal symptoms, with daily doses of between 60 mg and 120 mg being typical. Whilst the aim is to eliminate all use of heroin, for some this is a counsel of perfection. Studies have shown that the best methadone maintenance programmes can achieve an average reduction of up to 90 per cent of pre-treatment heroin use. Best results are from services that prescribe relatively high doses, have good support services, high staff-to-patient ratios, and retain patients in treatment for long periods.

Treatment with buprenorphine

High-dose buprenorphine has recently been licensed for use in treating opioid dependence. Buprenorphine has unusual properties, being a partial opioid agonist. This confers both advantages and disadvantages.

The chief advantage of buprenorphine is the drug's safety. This is because buprenorphine depresses respiration less than other opioids and increases in dose reach a plateau beyond which there is no further effect. Deaths from taking buprenorphine alone are extremely uncommon, even in those with no tolerance to opioids. Deaths caused by buprenorphine have been associated with injecting the drug and using it in combination with other drugs that depress the central nervous system.

Buprenorphine has a long duration of action so can be taken once daily with some people managing on alternate-day dosing. Buprenorphine is inactive if swallowed. It is absorbed sublingually by holding a tablet under the tongue until it dissolves. This can take several minutes which makes supervised consumption difficult. That tablets are easy to inject calls for particular vigilance. Also, specialist urine testing is required, as standard urine drug screens do not detect buprenorphine. A combination of buprenorphine and naloxone that deters injecting will soon become available. Naloxone is an opioid antagonist that causes immediate severe withdrawal symptoms if injected but is inactive when taken orally.

Changing treatment from methadone to buprenorphine is not straightforward. Daily doses of methadone must be reduced to 30 mg before starting buprenorphine in order to avoid a severe withdrawal reaction. For those heroin users newly presenting for treatment, buprenorphine should not be started before 4 hours after last heroin use. A typical starting dose is 2 mg on the first day, followed by 4 mg on the second day and 8 mg on the third day. A maintenance dose of buprenorphine is 8–16 mg daily. Buprenorphine appears to cause a milder withdrawal reaction than methadone. Dose reductions of 1 mg every four days are appropriate for outpatient detoxification. (See Table 11.1.)

High-dose buprenorphine provides an alternative to methadone in treating opioid dependence. Further research is needed to establish which patients are more suited to buprenorphine treatment and which are best treated with methadone. Buprenorphine should be seriously considered as a first-line treatment for those considering detoxification, those with no history of injecting, and where methadone maintenance treatment has previously failed. Extreme caution is needed before prescribing buprenorphine without supervised consumption because of the risk of tablets being injected.

Other treatments for opioid dependence using substitutes

A number of other drugs have been used in opioid substitution treatment although the evidence base supporting their effectiveness is less than for methadone and buprenorphine. In the UK reducing doses of dihydrocodeine, and in other European countries tramadol, have been widely used. In Austria, sustained-release morphine sulphate has been found to be as effective as methadone in maintenance treatment.

Table 11.1 Comparison of the relative advantages of buprenorphine and methadone

Advantages of methadone	*Advantages of buprenorphine*
More difficult to inject	Safety in overdose
Easier to supervise consumption	Ease of initiating treatment
Readily detectable in urine by standard tests	Relatively mild withdrawal symptoms

Treatment with injectable opioids is a controversial area. Clearly injecting carries long- and short-term dangers; even if the drug is sterile, pure and manufactured for intravenous administration. There are practical difficulties supervising injecting, risk of prescribed injectables being diverted, and basic psychological conditioning theory predicts that treatment with injectables is likely to further entrench injecting behaviour. Two rationales support treatment with injectables. One is to help those intractable injectors who have failed to benefit from treatment with an oral substitute. The other is to encourage into treatment those who are not attracted by services that provide only oral substitutes. The UK is unique in having a long history of prescribing injectable methadone and injectable heroin to a minority of those in treatment, but regrettably this has not been subjected to rigorous evaluation. Although prescribing injectable heroin to those not helped by methadone maintenance has shown benefits in Swiss programmes, the extensive range of support services available to those treated with injectables may be more responsible for subjects' improvement than the injectable heroin itself.

Symptomatic treatment of opioid withdrawal symptoms

A wide range of non-opioid medications is available for treating withdrawal symptoms. These may be used as the sole treatment for withdrawal or as adjuncts to gradual or rapid detoxification regimens. These include: antiemetics for nausea and vomiting, e.g. metoclopramide, prochlorperazine; antidiarhoeals, e.g. diphenoxylate, loperamide; antispasmodics for stomach cramps, e.g. hyoscine; analgesia for muscular cramps, e.g. paracetamol, ibuprofen.

Clonidine is an alpha$_2$-adrenergic agonist that has been shown to attenuate withdrawal symptoms caused by rebound over-activity of the autonomic nervous system. Its use has been restricted to inpatients because of clonidine's pronounced effect of lowering blood pressure. More recently lofexidine, a clonidine analogue, has shown similar benefits in reducing withdrawal symptoms with little effect on blood pressure. The dose of both clonidine and lofexidine must be gradually increased to therapeutic levels before opioids are stopped.

Usually the most persistent withdrawal symptom is insomnia. Some obtain good relief from sedative antihistamines (promethazine, diphenhydramine) or herbal remedies. For those that do not, sedative antidepressants, e.g. trazodone, low dose phenothiazines, e.g. chlorpromazine, or a short course of zopiclone or zolpidem could be tried. The most effective hypnotics are chloral derivatives and benzodiazepines but these should only be used as a last resort as they are prone to abuse and are dependence-forming.

Rapid detoxification from opioids

Using the opioid antagonists naltrexone or naloxone within an inpatient setting can shorten the duration of detoxification. Medication is needed to alleviate the severe withdrawal symptoms precipitated by antagonists. Typically, lofexidine or clonidine along with benzodiazepines and a range of other symptomatic treatments are given in generous doses. A controversial 'ultra-rapid' technique initiates detoxification under general anaesthetic, but mild to moderate withdrawal symptoms persist for seven to ten days after consciousness is regained.

Naltrexone in relapse prevention

Naltrexone is a long-acting opioid antagonist that is structurally related to naloxone and has enormous potential for preventing relapse. One 50 mg tablet taken once daily will block the effects of heroin, thus preventing relapse into opioid dependence. There are four drawbacks to naltrexone:

- Severe withdrawal symptoms occur unless all opioids have been eliminated. This will usually mean seven days after the last heroin use and ten days after last taking methadone. A 'naloxone challenge', comprising a 0.4 mg intravenous injection of naloxone is recommended before starting naltrexone. If naloxone does not precipitate withdrawal symptoms, naltrexone can be started.
- Opioid analgesia is rendered ineffective, so those taking naltrexone should carry a card warning emergency services that in case of an accident, alternative pain relief will be required.
- Those who are on naltrexone may be tempted to take enormous quantities of heroin to over-ride the block. This may result in a life-threatening overdose.
- Whether because of a desire to resume using or through misplaced confidence in ability to remain abstinent, compliance with naltrexone treatment for anything approaching the recommended six-month minimum is extremely poor. Compliance is improved if a family member or partner supervises administration. Tablets may be crushed and put in a drink to enhance compliance. Naltrexone may be given as single doses of 100 mg or 150 mg that last for two days and three days respectively.

Implantable and injectable sustained-release formulations of naltrexone that last one month or longer are in development.

Management of dependence on other opioids

A minority of those who present for treatment are dependent on opioids other than heroin. Examples include habitual users of codeine preparations in remedies for the common cold or diarrhoea, and those who have become dependent upon opioid analgesics prescribed to alleviate pain. In these instances treatment is usually aimed at withdrawal rather than maintenance. Dose reduction schedules should be agreed with the patient and daily dispensing should be considered for those likely to have difficulty restricting their use. Converting the original drug of dependence to an equivalent dose of methadone mixture can be helpful, particularly with short-acting drugs that need to be taken repeatedly through the day. Where the opioid was prescribed to relieve pain, alternative non-opioid analgesia may be required.

MEDICAL MANAGEMENT OF STIMULANT DEPENDENCE

Until the last decade or so, treatment for dependence on the stimulant drugs amphetamine and cocaine was largely ignored. Withdrawal from stimulants is not manifested by observable physical symptoms so that dependence has been dismissed as being merely a 'bad habit' that does not require medical treatment. It is now clear that both amphetamine and cocaine have profound and enduring neurochemical effects that may be amenable to pharmacotherapy. Both drugs act by potentiating the action of the neurotransmitter, dopamine, which suggests that an effective treatment for one may also be equally effective for the other.

Treatment of cocaine dependence

Treatment strategies for cocaine dependence have targeted the role of dopamine. Dopamine antagonists should block the stimulant and euphoric actions of cocaine in a similar fashion to the way naltrexone blocks the action of opioids. In practice, the dose of the dopamine antagonist haloperidol required to block the effects of cocaine produces severe side-effects that preclude its clinical use. Alternatively, dopamine agonists may attenuate withdrawal symptoms including drug craving. The dopamine agonist bromocriptine does bring some relief from withdrawal symptoms but the effect is minimal and short-lived. The amphetamine analogue methylphenidate has not proved beneficial and research using dexamphetamine as a cocaine substitute is currently underway. Antidepressants have also been evaluated on the basis that withdrawal symptoms are similar to symptoms of clinical depression. Although there is some reduction in withdrawal symptoms, this is slight and is not apparent until between ten days and two weeks after starting treatment.

Current research into the treatment of cocaine dependence includes evaluating the effect of anti-craving agents and developing peripheral cocaine blocking agents (PCBAs). The latter category includes inducing antibodies to cocaine by way of a cocaine vaccine.

Treatment of amphetamine dependence

In the UK, substitution treatment using dexamphetamine (the active amphetamine isomer) is widely practised. Several small-scale studies have shown impressive reductions in injecting and use of illicit amphetamine, but there have been no published reports of prospective randomised controlled trials. Dexamphetamine is prescribed in the form of either 5 mg tablets or a 1 mg per 1 ml mixture with daily doses ranging between 30 mg and 100 mg. The short half-life of dexamphetamine necessitates two or three daily doses thus making supervised consumption impractical and increasing the risk that prescribed dexamphetamine is sold on the street. There is a risk that instead of taking dexamphetamine in regular doses, patients can save up dexamphetamine in order to take high doses on an irregular basis, thus increasing the chance of experiencing psychotic reactions. Urine tests that discriminate between prescribed dexamphetamine and illicit amphetamine sulphate have only recently been developed. Dexamphetamine substitution is a controversial treatment and should only be undertaken by specialist centres. Small-scale uncontrolled studies using antidepressants have shown some benefit in reducing amphetamine use but require further evaluation.

As there are no medical treatments for stimulant dependence that have proved effective in randomised controlled trials, what should the therapist offer? Inpatient treatment, preferably at a specialist drug treatment unit, may confer a safe and therapeutic environment in which to withdraw. Antidepressants are commonly prescribed; they may be helpful in reducing anergia and low mood accompanying withdrawal and may help retain patients in treatment.

MEDICAL MANAGEMENT OF BENZODIAZEPINE DEPENDENCE

Those whose primary drug problem is with opioids or stimulants commonly take benzodiazepines. They may be taken as sleeping tablets, as anxiolytics, to enhance or modify the effect of other drugs, or to ease withdrawal symptoms. They may be taken at regular intervals or in binges, and they may be injected. It is important to establish at assessment if benzodiazepines are being taken, and if so, their precise pattern of use. Drug treatment services are under constant pressure from patients to prescribe benzodiazepines, but succumbing may cause more problems than it solves. Only a minority of those who request prescriptions for benzodiazepines are genuinely dependent on benzodiazepines and it is only these for whom medical treatment is indicated.

The general principle for treating benzodiazepine dependence is to prescribe reducing doses of a long-acting benzodiazepine, usually diazepam. Getting the dose right is difficult as a dose cannot be titrated against physically observable withdrawal symptoms and urine tests cannot establish whether patients are 'topping up' with additional benzodiazepines. Establishing a starting dose and an agreed rate of reduction probably has more to do with negotiating skills than medical expertise. Compliance is improved if prescriptions are made out for daily dispensing.

Commonly, reduction regimes fail and a repeated attempt in an inpatient setting should be considered. Maintenance prescribing of benzodiazepines should be a treatment of last resort. Research is currently underway evaluating the role of flumazenil, a benzodiazepine antagonist, in detoxification.

MANAGEMENT OF DEPENDENCE ON OTHER DRUGS

About 10 per cent of those who use cannabis develop dependence upon the drug. Cannabis dependence rarely presents for treatment; when it does, treatment is psychological rather than medical.

Dependence upon MDMA (Ecstasy) or one of the other methoxylated amphetamines, such as MDEA, is rare. Treatment is similar to that for amphetamine dependence.

Cases of dependence upon gamma-hyydroxybutyric acid (GHB) occasionally present for treatment. There are reports of successful treatment using reducing doses of benzodiazepines.

Volatile substance abuse (glue and gas sniffing) may lead to dependence. Admission to hospital may be needed to stop use of these substances. Where withdrawal symptoms are severe, reducing doses of benzodiazepines may be helpful.

GOOD PRACTICE IN THE TREATMENT OF DRUG DEPENDENCE

Supervised consumption and dispensing frequency

In marked contrast to the rest of the world, supervised consumption of prescribed drugs has not been a feature of treatment in the UK. Ensuring patients take substitute drugs under supervision at pharmacies or specialist treatment services has many advantages. It improves compliance, reduces the risk of prescribed drugs being taken by those for whom they were not intended, and enables increased interaction with the patient thus assisting monitoring of clinical progress. Supervised consumption is now recommended in the UK for at least the first three months of treatment with methadone.

Whether or not supervised consumption is available, initial prescriptions should be made out for dispensing on a daily basis (which usually necessitates dispensing for two days on Saturdays). As treatment progresses, gradually increasing dispensing intervals can reward clinical improvement. Similarly, deterioration in response to treatment would indicate resumption of daily dispensing/supervised consumption.

Urine testing

Urine drug testing provides a snapshot of recent drug use, encourages honesty in disclosing drug use, and is an essential adjunct for initial assessment and monitoring progress. Rigorous testing procedures that take samples at random intervals and observe the passing of urine into the specimen pot are rarely indicated. Analysis of hair is expensive but records drug use over time, a 1 centimetre sample from the head representing approximately one month.

Retention in treatment

Many research studies have shown the importance of retaining patients in treatment in order to maximise benefits. This applies to all forms of treatment for all types of drug problem. It is therefore no longer acceptable to stop prescribing methadone as soon as a sample of urine tests positive for heroin. Similarly, for those treatments where medication has little or no role to play, extensive efforts must be made to encourage patients' continued attendance and engagement in psychosocial treatment.

Shared care and prescribing restrictions

In the UK, it is recommended that the medical treatment of drug dependence be delivered through the principles of shared care. Family doctors should be able to treat most of their patients' drug problems with support from medical and non-medical staff from specialist drug services. Whilst the principles of shared care appear to make good sense, virtually all research showing the effectiveness of treatment for drug dependence has involved treatment delivered by specialist services.

The UK is unusual in encouraging family doctors to prescribe methadone. Indeed any doctor can prescribe any drug for the purpose of treating dependence with the exception of heroin, diconal (a combination of dipipanone and cyclizine) and cocaine, which require special licences from the Home Office. Plans are underway to extend the licensing system. In future, most doctors will be limited to prescribing only methadone mixture and buprenorphine for the treatment of opioid dependence.

Conclusion

Medical treatments for drug dependence are effective in reducing the physical, psychological and social harms associated with drug misuse. Treatments for opioid dependence are especially well established and have been subject to the most research. Advances in understanding the action of drugs on the brain are producing new treatment approaches. Outcomes from medical interventions are dependent upon the theoretical basis of the medical intervention, the practical manner in which it is delivered and the range and quality of psychosocial interventions available.

Summary

- Medical treatments for drug dependence have a central role in management and are becoming increasingly more important.
- Treatment approaches can be usefully viewed as three overlapping stages: detoxification, relapse prevention and, for some drugs, maintenance.
- The most established and effective treatments are those for heroin dependence.
- Successful treatment involves more than prescribing: practical measures to increase compliance, retain patients in treatment, and psychosocial interventions are essential to maximise benefits.

- An increased knowledge of the way drugs act on the brain will ensure the development of further effective medical treatments.

READER INPUT

(1) What factors (biological, psychological and social) contribute to drug users being reluctant to withdraw from maintenance treatment?
(2) Does the possibility of 'vaccination' against cocaine use raise any ethical questions for public health? In what ways is there a parallel with infectious diseases and how does it differ?
(3) How easy is it for somebody living in your catchment area to access prescribed drugs for the treatment of dependence? Is there a specialist service? Is there a shared care scheme with Primary Care? Are there Primary Care specialists? Do non-statutory/voluntary sector services arrange prescribing? What are the benefits and problems of prescribing drugs from different settings?
(4) What are the disadvantages of maintenance prescribing?

FURTHER READING

Carvey, P.M. (1998) *Drug Action in the Central Nervous System*, Oxford: Oxford University Press.
Department of Health (1999) *Drug Misuse and Dependence – Guidelines on Clinical Management*, London: The Stationery Office.
Seivewright, N. (2000) *Community Treatment of Drug Misuse: More than Methadone*, Cambridge: Cambridge University Press.
Ward, J., Mattick, R. and Hall, W. (1998) *Methadone Maintenance Treatment and Other Opioid Replacement Therapies*, Amsterdam: Harwood Academic Publishers.

CHAPTER 12

MEDICAL APPROACHES AND PRESCRIBING: ALCOHOL

Andrew McBride

LEARNING OBJECTIVES

After you have studied this chapter, you will be able to demonstrate an understanding of:

1 The basic principles of alcohol detoxification.

2 The main types of drug now in use to complement psychosocial interventions in maintaining abstinence after detoxification.

INTRODUCTION

Doctors, like other health and social care professionals, have an important role in identifying people with early and late alcohol related problems, making the link between excessive alcohol consumption and the problems presented and effectively communicating the link with the patient to facilitate change. As with other professional groups, the skills needed for assessment and communication should be in the armoury of well-trained doctors. The psychosocial interventions described in other chapters throughout this book are all potentially applicable to the doctor/patient relationship.

One aspect of treatment that doctors uniquely have access to through the prescription pad is the ability to prescribe medication. The use of drug treatments for alcohol related problems has received relatively little attention until recently, other than in detoxification. There is now an upsurge of interest in pharmacological treatment possibilities for the reasons outlined in Chapter 11. Although this chapter will deal only with pharmacological treatments, nursing care (whether this is provided in hospital, or at home by families) is essential to safe and effective detoxification; none of the other adjunctive drug treatments have been shown to work effectively in the absence of psychosocial intervention.

DETOXIFICATION

Any individual who drinks very heavily for more than a few weeks without periods of reduced consumption or abstinence, will develop withdrawal symptoms and signs on abstinence or abrupt reduction in the dosage of alcohol. The phenomena of the withdrawal syndrome are most readily understood and remembered as signs of psychological and physiological over-arousal.

Psychologically this shows itself as anxiety, panic attacks, depression, insomnia, and with increasing severity, hallucinations (usually simple visual hallucinations, sometimes complex auditory hallucinations in clear consciousness) through to the terrors of delirium tremens in which orientation in time, place and person is lost, and vivid hallucinations are experienced along with clouding of consciousness (akin to dreaming whilst awake).

Physically, tremor and sweating are accompanied by restlessness, agitation, raised pulse rate, blood pressure and temperature, and sometimes withdrawal fits (indistinguishable from grand mal epilepsy).

Severe symptoms are associated with a heavier pattern of drinking, ill health, poor nutrition, high pre-existing levels of anxiety, and some specific risk factors for withdrawal fits such as head injury, drug use and pre-existing epilepsy. Fortunately the majority of people will experience only mild or moderate withdrawal symptoms irrespective of how much and how long they have been drinking.

Identifying those who are at high risk of delirium tremens or withdrawal fits is not always possible. Also, each experience of withdrawal symptoms probably facilitates the development of more severe symptoms the next time round (so called 'kindling'). It is therefore always wise to minimise symptoms both in terms of severity and duration by appropriate treatment. The process of detoxification should minimise suffering and reduce the risks of severe morbidity and mortality.

The majority of alcohol withdrawal symptoms occur early on, usually developing within a matter of hours of abstinence and peaking within the first 72 hours. Concurrent use of other sedative drugs, such as benzodiazepines, may prolong the syndrome and make it more severe if the drug use is not disclosed and treated appropriately. The key message is that drug treatment needs to begin early if the maximum risk period for serious problems is not to have passed before adequate treatment is established.

Most people who drink excessively stop without any form of intervention. A minority deliberately undergo the process of detoxification either at home (see Chapter 15) or in hospital, and a further group, perhaps those at highest risk, are precipitated into abrupt abstinence by admission to hospital because of intercurrent illness or trauma. High levels of suspicion are therefore necessary among medical and nursing staff when an emergency admission begins to develop symptoms of anxiety and tremor.

During alcohol withdrawal substantial metabolic disturbance is identifiable in almost every measurable physiological system in the body (Glue and Nutt, 1990). Given this complex picture of endocrine, electrolyte and neuro-transmitter disturbances it is perhaps surprising that reassuring and calm nursing care, fluid balance monitoring, attention to diet and hygiene, delivered in comfortable relaxed surroundings, perhaps with some reality orientation, accompanied by a single drug treatment, will manage all but the most complicated of cases.

The trial evidence for the best drug treatment has been reviewed by Williams and McBride (1998). Although the evidence is generally of disappointing quality, the conclusion of the review is that a long-acting benzodiazepine is the most appropriate first line drug. Chlormethiazole has also shown to be effective, but has disadvantages in terms of side effects, routes of administration and toxicity if the patient begins to drink during the detoxification. Because of the potentially fatal interaction with alcohol, chlormethiazole should not be prescribed other than in a specialist in-patient setting. My preferred choice of drug is diazepam because it is safe, cheap, available to be given orally, rectally and intravenously and is generally the drug of choice should a withdrawal fit occur, therefore avoiding poly-pharmacy. Diazepam is the only drug that may have been shown to reduce the duration of delirium tremens, and is sufficiently familiar to doctors, nurses and patients, not to arouse suspicion or anxiety. Chlordiazepoxide (another long-acting benzodiazepine) is the preferred drug in some centres.

If a benzodiazepine is the drug used, then there are essentially two dosing regimes.

1 A relatively high initial dose (typically between 40 and 80 mg of diazepam per day in four divided doses) is given on day one and subsequently reduced over 7–10 days. Some flexibility is usually built into this regime, particularly early on, so that the dose can be increased if the patient reports severe withdrawal symptoms, or reduced if over-sedation is obvious. Experience and audit of specialist and non-specialist facilities alike suggest that unfortunately this regime is invariably arbitrary, and the starting dose unrelated to risk factors for severe withdrawal symptoms. The desirability of early abolition of withdrawal symptoms has already been mentioned, but the tendency of fixed dose tapering regimes is to maximise the effective level of diazepam and its metabolites at around the time the detoxification is theoretically drawing to a close.
2 The risks of under- or over-dosing the patient, lead me to use and recommend Symptom Triggered Therapy. In this regime, diazepam 20 mg is given every 90 minutes, for as long as the patient demonstrates significant withdrawal symptoms as rated by a trained observer, using a recognised withdrawal symptom scale such as the CIWA – Ar (Sullivan *et al.*, 1989). Using this system on my own in-patient unit, the average patient receives only around 80 mg diazepam, and is well enough (in terms of withdrawal symptoms) to begin some form of structured rehabilitation within two days of admission.

Patients with liver disease sometimes are prescribed a shorter-acting or more simply metabolised benzodiazepine such as oxazepam, to avoid accidental overdose. Symptom Triggered Therapy effectively avoids this because if diazepam is not effectively metabolised, accumulation abolishes symptoms earlier, the score falls more quickly and the medication is stopped. A very wide range of other drugs have been employed but their use cannot generally be recommended.

People with a past history of withdrawal fits can be prescribed an anti-convulsant in addition to the drug used for detoxification. Carbamazepine, which has been shown to be effective as the sole drug in mild to moderate alcohol withdrawal, is probably the drug of choice, but sodium valproate can also be used.

Supported detoxification by itself may be enough help for a minority of people. For others it simply allows a safe breathing space to recover enough health and strength to go back drinking. Anybody whose alcohol use has got to the point where they need pharmacological help to safely withdraw should at least be offered additional help, support and treatment that may lead on to a different and less toxic relationship with alcohol.

Treatment of vitamin deficiency

Poor nutrition is common in patients with severe alcohol dependence problems. The risk of developing severe neurological damage in the form of Wernicke Korsakoff syndrome (see Chapter 13) means that it is good practice to prescribe vitamin supplements, including intramuscular multivitamins which include thiamine. (In the UK the only preparation available is Pabrinex.) There is a very small risk of a severe allergic reaction (anaphylaxis) to parenteral vitamins, and appropriate treatment facilities need to be available. This very small risk needs to be balanced against the probable prevalence of severe cognitive impairment in perhaps one in eight dependent drinkers (Cook and Thomson, 1997).

DRUGS TO TREAT DEPENDENCE

Disulfiram

Disulfiram works in a similar way to having your own personal policeman driving along behind you to keep you to the speed limit. It is now the only drug of its kind available in the UK that can act as a deterrent to lapse and relapse.

If taken regularly at an adequate dose Disulfiram inhibits the enzyme acetaldehyde dehydrogenase. This allows the build-up of acetaldehyde when alcohol is consumed. Within a few moments of drinking alcohol the patient experiences an unpleasant sensation of warmth and flushing, headache, palpitations, breathlessness and nausea. Most of these symptoms are related to vasodilation and the consequent drop in blood pressure can be dangerous for those who have pre-existing cardiovascular disease (Chick, 1999).

Disulfiram is only of potential value in those whose intention is to abstain. There is little evidence as to who is most likely to benefit, but in practice I find it of particular value in those whose intention is to abstain but who lapse frequently and become disheartened and frustrated. For this group the knowledge that you have already taken the decision not to drink that day obviates the need for the rehearsal of all the arguments 'for' and 'against' every time the thought of having a drink enters your mind. Disulfiram should not be prescribed during pregnancy and great caution is needed in the elderly.

Within a week or two of taking Disulfiram many patients describe a reduction in craving which has nothing to do with pharmacological effects of the drug. The research evidence shows that supervision of the consumption of Disulfiram is essential for effectiveness. Varying degrees of coerciveness have been applied to this supervision. If the supervisor is not a professional or at least independent of the individual (such as an employer health nurse) then work needs to be done with the supervisor to maintain a constructive and positive attitude towards both the patient and the consumption of the drug.

Randomised controlled trials of Disulfiram have been undertaken, but there is a major methodological difficulty. If you (the patient) know that you have a less than 50 per cent chance of suffering a severe reaction (because of the placebo group), then the deterrent effect of taking the drug is perhaps too greatly reduced. In clinical practice if one tablet (200 mg) does not produce a deterrent effect the dose can be safely doubled.

The big advantage of Disulfiram is that it can provide a window of stability in which the patient can sort out their domestic problems, regain physical and mental health and take decisions about what they will do about their drinking in future. As a rule of thumb I usually suggest that people take Disulfiram for six months in the first instance, but shorter periods may be all that is necessary for some. A small number of people are very reluctant to give up Disulfiram even after a number of years, yet do so seemingly without ill effect.

The common side-effects of Disulfiram are drowsiness, headache, halitosis and an allergic skin reaction. These are all reversible and may occur in as many as one in ten patients to the extent that they require the withdrawal of the drug. Two severe side effects are liver hypersensitivity, in which fulminating liver failure occurs, usually during the first few weeks of treatment. This is exceptionally rare. More common is peripheral neuropathy, which is reversible but needs to be checked for at follow-up, as few patients, however well informed, associate tingling in the toes with medication that they may have been taking for months.

There are reports of Disulfiram being associated with psychosis, but again this is rare in people with no history of severe mental illness and in those with 'dual diagnosis' the risk needs to be weighed against possible benefits.

Naltrexone

Naltrexone is an opioid antagonist (see Chapter 11) which blocks the effects of the body's own natural opioid-like substances (endorphins) as well as the effects of other opioid drugs. One of the many effects of alcohol is to release natural endorphins into the brain; a positive and rewarding experience. The discovery that alcohol seeking behaviour in animals 'dependent' on alcohol is reduced when they are given Naltrexone therefore suggested a possible therapeutic use in humans.

Put simply, the theory is that if somebody with an alcohol dependence problem consumes Naltrexone before every drinking occasion, then the rewarding, pleasurable endorphin effects of alcohol will be blocked and over time the association between drinking alcohol and pleasurable effects will be extinguished and drinking will reduce (Sinclair, 2001).

There is little evidence as to the population of human drinkers most likely to benefit from Naltrexone, but the need to avoid giving the drug to those with liver disease is a significant limitation for clinical populations. Naltrexone should not be prescribed during pregnancy. High levels of craving may be one appropriate indication. Although the theoretical justification for Naltrexone is primarily the 'deconditioning' of alcohol use in those who continue to drink, the randomised controlled trial evidence relates mainly to those who have been detoxified and who are endeavouring to maintain abstinence. All published studies show an advantage to the group of patients randomised to Naltrexone, but the size of the effect is relatively modest (e.g. Bolpicelli *et al.*, 1995, Chick *et al.*, 2000a).

Naltrexone can cause nausea, which may be severe and persistent, headache, dizziness and weight loss. Depression and anhedonia have not been found to be problems in alcohol dependent patients. The patient needs to understand that in the event of trauma or other cause of severe pain, the effects of other opioid analgesics will be blocked. The attending doctors need to be made aware of this.

Naltrexone is usually commenced at half dose (25 mg) for a few days before increasing to 50 mg per day. There is evidence from some studies that Naltrexone is only effective if accompanied by skilled psychosocial intervention.

Acamprosate

Acamprosate (calcium acetyl homotaurinate) reduces the effects of the neurotransmitter glutamate. Persistent excessive glutamate activity has been reported in people with alcohol dependence for several months into abstinence. This may be a factor in the continued psychological and physical symptoms including mood and sleep disturbance. Acamprosate has shown potent effects in animal studies, both reducing 'relapse' and protecting against neurological damage during withdrawal.

In humans use is limited to those whose primary treatment goal is abstinence, but there is no evidence that any particular group of patients is more likely to benefit from Acamprosate. Several randomised placebo controlled trials have shown a significant advantage over placebo, approximately doubling the proportion maintaining abstinence after detoxification at six months. The one UK study (Chick *et al.*, 2000b) showed no advantage for the active treatment group, perhaps reflecting the high levels of morbidity in the sample studied and the less intensive psychosocial interventions available in the UK compared with other countries.

The only common side effect of Acamprosate is abdominal pain and diarrhoea. The drug has no psychological side effects and is free of dependence potential. It has no important drug interactions and can be taken with Disulfiram. In clinical practice Acamprosate can safely be given to anybody with alcohol dependence who expresses a preference for abstinence and who is willing to take the drug regularly three times a day. Severely impaired kidney function is the only contraindication to the drug. If Acamprosate has any effect it will do so during the first few months of treatment and there is little evidence to show any advantage to continuing the drug beyond six months.

Other drugs

There are few psychoactive drugs that have not at some point been recommended (and sometimes even investigated) for their effectiveness in 'treating' alcohol problems. In the absence of co-morbid mental health problems there is little evidence in favour of prescribing any psychotropic medication. In those with co-morbid mental health problems the use of any drug will need to be considered in the light of the enhanced risk of side effects and withdrawal effects if the patient continues to drink. Symptoms of anxiety and depression are unlikely to be successfully treated by anti-depressants or anxiolytics whilst the patient continues to drink.

Conclusions

Greater understanding of the pyschopharmacology of alcohol is leading to the developments of new pharmacological treatment alternatives for alcohol dependence. The evidence for the drug treatments available to date is that they should only be used in the context of broader psychosocial interventions. It is not possible to predict who will respond, and the drugs currently available can only be considered, at best, adjunctive to other necessary life changes. The search for new and more effective medication will no doubt continue, but the social and psychological complexities of alcohol use, problems and dependence mean that there is probably little true gold at the end of this particular therapeutic rainbow.

READER INPUT

(1) Find out what alcohol detoxification regimes are in use in your local services (primary care, acute hospital, mental health services and specialist services). How might the (very likely) differences be reduced to improve patient care?

(2) What factors contributing to alcohol misuse and dependence (biological, psychological and social) would you consider important in considering the realistic potential for new drug treatments for alcohol related problems?

(3) In the absence of good evidence for who should be prescribed each of the three treatments that might facilitate abstinence, consider the things that should be discussed with a patient you have seen recently to help them to consider their treatment options.

FURTHER READING

Kranzler, H.R. (2000) 'Pharmacotherapy of alcoholism: gaps in knowledge and opportunities for research', *Alcohol and Alcoholism* 35: 537–47.

Moncrieff, J. and Drummond, D.C. (1998) 'The quality of alcohol treatment research: an examination of influential controlled trials and development of a quality rating system', *Addiction* 93: 811–24.

Raistrick, D. (2000) 'Management of alcohol detoxification', *Advances in Psychiatric Treatment* 6(5): 348–55.

REFERENCES

Bolpicelli, J.R., Bolpicelli, R.A. and O'Brien, C.P. (1995) 'Medical management of alcohol dependence: clinical use and limitations of naltrexone treatment', *Alcohol and Alcoholism* 30: 789–98.

Chick, J. (1999) 'Safety issues concerning the use of disulfiram in treating alcohol dependence', *Drug Safety* 20: 427–35.

Chick, J., Anton, R., Checinski, K., Croop, R., Drummond, D.C., Farmer, R., Labriola, D., Marshall, J., Moncrieff, J., Morgan, M.Y., Peters, T. and Ritson, B. (2000a) 'A multicentre, randomised, double blind, placebo controlled trial of naltrexone in the treatment of alcohol dependence or abuse', *Alcohol and Alcoholism* 35: 587–93.

Chick, J., Howlett, H., Morgan, M.Y. and Ritson, B. (2000b) 'United Kingdom Multi Centre Acamprosate Study (UKMAS): a six month prospective study of acamprosate versus placebo in preventing relapse after withdrawal from alcohol', *Alcohol and Alcoholism* 35: 176–87.

Cook, C.C.H. and Thomson, A.D. (1997) 'B-complex vitamins in the prophylaxis and treatment of Wernicke-Korsakoff syndrome', *British Journal of Hospital Medicine* 57: 461–5.

Glue, P. and Nutt, D. (1990) 'Over excitement and disinhibition; dynamic neurotransmitter interactions in alcohol withdrawal', *British Journal of Psychiatry* 157: 491–9.

Sinclair, J.D. (2001) 'Evidence about the use of naltrexone and for different ways of using it in the treatment of alcoholism', *Alcohol and Alcoholism* 36(1): 2–10.

Sullivan, J.T., Sykora, K., Schneiderman, J., Naranjo, C.A. and Sellers, E.M. (1989) 'Assessment of alcohol withdrawal; the revised clinical institute withdrawal assessment alcohol scale (CIWA–Ar)', *British Journal of Addiction* 84: 1353–7.

Williams, D. and McBride, A.J. (1998) 'The drug treatment of alcohol withdrawal treatment; a systematic review', *Alcohol and Alcoholism* 33: 103–15.

CHAPTER 13

PHYSICAL HEALTH PROBLEMS

Ed Day and Ilana B. Crome

LEARNING OBJECTIVES

After you have studied this chapter you will:

1. Be aware of the wide range of potential physical problems associated with alcohol and drug use.
2. Understand the differences in the harm caused by different patterns of use.

INTRODUCTION

Use of drugs or alcohol is often associated with physical harm. The pattern of presenting problems depends on a variety of factors including:

- the combination of substances used
- the purity and strength of each substance
- the duration of use
- the mode of use
- individual susceptibility to harm (age, gender and genetic susceptibility)
- the environment of the substance user

This chapter will first examine the effects of alcohol in three broad patterns of usage defined in ICD-10 terms:

1 Acute intoxication.
2 Withdrawal.
3 Harmful use and dependence.

The physical effects of drugs of misuse are then considered in a second section.

ALCOHOL

Alcohol consumption is a major cause of health problems, and the mortality rate of heavy drinkers is at least twice that of the normal population. Alcohol is a small molecule soluble in both water and lipids, and so has effects on every system of the body. It can have a direct toxic effect on body tissues, but the by-products of its metabolism also cause problems (Lieber, 1995).

Acute intoxication

Acute intoxication with alcohol produces a steady progression through euphoria to incoordination, ataxia, stupor and even coma and death. Alcohol is the most common cause of road traffic accidents in the UK, with 1,500 deaths per year attributable to alcohol (a quarter of all deaths from road accidents) (Raistrick *et al.*, 1999). Intoxicated individuals are at increased risk of soft-tissue injuries, fractures, head injuries and other trauma. Apparent intoxication must always be regarded with caution as co-existent hypoglycaemia, subdural haematoma, systematic infection or chronic liver disease may also affect levels of consciousness. There is also a danger of aspiration pneumonia and cardiac arrhythmias. Acute gastritis associated with intoxication can lead to nausea, vomiting and pain. Alcoholic 'blackouts' are acute and transient episodes of memory loss associated with intoxication in both 'low-risk' and 'harmful' drinkers, particularly if alcohol is consumed in a 'binge'.

Withdrawal

Withdrawal effects may follow a bout of acute intoxication. It is difficult to predict the severity of symptoms, as variation occurs between one episode and the next, even in individuals. Weakness, faintness, sweating and insomnia may occur within a few hours of the blood alcohol levels reaching zero or declining sharply, and may be accompanied by a coarse tremor. Full recovery usually occurs in 24 to 72 hours.

In chronic heavy drinkers, or those with alcohol dependence, more severe withdrawal symptoms occur 12 to 36 hours after blood levels of alcohol begin to fall. In addition to the features mentioned above there may be:

- *illusions, misinterpretations and hallucinations* – usually auditory or visual with a frightening or threatening content
- *withdrawal seizures* – generalised tonic-clonic seizures occur 8 to 48 hours after cessation of drinking in 5–15 per cent of alcohol-dependent people

Acute intoxication	A transient condition following the administration of alcohol or other psychoactive substance, resulting in disturbances in level of consciousness, cognition, perception, affect or behaviour, or other psycho-physiological functions and responses.
Withdrawal state	A group of symptoms of variable clustering and severity occurring on absolute or relative withdrawal of a substance after repeated, and usually prolonged and/or high-dose, use of that substance.
Harmful use	A pattern of psychoactive substance use that is causing damage to health.
Dependence syndrome	Three or more of the following occurring during the previous month, or repeatedly together over a twelve month period:
	1. Strong desire or sense of compulsion to take the drug.
	2. Impaired capacity to control substance use in terms of its onset, termination or levels of use, as evidenced by the substance being often taken in larger amounts or over longer periods than intended, or by a persistent desire or unsuccessful efforts to reduce or control substance use.
	3. A physiological withdrawal state when the substance is reduced or stopped.
	4. Evidence of increased tolerance such that there is a need for significantly increased amounts to achieve intoxication or the desired effect, or a markedly diminished effect with the continued use of the same amount of substance.
	5. Preoccupation with substance use, as manifested by important alternative pleasures or interests being given up or reduced because of substance use.
	6. Persistent use despite evidence of harmful consequences, as evidenced by continued use when the individual is actually aware of the nature and extent of harm.
Definitions	
'Low risk' drinkers	0–14 units/week for women, 0–21 units/week for men
'Increasing risk' drinkers	15–35 units/week for women, 22–50 units/week
'Harmful' drinkers	>35 units/week for women, >50 units/week for men

Figure 13.1 Some alcohol problems (ICD-10 definitions)

Time after cessation of drinking	*Symptoms*
3–12 hours	Weakness Faintness Insomnia Tremor Sweating
8–48 hours	Illusions and fleeting hallucinations Seizures Cardiac dysrhythmias
>72 hours (Delirium Tremens)	Gross tremor Tachycardia Sweating Raised temperature Insomnia Agitation Restlessness Confusion Disorientation Delusions Hallucinations

Figure 13.2 Symptoms of alcohol withdrawal

- *cardiac dysrhythmias* – may be secondary to electrolyte imbalance or related to alcoholic cardiomyopathy

The most severe end of the withdrawal spectrum is known as delirium tremens, and is characterised by gross tremor, severe agitation, disorientation, confusion, sweating, tachycardia, delusional beliefs and visual hallucinations (Hall and Zador, 1997). The sufferer may be extremely frightened and this can lead to aggressive or self-destructive behaviour. These symptoms may last for up to 7 to 10 days and are associated with a fatal outcome in a small percentage of patients.

Since withdrawal seizures and delirium tremens are likely to recur during further withdrawal episodes, if such a history is elicited any future 'detoxification' process should usually take place in hospital.

Harmful or dependent use

Individuals drinking alcohol at levels categorised as 'increasing risk' or 'harmful' are susceptible to a wide range of physical problems.

Central and peripheral nervous system

The energy content of alcohol is relatively high and can account for a significant proportion of the calorific intake of dependent drinkers. Poor diet leads to nutrient deficiencies, and the problem is often compounded by malabsorption due to gastrointestinal, liver or pancreatic damage. Hypoxia, electrolyte imbalance or hypoglycaemia associated with intoxication or withdrawal may also combine with the direct toxic effect of alcohol to produce long-term damage to the brain (Lishman, 1990).

Thiamine (vitamin B_1) deficiency may lead to the development of Wernicke's encephalopathy or Korsakoff's syndrome (Cook and Thomson, 1997). Although described separately, both conditions share a common pathology, with post-mortem studies demonstrating severe neuronal loss in and around the aqueduct, fourth ventricle and mamillary bodies. Wernicke's encephalopathy is recognised by the triad of a confusional state, ocular abnormalities (nystagmus and ophthalmoplegia) and ataxia. The simultaneous presentation of all these symptoms is rare, and the diagnosis may be missed or misinterpreted as delirium tremens. If suspected it should be treated as a medical emergency, and as the problem responds well to parenteral thiamine it is important to retain a high index of suspicion.

The Korsakoff syndrome is characterised by a profound impairment of recent memory, relative preservation of remote memory and disorientation in time. There may also be apathy for mental and physical activity and distorted perceptual functions. It may directly follow the classical Wernicke syndrome, but can have an insidious onset and is often missed unless short-term memory testing is undertaken.

There is evidence for mild to moderate cognitive impairment in long-term 'high risk' drinkers. This may include deficits in both verbal and performance IQ and short-term memory. Recovery after abstinence appears to be slow, and problems may persist for several years.

Peripheral neuropathy is very common in alcohol misusers, and may range from subjective symptoms of paraesthesia to a severe distal sensory and motor neuropathy. The pathological mechanism is probably a combination of vitamin deficiency and direct alcohol toxicity. Co-existent autonomic neuropathy may contribute to hypotension and gastrointestinal motility problems. Proximal myopathy occurs in over 50 per cent of chronic alcohol abusers, usually with clinically detectable weakness (Peters and Preedy, 1999).

Effects on the hepatobiliary system

Alcohol misuse is the most common cause of liver damage in the developed world. The effects of alcohol on the liver follow a predictable course. The first stage is the development of fatty change (steatosis), which is usually asymptomatic and present in 90 per cent of heavy drinkers. In about 40 per cent of heavy drinkers it progresses to alcoholic hepatitis, which may present with pain in the right hypochondrium, jaundice or fever. This is the active phase of alcoholic liver disease in which an inflammatory process destroys liver cells, leaving a diffuse fibrosis with nodules of regenerating liver cells (cirrhosis). Cirrhosis develops in 8–30 per cent of drinkers with a 10 to 20 year history of daily heavy drinking, but susceptibility varies between individuals. Some important factors in determining outcome include (Day, 1998):

- *quantity of alcohol* – above a threshold of three standard drinks per day there is a steep dose-dependent increase in the relative risk of cirrhotic and non-cirrhotic liver disease
- *diet* – a good diet does not appear to prevent cirrhosis, but poor nutrition makes it worse. Both animal models and epidemiological studies in humans suggest that high dietary fat intake may increase the risk of cirrhosis
- *infection with hepatitis C virus* – even low levels of alcohol consumption increase the risk of progression of HCV disease
- *genetics* – women are more susceptible to alcoholic liver disease than men. Twin studies suggest that there is also a non-sex-linked genetic component to disease risk

There are a number of characteristic physical signs associated with cirrhotic liver disease. Cirrhosis may also be complicated by:

- *portal hypertension* – damage to the lobular structure of the liver causes raised portal venous blood pressure, so that collateral veins open between the portal and systemic systems to compensate. Rupture of the veins that run in the oesophageal wall (oesophageal varices) can lead to life-threatening bleeding (Krige and Beckingham, 2001)
- *ascites* – characterised initially by fullness in the flanks with dullness on percussion which shifts with a change of position. Later the abdomen becomes tense and uncomfortable, and there may be a right-sided pleural effusion and peripheral oedema. The condition may be complicated by spontaneous bacterial peritonitis (Jalan and Hayers, 1997)
- *hepatic encephalopathy* – is a chronic organic condition with intermittent exacerbations which can lead to impaired consciousness varying from mild confusion to coma. Anorexia, fatigue, apathy, slowness of response and a reversal of the sleep-wake cycle may also occur (Jalan and Hayes, 1997)
- *primary liver cancer* – some patients with long-standing cirrhosis develop hepatocarcinoma

A full assessment of the hepatic consequences of prolonged alcohol use involves clinical examination, blood tests and abdominal ultrasound scanning. Even a combination of all three cannot reliably distinguish the stage of liver disorder. Hepatic function is preserved with fatty liver, but there may be a slight increase in serum aspartate transaminase (AST), alanine transaminase (ALT) and gamma-glutamyl transpeptidase (γ-GT) (Drummond and Ghodse, 1999). Alcoholic hepatitis is characterised by a raised white cell count, raised ALT (relative to AST) and in severe cases by abnormal tests of blood coagulation (raised INR) and low serum albumin. A raised level of serum alpha fetoprotein is suggestive of primary liver cancer, and this may also be detected with an ultrasound scan. Liver biopsy is the only reliable way to stage alcohol related liver disease.

	Chronic liver disease	*Decompensated liver disease*
Face	Parotid enlargement Facial flushing	Fetor hepaticus Jaundice
Hands & body	Palmar erythema Telangiectasia Liver palms Finger clubbing Leuconychia Spider naevi Loss of body hair Gynaecomastia Muscle wasting	Asterixis ('liver flap') Peripheral oedema
CNS	Ophthalmoplegia Nystagmus	Encephalopthy
CVS	Dysrhythmias Hypertension	
Abdomen	Ascites Hepatomegaly Splenomegaly	Ascites Prominent veins on abdominal wall
Genitourinary	Testicular atrophy	

Figure 13.3 Signs of chronic liver disease on physical examination

Alcohol consumption is the main cause of acute pancreatitis, which usually presents with severe abdominal pain and which may become recurring or chronic (Mergener and Baillie, 1997). The patient is said to adopt a stooped or 'jack-knife' posture, and nausea and vomiting begin several hours after the onset of pain. The intensity and frequency of acute attacks usually decreases with abstinence and may stop. Major complications include pseudocysts, bile duct stenosis, and portal vein or splenic artery thrombosis. Chronic inflammation may disrupt either the endocrine or exocrine functions of the pancreas, leading to diabetes mellitus or malabsorbtion with steatorrhoea and malnutrition.

Gastrointestinal system

Prolonged alcohol consumption at 'harmful' levels may lead to smooth muscle dysfunction, resulting in gastro-oesophageal reflux and oesophagitis (usually presenting as heartburn). Alcohol misuse in conjunction with heavy smoking is associated with carcinoma of the oesophagus. Frequent vomiting may result in tears of the mucosa of the cardio-oesphageal junction (the Mallory-Weiss syndrome) leading to severe bleeding. Alcoholic gastritis occurs in more than 80 per cent of dependent alcohol users. A combination of damaged small bowel permeability and autonomic neuropathy may lead to poor small bowel functioning, diarrhoea and malabsorption.

Cardiovascular system

Population-based epidemiological studies suggest a 'J-shaped' relationship between alcohol consumption and the risk of coronary heart disease, with a 20–40 per cent lower rate among drinkers compared with non-drinkers. 'Low risk' alcohol consumption (up to 3 units per day) protects middle-aged men against coronary heart disease (CHD). Younger people and women have a lower incidence of CHD, and the effect of moderate drinking is less pronounced in these groups. Above 3 units per day in men and 2 units in women, mortality from all causes increases as alcohol consumption increases (Royal Colleges of Physicians, Psychiatrists and General Practitioners, 1995).

Heavy alcohol consumption increases the risk of cardiac dysrhythmias (a casualty presentation known as 'holiday heart'). Hypertension is linked to heavy drinking independently of age, body weight and smoking. It occurs in up to 25 per cent of those drinking at a 'harmful' level, so that alcohol is a common cause of reversible hypertension. Chronic 'harmful' drinkers are at greater risk of all forms of stroke (thromboembolic, haemorrhagic and subarachnoid haemorrhage). Alcoholic cardiomyopathy is probably a direct toxic action of alcohol. Although more common in men, women appear to be more susceptible.

Endocrine system

Liver damage leads to accumulation of oestrogen metabolites in men who develop gynaecomastia and testicular atrophy. Impotence occurs in up to 50 per cent of alcohol-dependent men, and women may experience amenorrhoea, subfertility and recurrent abortion. An alcoholic pseudo-Cushing's syndrome may develop due to excessive glucocorticoid production, leading to the characteristic 'moon' facial appearance, obesity and hypertension.

Skin

The classic skin signs of chronic alcohol misuse include palmar erythema, spider naevi and nail changes. Facial flushing is a common after-effect of alcohol use in dependent users. There is a distinct, alcohol-related, form of psoriasis that affects up to 15 per cent of alcohol misusers (Higgins and Vivier, 1992).

DRUGS

Opiates

Acute administration of opiates causes a feeling of euphoria and well being, followed by a state of drowsiness and poor concentration. Large doses can cause depression of the respiratory centres and respiratory arrest, but tolerance develops rapidly with repeated doses. Physical dependence becomes obvious when opiate administration stops, leading to a characteristic withdrawal syndrome. This peaks after 3 to 4 days and rarely lasts more than a week, although insomnia may persist for several weeks. Whilst unpleasant, opiate withdrawal is not life threatening.

Most problems with opiate use come not from the drug itself, but the unstable patterns of use. Once dependent, maintaining a supply of opiates is often a full-time occupation, leading to neglect of physical health. The drug suppresses appetite and causes constipation, leading to weight loss and nutritional deficiencies. Suppression of the respiratory centres and the cough reflex leads to an increased risk of respiratory problems including aspiration pneumonia. Tuberculosis is a growing problem among opiate users world-wide. Insomnia can be a debilitating problem, particularly when combined with the periodic break-through of withdrawal symptoms.

Sweating
Running eyes and nose
Sneezing
Yawning
Restlessness
Insomnia
Gooseflesh
Dilated pupils
Flushing
Shivering
Muscle twitching
Pains in muscles, bones and joints
Nausea and vomiting
Abdominal cramps
Diarrhoea
Tachycardia
Raised blood pressure
Low-grade fever

Figure 13.4 Opiate withdrawal syndrome

Overdose

Opiate overdose can be precipitated by poly-drug use and fluctuations in the purity of the drug bought on the street. It often follows a period of abstinence, when tolerance to the drug's respiratory depressant effects falls. The effects of overdose are slow, shallow breathing, low blood pressure, reduced levels of consciousness and ultimately coma and death. The effects of opiate overdose are rapidly reversed by the antagonist naloxone, which produces dramatic effects when given intravenously.

Stimulants

Amphetamines

Intoxication with amphetamines produces elevated mood and increased alertness and self-confidence (Gawin and Ellinwood, 1988). The pupils are dilated, the mouth is dry and the heart rate and blood pressure are increased, sometimes leading to palpitations. As the dose increases there may be restlessness, rapid speech, muscle twitching, nausea, vomiting and irregular respiration. Large doses may promote ataxia, insomnia and hyperthermia, and extreme hypertension may lead to cerebral haemorrhage and stroke. The beneficial mental effects of use and the depressant nature of withdrawal tend to promote binges. Large or frequent doses over 24 to 48 hours may lead to cardiac dysrhythmias, chest pain and grand-mal convulsions. Longer periods of use lead to malnutrition, vitamin deficiencies, weight loss, exhaustion and dental problems.

Cocaine

The effects produced by cocaine are similar to those described with amphetamine use. Chronic 'snorting' can lead to perforation of the nasal septum secondary to vasoconstriction and loss of blood supply.

Methylenedioxymethamphetamine (MDMA, 'Ecstasy')

Ecstasy enhances sensory perceptions and can produce states of altered consciousness and visual illusions, in combination with tachycardia, dry mouth, dilated pupils and facial muscle stiffness. Tiredness, muscle aching and headache may be present 24 hours after taking the drug. A number of deaths have been reported in occasional users of Ecstasy, many after taking only one tablet. The cause of death is variable, but hyperthermia is a characteristic feature.

Other stimulants

Khat is a naturally derived product of the shrub *Catha edulis* which is chewed to produce stimulant effects. It can produce physical effects similar to amphetamine.

Hypnotics and sedatives

Benzodiazepines

The benzodiazepines are effective anxiolytics, hypnotics, anticonvulsants and muscle relaxants (Lader, 1994). There is now a clearly documented association with the development of tolerance and a dependence syndrome, whereby unpleasant symptoms can develop following discontinuation. The pattern is highly variable, and the time course depends on the half-life of the benzodiazepine involved. The physical effects are combined with a wide range of neuropsychiatric complications and perceptual disturbances in all modalities, often leading to considerable disability. In high dose users there is a risk of fits during acute withdrawal, which can be particularly problematic with comorbid alcohol dependence.

Barbiturates

Intravenous barbiturate use was widespread in the 1970s, but is now less common. This is fortunate, in that they were commonly associated with physical problems and carried a high risk of causing respiratory depression or arrest.

Cannabis

Mild intoxication with cannabis produces an immediate feeling of light-headedness, often accompanied by ringing in the ears. The conjunctivae redden

Weakness
Headache
Dizziness
Sweating
Anorexia
Nausea
Abdominal discomfort
Diarrhoea
Insomnia
Tremor
Muscle twitching
Palpitations
Tachycardia
Postural hypotension
Psychomotor agitation

Figure 13.5 Sedative withdrawal symptoms

and photophobia and lachrymation may develop. The pulse and blood pressure are often increased, and some may experience tremors, twitching and ataxia (Ashton, 2001). In addition to a feeling of exhilaration and lightness of the limbs, there may be psychomotor overactivity with rapid speech or else a lethargic state approaching stupor. After-effects are uncommon, although the user may wake with fatigue or generalised aches and pains.

There is concern about the possibility of an increased risk of road traffic accidents due to psychomotor impairment whilst intoxicated with cannabis. Evidence for more chronic effects are also emerging, with respiratory diseases such as chronic bronchitis associated with smoking as the method of administration. Histopathological changes that may precede the development of lung malignancy may also occur, along with an increased risk of cancers of the oral cavity, pharynx and oesophagus. There is a risk of precipitating or exacerbating symptoms of cardiovascular disease such as hypertension and coronary artery disease, and subtle deficits in memory and attention may persist after periods of chronic intoxication.

Other drugs of abuse

Lysergic acid diethylamide (LSD) In addition to its hallucinogenic properties, LSD has a sympathomimetic action. Tachycardia, hypertension, pyrexia and dilated pupils occur shortly after ingestion.

Alkyl nitrites ('Poppers') These are used for their euphoric and relaxant properties. They have a vasodilatory effect which leads to rapid onset palpitations, tachycardia, hypotension, flushing, sweats, headache and dizziness.

Solvents Intoxication with solvents produces similar physical features as occur with sedative or hypnotic drugs. Regular users may have nasal or perioral sores, and sudden death may occur due to asphyxia or cardiac arrhythmia on exercise.

The risks of injecting

Many of the deleterious chronic physical effects of drugs of abuse are a direct result of injecting. Opiates, amphetamines, cocaine and benzodiazepines can be injected, and this mode of administration predominates when supplies of the drug are limited. The drive towards 'harm minimisation' aims to reduce the adverse health consequences of drug use by encouraging the use of safer injecting techniques and equipment, and ultimately to substitute it with another mode of drug administration.

Hyperpigmented scars or 'tracks' along the path of veins are due to repeated injection of drugs and adulterants using unsterile, contaminated equipment. This can lead to inflammation of the veins (thrombophlebitis) or local infections, abscesses and ulcers. Septicaemia may develop and 2 per cent of injecting drug users per year are estimated to develop endocarditis (a bacterial infection of the inner surfaces of the heart). Collapse of surface veins in the limbs can lead to persistent oedema.

The greatest public health concern arises from the transmission of a variety of blood-borne bacterial and viral infections via shared injecting equipment. These include hepatitis B, hepatitis C and HIV. The prevalence of HIV infection amongst intravenous drug users in the UK is approximately one in eighty for men and one in one hundred for women in London, with lower estimates elsewhere in the UK (Department of Health, 1999). Studies in the United States and the UK have suggested that over 60 per cent of heterosexually acquired HIV is related to injecting drugs. The problem may be compounded by difficulties in accessing health services, and involvement in other high risk activities such as prostitution.

There can be similarities between symptoms of HIV infection and other drug-related health problems (O'Connor *et al.*, 1994). Contaminants in street drugs can lead to lymphadenopathy, and symptoms of mild opiate withdrawal resemble the lethargy, fatigue and excessive sweating of HIV infection. Fever associated with HIV needs to be distinguished from that due to injection abscesses, septicaemia, pneumonia or endocarditis.

Hepatitis B is transmitted both parenterally and sexually. The incubation period varies from six weeks to six months, with a spectrum of severity between sub-clinical infection and fatal hepatic necrosis. Only 30 per cent of adult cases appear to result in jaundice, and many go unrecognised (Ryder and Beckingham, 2001a). About 5 per cent of those infected become chronic carriers of the virus, and around 15–25 per cent of carriers may develop an active hepatitis which progresses to cirrhosis (Ryder and Beckingham, 2001b). Chronic hepatitis B carriers with liver disease are at increased risk of developing hepatocellular carcinoma.

The commonest route of transmission of hepatitis C is by sharing blood-contaminated needles or injecting equipment during intravenous drug use. Between 30 and 80 per cent of past and current injecting drug misusers may be infected, and most acute infections fail to be diagnosed as jaundice rarely develops. The virus persists in 85 per cent of cases (Di Bisceglie, 1998), and virtually all patients with chronic infection develop some inflammatory liver changes. Again there is a range of severity, between slowly progressive, low-grade inflammation and chronic active hepatitis. About 20 per cent of those chronically infected develop cirrhosis, and 25 per cent of these may develop hepatocellular carcinoma. These serious complications can take 20 to 30 years to develop.

Conclusion

This chapter has given a broad overview of the physical consequences of alcohol and drug abuse. It is clear that no organ system of the body is unaffected. All health and social care professionals, whatever their speciality, must have a working knowledge of the serious health effects of substances of misuse and where to refer on for appropriate investigation and treatment.

FURTHER READING

Crome, I.B., Farrell, M. and Strang, J. (1996) Section 28. 'Alcohol and drug-related problems', in D.J. Weatherall, J.G.G. Ledingham and D.A. Warrell (eds) *Oxford Textbook of Medicine* (3rd edn) Vol. 3: 4263–317. Oxford: Oxford University Press.

Edwards, G., Marshall, E.J. and Cook, C.C.H. (1997) *The Treatment of Drinking Problems. A Guide for the Helping Professions* (3rd edn), Cambridge: Cambridge University Press.

Ghodse, A.H. (1997) *Drugs and Addictive Behaviour. A Guide to Treatment*, Oxford: Blackwell Science.

Lishman, W.A. (1998) *Organic Psychiatry. The Psychological Consequences of Cerebral Disorder* (3rd edn), Oxford: Blackwell Science.

The Tenth Revision of the International Classification of Diseases and Related Health Problems (ICD-10).

REFERENCES

Ashton, C.H. (2001) 'Pharmacology and effects of cannabis: a brief review', *British Journal of Psychiatry* 178: 101–6.

Cook, C.C.H. and Thomson, A.D. (1997) 'B-complex vitamins in the prophylaxis and treatment of Wernicke-Korsakoff syndrome', *British Journal of Hospital Medicine* 57: 461–5.

Day, C.P. (1998) 'Alcohol and the liver', *Medicine* 26: 19–22.

Department of Health (1999) *Drug Misuse and Dependence – Guidelines on Clinical Management*, London: Department of Health.

Di Bisceglie, A.M. (1998) 'Hepatitis C', *Lancet* 351: 351–5.

Drummond, C. and Ghodse, H. (1999) 'Use of investigations in the diagnosis and management of alcohol use disorders', *Advances in Psychiatric Treatment* 5: 366–75.

Gawin, F.H. and Ellinwood, E.H. (1988) 'Cocaine and other stimulants', *New England Journal of Medicine* 318: 1173–82.

Hall, W. and Zador, D. (1997) 'The alcohol withdrawal syndrome', *Lancet* 349: 1897–900.

Higgins, E.M. and Vivier, A.W.P.D. (1992) 'Alcohol and the skin', *Alcohol and Alcoholism* 27: 595–602.

Jalan, R. and Hayes, P.C. (1997) 'Hepatic encephalopathy and ascites', *Lancet* 350: 1309–15.

Krige, J.E.J. and Beckingham, I.J. (2001) 'ABC of diseases of liver, pancreas and biliary system. Portal hypertension – 1: varices', *British Medical Journal* 322: 348–51.

Lader, M. (1994) 'Benzodiazepines. A risk-benefit profile', *CNS Drugs* 1: 377–87.

Lieber, C.S. (1995) 'Medical disorders of alcoholism', *New England Journal of Medicine* 333: 1058–65.

Lishman, W.A. (1990) 'Alcohol and the brain', *British Journal of Psychiatry* 156: 635–44.

Mergener, K. and Baillie, J. (1997) 'Chronic pancreatitis', *Lancet* 350: 1379–85.

O'Connor, P.G., Selwyn, P.A. and Schottenfeld, R.S. (1994) 'Medical care for injection-drug users with Human Immunodeficiency Virus infection', *New England Journal of Medicine* 331: 450–9.

Peters, T.J. and Preedy, V.R. (1999) 'Chronic alcohol abuse: effects on the body', *Medicine* 27: 11–15.

Raistrick, D., Hodgson, R. and Ritson, B. (1999) *Tackling Alcohol Together*, London: Free Association Books.

Royal Colleges of Physicians, Psychiatrists and General Practitioners (1995) *Alcohol and the Heart in Perspective: Sensible Limits Reaffirmed* (Report of a joint working group CR42), London.

Ryder, S.D. and Beckingham, I.J. (2001a) 'ABC of diseases of liver, pancreas, and biliary system. Acute hepatitis', *British Medical Journal*, 322: 151–3.

Ryder, S.D. and Beckingham, I.J. (2001b) 'ABC of diseases of liver, pancreas, and biliary system. Chronic viral hepatitis', *British Medical Journal* 322: 219–21.

Vale, A. (1999) 'Alcohol withdrawal', *Medicine* 27: 18–19.

CHAPTER 14

RELAPSE PREVENTION

Michael Gossop

LEARNING OBJECTIVES

After you have studied this chapter you will:

1 Understand the importance of relapse as a key issue in the assessment and treatment of addictive disorders.

2 Understand the basic model of Relapse Prevention.

INTRODUCTION

Two essential elements of an addiction are a strong desire or feeling of compulsion to engage in the particular behaviour, and impaired capacity to control the behaviour (Gossop, 1989). The inability to stop using drugs and especially the inability to avoid returning to use are at the heart of what we mean by an addiction. In this respect, the problem of relapse is one of the defining features of the addictive disorders. Even for the heavily dependent drug user it is relatively easy to stop taking drugs: it is more difficult to remain drug-free. The problem of relapse is how to maintain habit change. As such, relapse is central to our understanding of, and ability to treat addictive behaviours.

The Relapse Prevention (RP) model regards addiction as a collection of maladaptive habit patterns. Relapse Prevention is seen as: 'a generic term that refers to a wide range of strategies . . . the primary focus of RP is on the area of maintenance in the habit-change process. The purpose is twofold: to prevent the occurrence of initial lapses . . . and/or to prevent any lapse from escalating into a total relapse' (Marlatt and Gordon, 1985).

Relapse Prevention models and treatment interventions have been applied to a range of addictive behaviour problems, including drug addiction, alcoholism, HIV risk behaviours, eating disorders, compulsive sexual disorders, anger control, gambling, and other problems of 'impulse control'.

THEORETICAL UNDERPINNING

One paper played an important role in drawing attention to the problem of relapse. This is the review article of Hunt *et al.* (1971). The seminal effect of this paper in drawing attention to relapse and to the similarities between the relapse (cumulative survival) curves for people trying to give up using heroin, alcohol and cigarettes, and its effects can be traced through dozens of later papers on relapse.

The early studies of Litman and her colleagues in London during the 1970s (Litman *et al.*, 1977, 1979) helped to identify and legitimise relapse as an important problem in its own right, and to establish some of the key concepts within the understanding of relapse. Subsequently, this work was overshadowed by the work of Marlatt (e.g. Marlatt and Gordon, 1985), and this has come to be seen as central to the development, or at least to the popularisation, of Relapse Prevention.

Marlatt's cognitive-behavioural model and interventions (Marlatt and Gordon, 1980; Marlatt, 1982; Marlatt and George, 1984; Marlatt and Gordon, 1985) provided an integrative statement of the theoretical perspectives and treatment approaches. Conceptually this includes elements of classical and operant conditioning, social learning theory, and social and cognitive psychology. A common thread which underpins most Relapse Prevention models is the social learning theory of Bandura (1977, 1982).

Recognition of the commonalities between different addictive behaviours was one of the interesting conceptual developments which occurred in addictions research during the 1980s (Brownell *et al.*, 1986; Donovan and Marlatt, 1988). The potential application of relapse to the understanding and treatment of heroin addiction, alcohol problems, cigarette smoking, compulsive sexual disorders, eating disorders, and gambling has been explored in several works (e.g. Gossop, 1989).

Theory and practice

The key components of Relapse Prevention are:

- high risk situations for relapse
- instruction and rehearsal of coping strategies
- self-monitoring and behavioural analysis of substance use
- planning for emergencies and lapses

The two central concepts are those of *High Risk Situations* and *Coping Strategies*. High Risk Situations may be situations, events, objects, cognitions or mood states which have become associated with drug use and/or relapse. They may include negative mood states, social pressure, social networks, inter-personal conflicts, negative physical states and some positive emotional states (Litman *et al.*, 1983; Gossop *et al.*, 1990; Unnithan *et al.*, 1992). Risk factors often occur together, either in clusters or in sequence (Bradley *et al.*, 1989). In treatment clients are taught to recognise the particular factors which increase the risk of their returning to the probematic behaviour, and to avoid or to cope with these factors.

To support the maintenance of change, RP requires the development of *Specific Coping Strategies* to deal with High Risk Situations. These may include skills training and the development or strengthening of more *Global Coping Strategies* that address issues of life style imbalance and antecedents of relapse.

Different Relapse Prevention models have been developed. These have much in common, though they differ in points of detail. The model of Annis and colleagues, for instance, gives greater weight than Marlatt to cognitions and especially to the issue of self-efficacy (Annis, 1986; Annis and Davis, 1988).

EVIDENCE BASE

A substantial body of evidence exists regarding the effectiveness of Relapse Prevention interventions. In a review of twenty-four controlled clinical trials of RP, Carroll (1996) found good evidence for the effectiveness of RP approaches when compared to no-treatment controls. The evidence was less consistent when RP approaches were compared with other active treatments. In this respect, the evidence regarding RP is very similar to that for most other addiction treatment interventions where the research literature has tended to show that treatment interventions are more effective than no intervention, but that no specific treatment type is consistently found to be superior to others.

The failure to demonstrate consistency of treatment effectiveness may be due partly to methodological differences between studies. It may also be due to the extremely complex nature of the addictive disorders. Among the complications are whether Relapse Prevention methods are equally applicable to different types of substance misuse, whether they are applicable to all clients, whether they are more effective as individual or group treatments, and whether in residential or in community settings.

A study of marital therapy for male alcoholics (O'Farrell *et al.*, 1998) found that marital therapy with couples was more effective when complemented by Relapse Prevention. Marital therapy plus RP led to more days abstinent and to better compliance with medication than marital therapy alone. Rawson *et al.* (1993) concluded that the evidence regarding the role of RP for the treatment of alcoholism did not support the use of such methods as stand-alone treatments, but that they should be used within a comprehensive treatment package to maximise their therapeutic benefit.

Carroll *et al.* (1991) compared RP versus inter-personal psychotherapy for cocaine misusers. Although no differences in main treatment effects were detected, a significant patient × treatment interaction was found, with the more severely dependent cocaine users being more likely to achieve abstinence after RP. A similar finding, with more severely dependent cocaine users responding better to RP, was also found in a subsequent study (Carroll *et al.*, 1994). In a controlled study of patients randomly assigned either to RP or to a community-based aftercare programme, McAuliffe (1990) found that patients who received RP achieved better abstinence rates at both six-month and twelve-month follow-up, better employment rates, and reduced criminal activity.

EXAMPLES OF GOOD PRACTICE

Efforts to ensure good practice are a priority within the addictions. Having spent many years working within and observing the processes and procedures of drug misuse treatment, it is difficult for me to avoid the conclusion that treatments are often delivered in ways which could politely be described as 'sub-optimal'. Treatment services which apparently provide similar interventions vary greatly both in their treatment practices and in their clients' treatment outcomes.

One of the ways in which clinical psychology has sought to improve treatment provision is through manual based therapies. An important distinction to be made here is that between the ideals of 'best practice' and the reality of treatment interventions delivered under day-to-day conditions in existing services. Treatment manuals provide direction about the key methods and procedures for the delivery of an intervention by specifying what the therapist should do within sessions and how the sessions should proceed. Manuals are particularly useful where interventions are delivered by therapists with limited training and expertise (as is typically the case in addiction treatment services).

Specifying the rationale and goals of therapy, the mutual agreement of these between therapist and client, delineating treatment procedures, and providing feedback about progress are core features of cognitive-behavioural therapies such as RP, but they are probably also common features of all effective psychological treatments. The marked and often unacceptable variation in programme delivery leads to a situation in which key elements of treatment may be neglected or even omitted. The use of treatment manuals helps to improve treatment integrity.

Manual based therapies have been widely discussed within clinical psychology (e.g. Wilson, 1996; Kazdin, 1998), and this is not the appropriate place to enter a full discussion of the merits of possible limitations of such methods. However, it is likely that the use of manuals for RP will be of direct relevance to many of the problems that lead to the sub-optimal provision of treatments for addictive disorders. No single manual has established itself for this purpose, though manuals have been developed for training purposes (Wanigaratne *et al.*, 1990) and manual based therapies have also been used in clinical trials (e.g. McAuliffe, 1990).

Conclusion

RP has made three important contributions to our understanding and ability to treat the addictive disorders:

- RP has altered the former view of relapse as merely a poor outcome to treatment, and redirected attention to relapse as a process which can be understood, anticipated and avoided.
- RP has given direction and purpose to treatment in the day-to-day clinical setting by showing how assessment should be conducted and targeted to key problem areas.
- RP has provided a model for treatment intervention and encouraged a cognitive-social-behavioural approach to addiction treatment.

There has been some controversy regarding the use of the term 'relapse' in the addictions (Grabowski, 1986; Saunders and Allsop, 1989). The term has been criticised because of its perceived connotations of a disease model. In the United States, RP approaches, and the notion of accepting and working with 'lapses', in particular, have often been seen as in conflict with Twelve Step treatment models which insist upon working towards complete abstinence.

Brown (1998) has argued that although relapse is of central importance within the addictions, addiction should not itself be defined as a 'chronic relapsing condition' (e.g. Institute of Medicine, 1996) since many dependent drug misusers achieve and maintain abstinence from drugs (Simpson and Sells, 1990; Hubbard *et al.*, 1997; Gossop *et al.*, 1997). The view of addiction as a relapsing disorder is seen as supporting a pessimistic view of drug misusers' capacity for change. The therapeutic nihilism of some commentators has been a powerfully demotivating factor for clinicians in this field. However, the relapse prevention model need not support this negative view of addiction, and can be seen as a practical and useful way of redressing such pessimism.

One challenge for the model is that relapses may happen not because of a failure of coping skills but because the individual has actively decided to seek a relapse. Such 'relapses by choice' or 'volitional relapses' are not infrequent (Bradley *et al.*, 1989; Saunders and Allsop, 1987). From a Relapse Prevention perspective it is still possible to consider this decision and its antecedents as part of a relapse process rather than an unpredictable event, and to identify factors associated with deciding to use drugs again.

The validity of the concept of High Risk Situations has been questioned (Sutton, 1993). For example, someone trying to maintain habit change may quite frequently experience negative mood states but each occurrence may not produce a lapse. Precisely when and how a potential risk factor becomes active is unclear, except in retrospect. A detailed and often critical analysis of Marlatt's typology of relapse was published by a number of authors in a 1996 supplement to *Addiction*.

RP methods are not intended to be a complete treatment for all clients with addiction problems. For users who are not aware of their need to change, RP may not be the treatment of choice, or it may need to be supplemented by motivational enhancement therapies. However, it is clear that many of the most important factors which determine the success or otherwise of an attempt to change behavioural habits happen during the maintenance-of-change phase and the RP model has particular relevance and applicability to this stage of change.

To what extent should the RP approach be widened beyond what is essentially a cognitive-behavioural approach to treatment? RP has sometimes paid insufficient attention to the potentially supportive role of pharmacotherapies. The development of antagonist drugs and anti-craving drugs could be seen to offer forms of medication which might be incorporated within RP packages. Although this has been resisted by some RP providers, pharmacotherapeutic agents such as naltrexone and acamprosate can be used as adjuncts to RP. In a meta-analysis of studies on the efficacy of RP, Irwin *et al.* (1999) identified three studies which had used combined RP plus adjunctive medication treatments with problem drinkers and one study with cocaine misusers: the results of these studies suggested that the combined use of RP with adjunctive medication was more effective than RP alone.

Despite the criticisms of the model and its application, the identification of relapse as a process and not just an event has been important in the current formulation of addictive disorders. It is an interesting paradox that the increased attention directed towards relapse provided an important stimulus to research into processes of recovery. Indeed, some of the research which was designed to address questions of relapse has subsequently developed into research into recovery processes. One of the important consequences of the work on relapse has been the identification of relapse as a process which can be understood, anticipated and avoided, rather than as an unpredictable event. Paradoxically, the attention to relapse has also provided an important stimulus to research into processes of recovery. Indeed, some of the research which was designed to address questions of relapse has subsequently developed into research into recovery processes.

One of the great merits of the RP model is that it provides clear guidance for the clinician about how to conduct a relevant individual assessment. The identification and explication of high risk situations, relapse precipitants and coping strategies had an important but relatively non-specific impact upon the delivery of treatment interventions in the treatment services of many countries. This is reflected not so much in the provision of formal Relapse Prevention programmes, but in a rather more general manner, with the concepts being used as guidelines for the planning and delivery of treatment. To some extent, this is not surprising since Relapse Prevention methods are often seen not so much as an alternative to existing treatment methods but rather as a focused application of conventional techniques which are widely used in current clinical psychology practice.

READER INPUT

(1) What are the key elements of Relapse Prevention for substance misuse? To what extent might the same principles be applied to other problematic behaviours and health problems?

(2) How should lapses be dealt with in the setting of a Relapse Prevention programme?

(3) To what extent are Relapse Prevention strategies employed in your local services? Are they identified specifically as Relapse Prevention? What are the advantages and disadvantages of having a programme rather than a general approach that is mindful of Relapse Prevention thinking?

FURTHER READING

Annis, H.M. and Davis, C.S. (1989). 'Relapse prevention training: a cognitive-behavioural approach based on self efficacy theory', *Journal of Chemical Dependency Treatment* 2(2): 81–103.

Bradley, B.P., Philips, G., Green, L. and Gossop, M. (1989) 'Circumstances surrounding the initial lapse to opiate use following detoxification', *British Journal of Psychiatry* 154: 354–9.

Brown, B.S. (1998) 'Drug use – chronic and relapsing or a treatable condition?' *Substance Use and Misuse* 33(12): 2515–20.

Gossop, M. (ed.) (1989) *Relapse and Addictive Behaviour*, London: Tavistock/Routledge.

Hunt, W.A., Barnett, L.W. and Branch, L.G. (1971) 'Relapse rates in addiction programs', *Journal of Clinical Psychology* 27: 455–6.

Marlatt, G.A. and George, W.H. (1984) 'Relapse prevention: introduction to and overview of the model', *British Journal of Addiction* 79: 261–73.

Marlatt, G.A. and Gordon, J.R. (1985) *Relapse Prevention: Maintenance Strategies in the Treatment of Addictive Behaviours*, New York: Guilford Press.

REFERENCES

Annis, H.K. (1986). 'A relapse prevention model for treatment of alcoholics', in D. Curson, H. Rankin and E. Shepard (eds) *Relapse in Alcoholism*, Northampton: Alcohol and Counselling Information Service.

Annis, H., and Davis, C.S. (1988) 'Self-efficacy and the prevention of alcoholic relapse: initial findings from a treatment trial', in T.B. Baker, and D.S. Cannon, (eds) *Assessment and Treatment of Addictive Disorders*, New York: Pergamon Press.

Bandura, A. (1977) *Social Learning Theory*, Englewood Cliffs, NJ: Prentice-Hall.

Bandura, A. (1982) 'Self efficacy mechanism in human agency', *American Psychologist* 37: 122–47.

Brownell, K., Marlatt, G., Lichtenstein, E. and Wilson, G. (1986) 'Understanding and preventing relapse', *American Psychologist* July: 765–82.

Carroll, K.M. (1996) 'Relapse prevention as a psychosocial treatment: a review of controlled clinical trials', *Experimental and Clinical Psychopharmacology* 4(1): 46–54.

Carroll, K.M., Rounsaville, B.J. and Gawin, F.H. (1991) 'A comparative trial of psychotherapies for ambulatory cocaine abusers: relapse prevention and interpersonal psychotherapy', *American Journal of Drug and Alcohol Abuse* 17(3): 229–47.

Carroll, K.M., Rounsaville, B.J., Nich, C. and Gordon, L.T. (1994) 'One year follow up of psychotherapy and pharmacotherapy for cocaine dependence: delayed emergence of psychotherapy effects', *Archives of General Psychiatry* 51(12): 989–97.

Donovan, D.M. and Marlatt, G.A. (ed). (1988) *Assessment of Addictive Behaviours*, New York: Guildford Press.

Gossop, M., Green, L., Philips, G. and Bradley, B.P. (1990) 'Factors predicting outcome among opiate addicts after treatment', *British Journal of Clinical Psychology* 29(2): 209–16.

Gossop, M., Marsden, J., Stewart, D., Edwards, C., Lehmann, P., Wilson, A., and Segar, G. (1997) 'The National Treatment Outcome Research Study in the United Kingdom: six month follow up outcomes', *Psychology of Addictive Behaviours* 11(4): 324–37.

Grabowski, J. (1986). 'Acquisition, maintenance, cessation and reacquisition:an overview and behavioral perspective of relapse to tobacco use', in F.M. Tims and

C.G. Leukefeld (eds) *Relapse and Recovery in Drug Abuse*. National Institute on Drug Abuse Research Monograph 72, Rockville, Maryland: Department of Health and Human Services.

Hubbard, R.L., Craddock, S.G., Flynn, P.M., Anderson, J. and Etheridge, R.M. (1997) 'Outcomes of one year follow up outcomes in the Drug Abuse Treatment Outcome Study (DATOS)', *Psychology of Addictive Behaviour* 11: 261–78.

Institute of Medicine (1996) *Pathways of Addiction. Opportunities in Drug Abuse Research*. Washington, USA: National Academy Press.

Irwin, J., Bowers, C., Dunn, M. and Wang, M. (1999) 'Efficacy of relapse prevention: a meta-analytic review, *Journal of Consulting and Clinical Psychology* 67: 563–70.

Kazdin, A.E. (ed.) (1998) *Methodological Issues and Strategies in Clinical Research* (2nd edn), Washington DC, USA: American Psychological Association.

Litman, G.K., Eiser, J.R., Rawson, N.S.B. and Oppenheim A.N. (1977) 'Towards a typology of relapse: a preliminary report', *Drug and Alcohol Dependence* 2: 157–62.

Litman, G.K., Eiser, J.R., Rawson, N.S.B. and Oppenheim, A.N. (1979) 'Differences in relapse precipitants and coping behaviours between alcohol relapsers and survivors', *Behaviour Research and Therapy* 17: 89–94.

Litman, G.K., Stapleton, J., Oppenheim, A.N., Peleg, M. and Jackson, P. (1983) 'Situations related to alcoholism relapse', *British Journal of Addiction* 78: 381–9.

Marlatt, G.A. (1982) 'Relapse prevention: a self control program for the treatment of addictive behaviours', in R.B. Stuart (ed.) *Adherence, Compliance, and Generalisation in Behavioural Medicine*, New York: Brunner/Mazel.

Marlatt, G.A. and Gordon, J.R. (1980) 'Determinants of relapse: implications for the maintenance of behaviour change', in P.O. Davidson and S.M. Davidson (eds) *Behavioural Medicine: Changing Health Lifestyles*, New York: Brunner/Mazel.

McAuliffe, W.E. (1990) 'A randomized controlled trial of recovery training and self help for opioid addicts in New England and Hong Kong', *Journal of Psychoactive Drugs* 22(2): 197–209.

O'Farrell, T.J., Choquette, K.A. and Cutter, H.S.G. (1998) 'Couples relapse prevention sessions after behavioural marital therapy for male alcoholics: Outcomes during the three years after starting treatment', *Journal of Studies on Alcohol* 59(4): 357–70.

Rawson, R.A., Obert, J.L., McCann, M.J., Marinelli-Casey, P. (1993) 'Relapse prevention strategies in out-patient substance abuse treatment', *Psychology of Addictive Behaviours* 7(2): 85–95.

Saunders, B. and Allsop, S.J. (1987) 'Relapse: a psychological perspective', *British Journal of Addiction* 82: 417–29.

Saunders, B. and Allsop, S.J. (1989) 'Relapse: A critique', in M. Gossop (ed.) *Relapse and Addictive Behaviour*, London: Tavistock/Routledge.

Simpson, D.D. and Sells, S.B. (1990) *Opioid Addiction and Treatment: a 12 year follow-up*, Malabar: Krieger.

Sutton, S. (1993) 'Is wearing clothes a high risk situation for relapse? The base rate problem in relapse research', *Addiction* 88(6): 752–27.

Unnithan, S., Gossop, M. and Strang, J. (1992) 'Factors associated with relapse among opiate addicts in an out-patient detoxification programme', *British Journal of Psychiatry* 161: 654–7.

Wanigaratne, S., Wallace, W., Pullin, J., Keaney, F. and Farmer, R. (1990) *Relapse Prevention for Addictive Behaviours. A manual for therapists*, Oxford, Blackwell Science.

Wilson, G.T. (1996) 'Manual-based treatments: the clinical applications of research findings', *Behaviour Research and Therapy* 34(4): 295–314.

CHAPTER 15

HOME DETOXIFICATION

Julia Lewis and Simon Williams

LEARNING OBJECTIVES

After reading this chapter you will understand:

1. Why home detoxification has advantages because of treating patients in their own environment.
2. Why comprehensive assessment is vital before embarking on a home detoxification regime (this includes a risk assessment).
3. That home detoxification has the same safety and efficacy as inpatient detoxification and can be more cost effective.
4. That it is important to tailor the detoxification environment to the needs of the patient.

INTRODUCTION

Before considering the topic in detail, we need to clarify what we mean by the term 'home detoxification'. Detoxification is the gradual or controlled withdrawal of a substance of dependence. The treatment process aims to alleviate subjective discomfort, minimise objective withdrawal signs and prevent the morbidity and mortality which may follow sudden cessation of use of the substance. The criteria used for assessing effectiveness are the severity of withdrawal symptoms and the presence of medical complications. Traditionally, the treatment of patients requiring controlled withdrawal remained within the remit of inpatient units, but in 1951 the World Health Organisation produced a report which placed the emphasis on an outpatient setting (WHO, 1951). Despite this message, the Ministry of Health in 1962 proposed that in the United Kingdom (UK) the inpatient unit should remain the focus of alcohol detoxification. Community alcohol detoxification teams were developed following the recommendations of a study by Stockwell *et al.* (1986), conducted with GPs in the Exeter Health District. Around this time Community Drug Teams (CDTs) were also being established, following a report by the Advisory Council on the Misuse of Drugs. Most CDTs are located in community premises which are managed either by the NHS or Local Authority. A one-year analysis of new referrals to one CDT showed that 66 per cent of referrals were treated for opiate misuse, 17 per cent for benzodiazepines and 6 per cent for amphetamines. The remaining 11 per cent were described as using other drugs (Strang *et al.*, 1992). It is now common practice for both these services to be merged as Community Substance Misuse Teams. These teams are usually multidisciplinary and offer a wide range of services including home detoxification.

Home detoxification in the UK tends to mean the treatment of the patient in their own home, with daily visits to a specialist clinic or daily home visits from a community nurse (Cooper, 1994). The former could also be described as an outpatient detoxification programme. In some areas the term 'home detoxification' is used to describe a treatment regime carried out under the guidance of the GP alone, without the involvement of specialist services (Stockwell *et al.*, 1986). Whatever the precise method, the rationale is that as most of the social cues which precede drug or alcohol misuse are in an individual's environment, treating people in their own homes will have therapeutic advantages. Wetherill *et al.* (1987) found that patients feel more comfortable in their own homes when divulging confidential information.

TYPES OF PROGRAMMES AVAILABLE AND SELECTION CRITERIA

Withdrawal management in a community setting is primarily focused on alcohol, opiates, benzodiazepines and stimulants. Prior to a home detoxification programme, it is essential that a thorough assessment is completed and clients meet agreed criteria for home treatment. Unfortunately authors cite different criteria; for example, Abbott (1996) suggests the following:

- an interest in long-term rehabilitation
- minimal involvement with other drugs
- absence of severe medical complications
- not acutely suicidal, depressed or psychotic
- good impulse control
- socio-economic stability

He also suggests that, with careful screening, less than 10 per cent of patients will need to be admitted for detoxification. Of course, patient preference should always be borne in mind when considering the ideal location for detoxification. Rates of withdrawal should be tailored to suit the individual, and only planned after a detailed assessment. Unlike opiate and stimulant detoxification, rapid reduction in dosage of benzodiazepines can result in life-threatening seizures, so it is prudent to err on the side of caution when negotiating cuts in medication.

Before commencing a community detoxification it is important that:

- a risk assessment for the process, the proposed setting, the client and the visiting substance misuse worker are undertaken
- the treatment programme is tailored to suit the individual's needs
- a supportive network of family and friends is arranged prior to treatment
- a contract is set up stating what the keyworker expects from the client and what the client can expect from the keyworker: this should include appointment keeping, the provision of regular samples for toxicology and estimated timescale for the reduction programme

ALCOHOL DETOXIFICATION (SEE CHAPTERS 12 AND 13)

Alcohol detoxification in the UK is not standardised and treatment is usually determined by local policies. A systematic review of drug treatment for the alcohol withdrawal syndrome carried out by Williams and McBride (1998) recommends a long-acting benzodiazepine as the drug of choice. Studies of the pharmacokinetics of diazepam have shown it to be safe and effective in the treatment of alcohol withdrawal (Mayo-Smith, 1997). Diazepam has substantial cross-tolerance with alcohol and is less likely to interact with any other drugs that the patient might be prescribed. Diazepam has other useful properties when used in alcohol detoxification:

- anxiolytic
- anti-emetic
- muscle relaxant
- anti-convulsant
- sedative/hypnotic

Patients are commenced on a reducing dose of a benzodiazepine over a period of five to ten days. For example, they may be started on 10 mg of diazepam four times a day (day one 40 mg) which is then reduced by 5 mg each day (day two 35 mg, day three 30 mg, etc.). An alternative regime uses 25–100 mg of chlordiazepoxide (another long-acting benzodiazepine), three to four times a day, reducing over a five to nine day period.

These doses are to some degree arbitrary and as withdrawal severity varies greatly, treatment should allow for a degree of individualisation if larger amounts of medication are needed (Mayo-Smith, 1997). The symptom triggered, or 'loading' method of managing the alcohol withdrawal syndrome is not yet commonplace in the community. An objective rating scale, such as the Clinical

Institute Withdrawal Assessment for Alcohol (CIWA-Ar) (Sullivan *et al.*, 1989) can usefully be employed during a home detoxification programme in the initial stages to ensure that the patient is receiving an adequate amount of diazepam.

HOME DETOXIFICATION FROM PSYCHOACTIVE DRUGS

As with alcohol detoxification a detailed assessment is essential before any treatment for drug misuse can be commenced. Home detoxification from psychoactive drugs such as opiates, amphetamines and benzodiazepines usually entails an individual attending their local community service on a regular basis. In certain circumstances it is possible to undertake a community detoxification from psychoactive drugs at home, with regular visits from a member of the service. Prior to detoxification individuals will usually be offered practical support and given harm reduction information. Community detoxification is usually undertaken by substituting illicit substances with prescribed medication. The rationale behind this is that by being prescribed a drug along with therapeutic input, the individual is less likely to crave or take illicit substances. There is still debate whether successful treatment is dependent on prescribing or on other therapeutic interventions (Farrell *et al.*, 1994). The amount of medication required will differ in each individual case, and will depend on tolerance, duration of use and amount of drugs used prior to treatment. The ideal dose should ensure that the individual is comfortable, not in a state of withdrawal and unlikely to overdose (see Chapter 11).

During the detoxification process the individual's illicit drug use and injecting behaviour must be monitored. Continued use of illicit drugs suggests that the patient is either not receiving enough medication or is not ready to undertake a detoxification programme. Many patients who request detoxification may be more suitable for maintenance treatment, and it may take months, or years before detoxification is appropriate (DOH, 1999).

Opiates

Within the UK methadone is considered the main treatment for opiate detoxification (Seivewright, 2000). Methadone prescribing is an effective form of treatment to assist individuals in the cessation of illicit intravenous heroin use (Strang *et al.*, 1992). The most common type of withdrawal programme is that using decreasing amounts of oral methadone (Gossop *et al.*, 1986). Government guidelines (DOH, 1999) suggest methadone mixture 1 mg/ml as the drug of choice in opiate dependence. Once an individual has been converted to and stabilised on methadone mixture, then negotiations over a reduction regime can begin. As with alcohol detoxification, rates of reduction in medication can vary. Some favour a rapid reduction, so that an individual can move on and address issues around their drug use, while longer-term detoxification programmes can last for up to six months.

Buprenorphine use is now on the increase, and it offers a heroin user a greater range of treatment. It has a few advantages over methadone, it is less addictive, withdrawal symptoms are milder, and it is less likely to interact with other drugs. Conversely methadone is cheaper and readily detectable in standard urine tests. There have been many trials in the United States comparing buprenorphine to methadone in opiate detoxification and it has recently been subject to a Cochrane Review (Gowling *et al.*, 2000).

Stimulants

After cannabis, amphetamine sulphate is the most widely used illicit drug in the UK. Amphetamine prescribing is second only to methadone in the management of drug misuse within England and Wales (Strang and Sheridan, 1997). A recent study highlighted the attempts that dependent amphetamine users make when they attempt a 'self-detoxification' (Cantwell and McBride, 1998). Unlike opiate detoxification, these attempts at withdrawal do not usually involve a gradual reduction of amphetamine or a related substitute. Cantwell and McBride (1998) found that the three most common types of drugs used after cessation of amphetamines were benzodiazepines, alcohol and cannabis (all central nervous system depressants). There is a paucity of studies on amphetamine detoxification and it is generally agreed that the whole area of amphetamine use is neglected. Treatment can range from counselling to substitute prescribing of dexamphetamine. It has been estimated that there are between 900 and 1,000 individuals receiving a dexamphetamine prescription in the UK at any one time (Strang and Sheridan, 1997). Dexamphetamine prescribing is indicated only in severe amphetamine misuse. Suitable subjects should have a long history of intravenous use and should be using more than 1 g of amphetamine a day (DOH, 1999). It is widely agreed that long-term prescribing should be avoided. As with methadone prescribing, when an individual is stabilised on dexamphetamine a reduction regime can be commenced. Dexamphetamine detoxification programmes are not standardised and dosage will be dependent on the amount of illicit drug that is misused. Strang and Sheridan (1997) in their survey of community pharmacists, found that daily doses ranged from between 5.0 mg and 200 mg (mean 40 mg). Individuals receiving 40 mg of dexamphetamine a day, could be comfortably reduced by 5 mg a week in a community setting. This would have to be combined with weekly or more frequent support from their keyworker, who should carefully monitor blood pressure, weight and progress. Stimulant withdrawal (illicit or prescribed) can result in mood disturbances, ranging from mild anxiety to psychosis. Depression is the most common and the individual's mental state should be regularly assessed for suicidal ideation. Anti-depressants may be indicated, although there is little evidence as to choice or even benefit, along with a short-term hypnotic for insomnia.

Benzodiazepines

Benzodiazepines are the most commonly prescribed drugs in Britain. Whilst hospital admission for detoxification is indicated in some cases, most individuals who are prescribed benzodiazepines are best treated in the community. Reduction regimes will depend on the dose, duration of use and the individual's ability to cope with the benzodiazepine withdrawal syndrome.

It is often recommended that benzodiazepines be converted to the equivalent dose of diazepam, as it has a rapid onset and is an effective hypnotic. It is available in scored tablets of 2 mg, 5 mg and 10 mg strength which allows it to be more flexibly adjusted than other benzodiazepines. Typical reduction programmes reduce the dosage by between 5 mg and 10 mg a month. This can be slowed down during the final stages of withdrawal if necessary.

Advantages and disadvantages of home detoxification

It is important not to be too rigid with guidelines for outpatient detoxification. It can be tempting to draw up protocols in such circumstances but it is important to match treatment strategies to individual patients. There are advantages and disadvantages to undertaking a home detoxification programme and certain criteria should be met prior to the commencement of treatment. A family member or friend should be willing to act as a supporter during treatment. This person needs to be educated about the process, the medication, the possible withdrawal symptoms, what to do about them and a contact telephone number for help if problems arise. The patient's GP must be aware of the management plan and prescribing regime. There should be no recent history of convulsions or delirium tremens and no concurrent physical or mental illness which would make admission to hospital a sensible precaution before embarking on a detoxification process. Home detoxification can be as safe and effective as hospital based care as long as standards and policies are adhered to.

Advantages of home detoxification

Those to the patient: It does not remove the patient from the family environment and its inherent support (Stinnett, 1982).
It tests the patient's resolve against temptations within the community, leading to the development of appropriate coping strategies (Cue exposure).
The patient can develop a working relationship with the community team who will take forward the rehabilitation part of treatment (Edwards and Guthrie, 1967).

Those to the family: It does not remove the family member from the home (Stinnett, 1982).

Those to service providers: A rapid response can be given to referrals (Cooper, 1994) helping to reduce the frustration of health-care workers who are so often unable to respond to the 'window' of motivation displayed by their patients.

Those to referrers:	GPs, who undertake approximately 50 per cent of all home detoxification, have been shown to prefer to have some specialist support (Kaner and Masterson, 1996). Home detoxification programmes aid the development of an effective partnership between primary and secondary care.

Disadvantages of home detoxification

Those to the patient:	Some patients would prefer to be removed from the temptations within the community during their period of detoxification.
Those to the family:	Detoxification can amplify problems of family dynamics, although this can work both ways.
Those to service providers:	Concerns have been raised over the monitoring of medication (Stockwell *et al.*, 1986) as medical assistance can sometimes be difficult to obtain should an emergency occur (Stinnett, 1982).
Those to referrers:	Issues of medical responsibility can arise. More primary care teams might be willing to get involved if responsibility is shared between professionals (Stockwell *et al.*, 1990).

Efficacy and safety of drug alcohol home detoxification

The pioneers of alcohol home detoxification, Edwards and Guthrie (1967), performed a randomised controlled trial of inpatient versus outpatient detoxification and rehabilitation. They found no significant differences in outcome between the two groups at the end of one year. In 1990, Collins *et al.* followed up a group of patients from the emergency psychiatric clinic of St George's Hospital in London, who took part in an outpatient detoxification regime. Seventy-nine per cent of the patients completed successfully and, during that time, there was a 50 per cent fall in the total number of patients admitted for detoxification. Overall the various studies show that, although initial completion rates tend to be lower than for inpatient detoxification, the longer-term abstinence rates are equal. Most studies of home detoxification report no differences in the rates of complications compared with inpatient detoxification (Stinnett, 1982). Even in an 'at-risk' population it can be argued that safety can be monitored and maintained satisfactorily for most patients.

The research findings for community drug treatment programmes are not so encouraging. In a randomised controlled trial of inpatient and outpatient methadone detoxification (Gossop *et al.*, 1986), twenty-five of thirty-one inpatients achieved complete withdrawal, whilst in the outpatient group only five out of nineteen were successful. The study found that the main reason for failure in the outpatient group was pressure from other drug users.

Summary

The development of programmes for alcohol and drug detoxification represents an important challenge for community health services. Research has shown that not only can such services match inpatient ones in terms of safety and efficacy, but that they are also more cost effective. Unfortunately, there is a tendency within the literature to use the blanket term 'outpatient detoxification' to describe a variety of different intensities of support (the more intensive programmes often being seen in America). What is clear is that there are advantages and disadvantages to inpatient and outpatient detoxification and the chosen environment should be tailored to the needs and preferences of the patient. Detoxification can give an individual a chance to reflect on their drug and alcohol use and make decisions about their future. A successful detoxification does not automatically indicate that an individual is going to remain abstinent for a long period of time; however, it should be seen as an introduction to a structured programme of treatment.

READER INPUT

(1) What factors make it difficult to compare inpatient (or residential) detoxification with home detoxification in terms of cost and effectiveness?

(2) How are (should) home detoxification services (be) integrated with other elements of an holistic treatment package in your area?

(3) What impact might enhanced home detoxification services have on the need for inpatient or residential treatment in your area? Consider specialist, mental health and acute medical/surgical facilities.

(4) Review some of the patients you have seen recently (or look at some of the cases in Part V), considering how home detoxification could be tailored to their needs. If it cannot be, why not?

(5) What elements of risk assessment are particularly relevant to home based treatment? Consider the patient, the family (or others) and the staff involved.

FURTHER READING

Cooper, D. (1994) *Alcohol Home Detoxification and Assessment*, Oxford and New York: Radcliffe Medical Press.

Cooper, D. (1995) 'Alcohol home detoxification: a way forward', *British Journal of Nursing* 4(22): 1315–18.

Fleeman, N. (1997) 'Alcohol home detoxification: A literature review', *Alcohol and Alcoholism* 32(6): 649–56.

Seivewright, N. (1999) *Community Treatment of Drug Misuse*, Cambridge: Cambridge University Press.

REFERENCES

Abbott, P. (1996) 'Admission criteria and patient placement guidelines for ambulatory alcohol medical detoxification', *Alcoholism Treatment Quarterly* 14(2): 15–27.

Cantwell, B. and McBride, A. (1998) 'Self-detoxification by amphetamine dependent patients: a pilot study', *Drug & Alcohol Dependence* 49(2): 157–63.

Collins, M., Burns, T., Van Den Berk, H. and Tubman, G. (1990) 'A structured programme for outpatient alcohol detoxification', *British Journal of Psychiatry* 156: 871–4.

Cooper, D. (1994) *Alcohol Home Detoxification and Assessment*, Oxford and New York: Radcliffe Medical Press.

Department of Health (1999) *Drug Misuse and Dependence – Guidelines on Clinical Management*, London: The Stationery Office.

Edwards, G. and Guthrie, S. (1967) 'A controlled trial of inpatient and outpatient treatment of alcohol dependency', *The Lancet* 1: 555–9.

Farrell, M., Ward, J., Mattick, R., Hall, W., Stimson, G., Jarlais, D., Gossop, M. and Strang, J. (1994) 'Methadone maintenance treatment in opiate dependence: a review', *British Medical Journal* 309: 997–1001.

Gossop, M., Johns, A. and Green, L. (1986) 'Opiate withdrawal: inpatient versus outpatient programmes and preferred versus random assignment to treatment', *British Medical Journal* 295: 103–4.

Gowling, L., Ali, R. and White, J. (2000) 'Buprenorphine for the management of opiod withdrawal (Cochrane Review)', in *The Cochrane Library*, Issue 4, Oxford: Update Software.

Kaner, E. and Masterson, B. (1996) 'The role of general practitioners in treating alcohol dependent patients in the community', *Journal of Substance Misuse* 1: 132–6.

Mayo-Smith, M. (1997) 'Pharmacological management of alcohol withdrawal: a meta-analysis and evidence-based practice guideline', *Journal of the American Medical Association* 278(2): 145–51.

Seivewright, N. (1999) *Community Treatment of Drug Misuse*, Cambridge: Cambridge University Press.

Stinnett, J. (1982) 'Outpatient detoxification of the alcoholic', *The International Journal of Addictions* 17(6): 1031–46.

Stockwell, T., Bolt, E. and Hooper, J. (1986) 'Detoxification from alcohol at home managed by general practitioners', *British Medical Journal* 292: 733–6.

Stockwell, T., Bolt, L., Milner, I., Pugh, P. and Young, I. (1990) 'Home detoxification for problem drinkers: acceptability to clients, relatives, general practitioners and outcome after 60 days', *British Journal of Addiction* 85: 61–70.

Strang, J. and Sheridan, J. (1997) 'Prescribing amphetamines to drug misusers: data from the 1995 national survey of community pharmacies in England and Wales', *Addiction* 92: 833–38.

Strang, J., Smith, M. and Spurrell, S. (1992) 'The community drug team', *British Journal of Addiction* 87: 169–78.

Sullivan, J., Sykora, K., Scheiderman, J., Naranjo, C. and Sellers, E. (1989) 'Assessment of alcohol withdrawal: the revised clinical institute withdrawal assessment for alcohol scale (CIWA-Ar)', *British Journal of Addiction* 84: 1353–7.

Wetherill, J., Kelly, T., and Hore, B. (1987) 'The role of the community nurse in improving treatment compliance in alcoholics', *Journal of Advanced Nursing* 12: 707–11.

Williams, D. and McBride, A. (1998) 'The drug treatment of alcohol withdrawal symptoms: a systematic review', *Alcohol and Alcoholism* 33(2): 103–15.

World Health Organisation (1951) 'Nomenclature and classification of drug- and alcohol-related problems: a WHO memorandum', *Bulletin of the World Health Organisation* 59(2): 225–42.

CHAPTER 16

COMPLEMENTARY OR ALTERNATIVE MEDICINE FOR SUBSTANCE MISUSE

Adrian White and Edzard Ernst

LEARNING OBJECTIVES

After having studied this chapter, you will understand:

1 The range of alternative therapies that have been researched in the treatment of substance misuse problems.

2 What rigorous research has revealed about the efficacy of various complementary therapies in the treatment of substance misuse problems.

INTRODUCTION

Complementary/alternative medicine (CAM) is defined as diagnosis, treatment and/or prevention which complements mainstream medicine by contributing to a common whole, by satisfying a demand not met by orthodoxy or by diversifying the conceptual frameworks of medicine [1]. CAM has become an important subject not least because of its growing popularity. Survey data from the US show that CAM-use within the general population has increased from 33 per cent in 1990 to 42 per cent in 1997 [2]. In the UK, its prevalence in 1999 amounted to a more modest 20 per cent [3]. A significant proportion of this use is directed towards substance misuse. This chapter is an attempt to assess the efficacy of CAM for this indication.

METHODS

Medline and Embase searches were conducted to identify all controlled clinical trials in this area. In addition, our own files were searched for such papers. The bibliographies of the articles thus found were scanned for further references. Hard copies of all articles thus located were obtained and read by both authors. The information contained in these articles was extracted in a pre-defined manner (Table 16.1).

RESULTS

The following CAM therapies have been tested most extensively in controlled clinical trials: acupuncture, biofeedback, electrostimulation, herbal medicine and hypnotherapy. These are discussed in the following paragraphs.

Acupuncture

Traditional acupuncture has a long history, some of the earliest descriptions being found in Chinese texts dating from the second century BC. Acupuncture needles were believed to balance the energy flowing throughout the body in channels,

Table 16.1 Sham-controlled RCTs of acupuncture for alcohol dependence

Reference	*Sample size*	*Intervention [regimen]*	*Result*	*Comment*
Alcoholism: Clin & Exp Research 1987; 11: 292–5	54	(A) Acupuncture [5 sessions/w initially, total 30] (B) Placebo acupuncture	A better than B	High dropout rate in controls
Lancet 1989;1: 1435–9	80	(A) Acupuncture [5 sessions/w initially, total 26] (B) Placebo acupuncture	A better than B	High dropout rate in controls
Drug & Alcohol Dependence 1992; 30: 169–73	56	(A) Acupuncture [5 sessions/w initially, total 39] (B) Placebo acupuncture	A no different from B	
Am J Acup 1996; 24: 19–25	118	(A) Acupuncture [12–15 sessions] (B) Standard care	A better than B	Subjects already withdrawn from alcohol
Complement Ther Med 1997; 5: 19–26	59	(A) Acupuncture [weekly for 6] (B) Placebo acupuncture (C) Standard care	A no different from B or C	
Alcohol & Alcoholism 1999; 34: 629–35	72	(A) Acupuncture [5 sessions/w initially, total 30] (B) Placebo acupuncture	A no different from B	

though more recently it has been realised that they can stimulate the nervous system and alter the release of various transmitters in the brain. A simplified form of acupuncture, known as auriculoacupuncture, is commonly used to treat dependence. Four or five needles are inserted into particular sites in the ears (usually both) while the client sits quietly for 30 to 45 minutes. The treatment is usually repeated frequently, and the resultant calming effect helps reduce withdrawal symptoms. Clearly, acupuncture needles cannot replace other treatments such as counselling and should be used as part of a wider management strategy.

For alcohol dependence, after some early positive RCTs, the balance of evidence (Table 1) now suggests that acupuncture has no great value in achieving or maintaining abstinence. If it does have any role, it may be to help keep the patient in contact with therapy services, though this may not be a specific acupuncture effect. In cocaine and opiate treatment programmes, uncontrolled analyses of acupuncture as an adjunct [e.g. 4] have been promising. However, these results have been contradicted by most of the rigorous RCTs that have been conducted. For example, in one RCT involving sixty subjects entering a methadone maintenance programme, cravings were greater in the group that had real acupuncture compared with those given placebo acupuncture [5]. In another RCT involving 100 subjects with heroin dependence, acupuncture increased the rate of continuation in treatment, although only six subjects remained in the study at twenty-one days [6]. In cocaine dependence, an RCT of 236 cocaine addicts found no difference in the outcomes after acupuncture compared with placebo acupuncture [7], and the same negative results were achieved using acupuncture as an adjunct to standard cognitive-behavioural therapy in 277 cocaine dependants [8]. In a very recent RCT involving eighty-two cocaine-dependent patients maintained on methadone in America, an eight-week course of genuine acupuncture was superior to acupuncture with the needles in the wrong site, and also superior to relaxation therapy alone [9].

Biofeedback

Biofeedback is a method used to help learn relaxation. The skin's electrical resistance changes with emotional tension and can be measured by a pair of electrodes placed on the skin. The resistance is converted into an audible signal by a small, portable apparatus. As patients concentrate on changing the signal to the relaxed state, so they themselves become more relaxed. Other signals from the body can be used in the same way, such as the electrical activity of the brain (EEG). The procedure needs to be repeated regularly to have any long-lasting effect.

A group of 277 cocaine addicts, predominantly African-Americans, were given either EEG biofeedback, or acupuncture, or medication, in addition to standard cognitive-behavioural therapy [8]. All three additional therapies improved the retention of clients in the treatment programme, although this in itself was not associated with a higher incidence of abstinence. The standard therapy, but not any of the three additional treatments, appeared to be associated with success as measured by the number of negative urine tests. In another RCT in alcohol dependent young adults, biofeedback training with relaxation increased the 'internal locus of control' (the sense that one feels responsible for one's health and behaviour) compared with no intervention, which is a change that is associated with improved control over drinking habits [10]. Another RCT found lower relapse rates with EEG biofeedback in chronic alcohol dependency compared with the standard Alcoholic Anonymous 12-step programme, as well as reductions in psychopathology [11].

Electrostimulation

Electrostimulation involves passing very small electrical currents into the body from a battery-operated apparatus, and different forms are often given individual names by their inventors. The electrodes are stuck temporarily to the skin, often around the skull, and in most cases the current is too low to be felt.

Various forms of cranial electrostimulation (using a range of terms including transcranial electrical therapy and neuroelectric therapy) have been applied to patients with drug or alcohol dependency, mainly with the aim of reducing their withdrawal symptoms. A review paper of the RCTs available in 1990 [12] found that the wide variety of electrical parameters and treatment regimens used in different studies meant that no meaningful conclusions could be made. Several double-blind RCTs had positive results but certain problems in them (usually the large proportion of patients who dropped out) make them unconvincing. Since that time, more rigorous, double-blind RCTs with negative results have been published in the treatment of cocaine/opiate dependence [13]. However, one author argues that a particular intensity, wave-form and frequency need to be chosen, depending on which drug is being withdrawn – although the evidence for this is not very convincing – and states that the negative results are due to failure to appreciate this fact [14].

Herbal medicine

Plants have been used since the dawn of humanity for medical purposes and are the source of many modern drugs. Whole plants may be used or particular parts of the plant or extracts. Herbs are still used in many medical environments, and each culture has its own typical approach, such as the Ayurvedic tradition in India or modern phytomedicine in Germany. As well as producing therapeutic effects, it is well recognised that plants are capable of producing serious side effects.

Some withdrawal programmes in China involve bowel irrigation with Chinese herbs as a method of detoxification. Only one RCT was found using this method, and the study was badly designed so no meaningful conclusion can be drawn [15]. *Kudzu* (*Pueraria lobata*) is a long-established Chinese herbal remedy, taken by mouth, which has been used for treatment of alcohol dependency. It has been shown to reduce voluntary alcohol intake in hamsters [16], but a small RCT in thirty-eight humans found no effect on craving or sobriety scores compared with placebo [17].

Hypnotherapy

Hypnotherapy is the use of a trance-like state to produce deep relaxation of the conscious mind in which it becomes much more suggestible. Ideas can be implanted which affect behaviour subsequently, and patients may allow access to their subconscious problems. Nobody can be hypnotised against their will, and individuals vary in the ease with which they can be hypnotised. Clearly, anyone in a trance state is vulnerable and only highly regulated and reputable practitioners should practise hypnotherapy.

For treatment of alcohol dependence, one review of the research found that the total rigorous evidence about hypnotherapy amounted to just one RCT. It had a negative outcome, but this was not a good study as it failed to distinguish between participants who were susceptible to hypnosis and those who were not [18]. There have been no rigorous investigations since the date of this review.

Other therapies

Exercise is known to have various positive mental benefits, and in one controlled trial in a group of alcohol dependent patients, those who exercised experienced reduced craving compared with those who received standard rehabilitation treatment [19].

The use of restricted environmental stimulation therapy (REST) involving twelve or twenty-four hour residence in special chambers with repeated recorded messages has produced promising results in alcohol dependants, but no controlled studies are available.

Intercessory prayer was found to be of no benefit for alcohol dependency in an RCT of forty subjects in which it was compared with no additional treatment [20].

Appetite and quality of nutritional intake are both very often poor in people with drug dependence, and excessive alcohol use can cause severe disturbance to the body's metabolism. It is clearly important to consider giving nutritional supplements (particularly vitamins) during withdrawal and recovery [21]. In addition, particular amino acid supplements may specifically restore brain neurotransmitter concentrations. They proved to be superior to placebo supplements in a controlled trial of sixty-two alcohol dependent patients, improving retention in the programme, reducing stress and easing detoxification [22]. In another double-blind controlled trial, a supplement known as gamma-hydroxybutyric acid reduced symptoms of alcohol withdrawal more effectively than placebo control [23]. These studies are exploratory, and more evidence from other research groups is required before these forms of treatment can be recommended.

Relaxation has been used alone as the control method in several controlled trials and found to be of little benefit (though it may not have been applied in the best form) [e.g. 24]. Yoga was not superior to dynamic group psychotherapy in an RCT of sixty-one patients undergoing methadone maintenance therapy, as assessed by a range of psychological, sociological and biological measures [25]. There is no reliable evidence available on the efficacy of aromatherapy or reflexology in drug withdrawal or rehabilitation.

Conclusions

CAM therapies are increasingly popular. Some are used purely as support and make no particular claims to treat withdrawal symptoms except in the general sense of making the client feel more comfortable. Of the therapies that make claims to reduce the withdrawal symptoms and therefore to have a valuable place in treatment programmes, auricular acupuncture is most widely used and is supported by a small amount of evidence. Mind–body therapies such as biofeedback, relaxation and hypnotherapy are also common, but more supporting evidence is needed before their exact role in drug dependence management can be defined.

READER INPUT

(1) The evidence reviewed here is limited in both its quantity and quality. What factors may account for this?

(2) When you have read Chapter 21, return to this question and, using the methods discussed in Chapter 21, consider how you might try to evaluate the *effectiveness* of acupuncture for the treatment of the drug dependence of your choice? If you were involved in running a *service* providing acupuncture service for cocaine users, how do you think such a service might be evaluated?

(3) If it is the case that there is only limited evidence for the effectiveness of complementary therapies for helping people with substance misuse problems, what factors could account for its apparent popularity among those who suffer from these problems and with those providing services?

(4) Who should provide alternative therapies for people with substance misuse problems? How might access be improved?

(5) How important is it to understand the theoretical background and tradition of any given treatment? Does it matter more or less for the psychological and pharmacological approaches discussed in other chapters?

REFERENCES

1 Ernst, E., Resch, K.L., Mills, S., Hill, R., Mitchell, A., Willoughby, M. and White, A. (1995) 'Complementary medicine – a definition', *Br J Gen Pract* 45: 506.

2 Eisenberg, D.M., David, R.B., Ettner, S.L., *et al.* (1998) 'Trends in alternative medicine use in the United States, 1990–1997', *JAMA* 280: 1569–75.

3 Ernst, E. and White, A. (2000) 'The BBC survey of complementary medicine use in the UK', *Complement Ther Med* 8: 32–6.

4 Schwartz, M., Saitz, R., Mulvey, K. *et al.* (1999) 'The value of acupuncture detoxification programs in a substance abuse treatment system', *J Subst Abuse Treat* 17: 305–12.

5 Wells, E.A., Jackson, R., Dias, O.R. *et al.* (1995) 'Acupuncture as an adjunct to methadone treatment services', *Am J Addictions* 4: 169–214.

6 Washburn, A.M., Fullilove, R.E., Fullilove, M.T. *et al.* (1993) 'Acupuncture heroin detoxification: a single-blind clinical trial', *J Subst Abuse Treat* 10: 345–51.
7 Bullock, M.L., Kiresuk, T.J., Pheley, A.M., *et al.* (1999) 'Auricular acupuncture in the treatment of cocaine abuse', *J Subst Abuse Treatment* 16: 31–8.
8 Richard, A.J., Montoya, I.D., Nelson, R., Spence, R.T. (1995) 'Effectiveness of adjunct therapies in crack cocaine treatment', *J Subst Abuse Treat* 12: 401–13.
9 Avants, S.K., Margolin, A., Holford, T.R., Kosten, T.R. (2000) 'A randomized controlled trial of auricular acupuncture for cocaine dependence', *Arch Intern Med* 160: 2305–12.
10 Sharp, C., Hurford, D.P., Allison, J., Sparks, R., Cameron, B.P. (1997) 'Facilitation of internal locus of control in adolescent alcoholics through a brief biofeedback-assisted autogenic relaxation training procedure', *J Subst Abuse Treat* 14: 55–60.
11 Peniston, E.G., Kulkosky, P.J. (1989) 'Alpha-theta brainwave training and beta-endorphin levels in alcoholics', *Alcoholism: Clin Exp Res* 13: 271–79.
12 Alling, F.A., Johnson, B.D., Eldoghazy, E. (1990) 'Cranial electrostimulation (CES) use in the detoxification of opiate-dependent patients', *J Subst Abuse Treat* 7: 173–80.
13 Gariti, P., Auriacombe, M., Incmikoski, R., McLellan, A.T., Patterson, L., Dhopesh, V., Mezochow, J., Patterson, M., O'Brien, C. (1992) 'A randomized double-blind study of neuroelectric therapy in opiate and cocaine detoxification', *J Subst Abuse* 4: 299–308.
14 Patterson, M.A., Patterson, L., Flood, N.V. *et al.* (1993) 'Electrostimulation in drug and alcohol detoxification: significance of stimulation criteria in clinical success', *Addiction Res* 1: 130–44.
15 Sha, L.J., Zhang, Z.X., Cheng, L.X. (1997) 'Colonic dialysis therapy of Chinese herbal medicine in abstinence of heroin addicts – report of 75 cases', [Chinese], *Chung-Kuo Chung Hsi i Chieh Ho Tsa Chih* 17: 76–8.
16 Keung, W.M., Vallee, B.L. (1998) 'Kudzu root: an ancient Chinese source of modern antidipsotropic agents', *Phytochemistry* 47: 499–506.
17 Shebek, J., Rindone, J.P. (2000) 'A pilot study exploring the effect of kudzu root on the drinking habits of patients with chronic alcoholism', *J Altern Complement Med* 6: 45–8.
18 Wadden, T.A. and Penrod, J.H. (1981) 'Hypnosis in the treatment of alcoholism: a review and appraisal', *Am J Clin Hypnosis* 24: 41–7.
19 Ermalinski, R., Hanson, P.G., Lubin, B., Thornby, J.I., Nahormek, P.A. (1997) 'Impact of a body–mind treatment component on alcoholic inpatients', *J Psychosoc Nursing & Mental Health Services* 35: 39–45.
20 Walker, S.R., Tonigan, J.S., Miller, W.R., Corner, S. and Kahlich, L. (1997) 'Intercessory prayer in the treatment of alcohol abuse and dependence: a pilot investigation', *Altern Ther Health Med* 3: 79–86.
21 Beckley-Barrett, L.M. and Mutch, P.B. (1990) 'Position of the American Dietetic Association: nutrition intervention in treatment and recovery from chemical dependence', *ADA Reports* 90: 1274–7.
22 Blum, K., Trachtenberg, M.C. and Ramsay, J.C. (1988) 'Improvement of inpatient treatment of the alcoholic as a function of neurotransmitter restoration: a pilot study', *Int J Addictions* 23: 991–8.
23 Gallimberti, L., Canton, G., Gentile, N. *et al.* (1989) 'Gamma-hydroxybutyric acid for treatment of alcohol withdrawal syndrome', *Lancet* 2: 787–9.
24 Brown, R.A., Evans, D.M., Miller, I.W., Burgess, E.S. and Mueller, T.I. (1997) 'Cognitive-behavioral treatment for depression in alcoholism', *J Consult Clin Psychol* 65: 715–26.
25 Shaffer, H.J. and Lasalvia, T.A. (1997) 'Comparing Hatha yoga with dynamic group psychotherapy for enhancing methadone maintenance treatment: a randomized clinical trial', *Altern Ther Health Med* 3: 57–66.

PART III

ORGANISATIONAL AND POLICY ISSUES

CHAPTER 17

A SUITABLE CASE FOR TREATMENT: AN INTRODUCTION TO BRITISH DRUG POLICY

Mike Blank

LEARNING OBJECTIVES

After you have studied this chapter you will be able to demonstrate an understanding of:

1 Some of the process of drug policy development and implementation.

2 Some of the forces which shape drug policy including a recognition of the importance and impact of historical factors.

INTRODUCTION

A senior civil servant once famously explained social policy as being rather like an elephant – you know one when you see one but it is impossible to describe one. This chapter sets out to describe the elephant of British drug policy and place today's initiatives and strategies 'combating' illicit drug use in context.

Why is it important to understand policy? Because policy, largely developed by government, increasingly dictates how practitioners will deliver services that are designed to prevent drug use, police the availability of drugs and treat the unpleasant effects that may arise from drug use. In a nutshell, those who work in publicly funded frontline services in contact with drug users are doing the government's bidding – they are implementing drug policy.

Policy can be roughly divided into two separate but linked fields. First, there is policy development which is, as the phrase implies, concerned with the creation of policy by government. The second is implementation, which is when policy is put in to practice.

HOW POLICY IS DEVELOPED

Perhaps the most important influence on any policy – and this is as true of drug policy as any other – is past policy. Today's drug policy is built upon yesterday's; it is 'a policy arena formed by its history' (Berridge, 1999). Of course there are other influences too: pressure groups, the media, individuals, politicians' personal convictions, and not least this country's 'permanent government', the Civil Service – can all play a significant role in the development of policy.

Today's British drug policy is rooted in the attempts of the last 150 years or so to control drug use. This type of policy, which develops from what has gone before, is most commonly known as an 'incremental policy'. In other words, policy which has already been implemented is refined and improved and mistakes are removed or adjusted. At least, that is the theory. The policy makers may be influenced by feedback from individuals and groups or by political interests. Other important factors also contribute to the development of policy: How much will it cost? Who will implement the policy? Is it acceptable to the population and to a government's supporters? Will it impact on the target group?

Implementation of policy

Policy is implemented when somebody does something to or for somebody else. So for instance, the clerk in the Benefits Office who calculates a claimant's benefit entitlement and then arranges payment is implementing welfare policy. Unfortunately for governments, all too often the people who are meant to implement policy find that the policy they are implementing is badly thought through and therefore can't be done (or at least not as intended), find themselves constrained by resources, get it wrong, or simply don't do it at all. The poll tax of the late 1980s is an example of a policy which was difficult to implement. It cost a fortune, it was hugely unpopular with the electorate and very difficult to collect, so it failed. On the other hand, child benefit is an example of a successful policy: uptake is high, it is popular and the money generally gets to its target group – mothers with children. Perhaps it is also worth noting from these two examples that policies which give tangible benefits to people tend to be popular and are therefore generally easier to implement.

Policy development and implementation are tangled together. Well thought out policy which is developed with implementation in mind is more likely to succeed than poorly constructed policy. Policy implementation over which central government has a degree of control is more likely to be implemented to government satisfaction than policy which is implemented by third parties over which it has less control.

Developing British drug policy

The history of British drug policy has swung between the perception of drug use as a moral failing controllable by legal sanctions and drug use as a condition susceptible to medical treatment or other interventions albeit within a legal framework. Attempts to control opium in the latter part of the nineteenth and early twentieth centuries probably mark the beginnings of modern drug policy in the UK, but there have been attempts to control the use of various drugs including alcohol throughout the world for many hundreds of years. Until their recent reform, the British laws governing the sale and consumption of alcohol were relics of the First World War. The government of the day restricted alcohol sale and use in order to prevent ammunition workers drinking when it felt they should have been making shells (Gossop, 1993). The USA has a long tradition of prohibition of both alcohol and drugs culminating (at the moment but who knows what may come?) in the current 'three strikes and you're out' regime. Three convictions for the possession of small amounts of cannabis for personal use may potentially mean life imprisonment.

It was the latter part of the nineteenth century that saw real changes in the way British society regulated the use of drugs. Until then there had been little if any distinction between the social and medical uses of drugs. Addiction as a concept did not really exist, and many people used drugs such as opium both for the treatment of illness and for pleasure. Indeed opium was one of the few treatments then available that is now accepted as effective. It alleviated symptoms and was widely and cheaply available. Starting with attempts to control opium use, drug policy developed through the nineteenth and twentieth centuries as a result of complex pressures, some of which are outlined below.

The medical profession

Doctors began to organise themselves as a professional group during the latter part of the nineteenth century and started to exert control over the prescription and distribution of certain drugs. At the same time the concept of addiction became more widely accepted and treatment of addiction as a 'medical' speciality developed.

New UK laws

A series of new laws, notably the Defence of the Realm Act introduced in the First World War and the 1920 Dangerous Drugs Act, placed control upon possession and supply of drugs such as morphine and cocaine and marked a 'penal reaction to drug use' (Berridge, 1994). A succession of Acts of Parliament controlling various aspects of drug use followed through the twentieth century with perhaps the most significant being the 1971 Misuse of Drugs Act. This Act is the prime piece of legislation on drug use and articulation of British drug policy. It outlaws the possession of various drugs and their supply (or the intention to supply) to third parties and gives the courts powers to impose long prison sentences on those people convicted of offences under the Act.

The British system

Although Acts of Parliament introduced the penalisation of the sale and use of some drugs, the pendulum swung back to a medical perspective on the management and treatment of addiction with the publication of the ground-breaking Rolleston report of 1926. This report recommended the prescription of opiates to those who were addicted and the treatment of addiction as an illness rather than a moral failing. It became the template for the management of addiction problems for the following half-century. It was not until the 1990s that the notion of the need to treat rather than punish addiction was seriously challenged.

AIDS

In the mid-1980s injecting drug users (IDUs) came to be seen as a route by which HIV might spread to the general population. This fear moved the health of drug users to the top of the policy agenda. From government down the emphasis was to ensure that as many IDUs as possible were alerted to the risks of infection and encouraged to protect their health and that of others through the use of needle and syringe exchanges and safer sex practices. This policy development and its implementation were very successful. The HIV infection rate amongst IDUs with access to exchanges was very low indeed. This shift in emphasis marked the phase of drug policy known as harm-reduction – the idea that abstinence might not be possible for many drug users but that steps could be taken to reduce the harm linked with drug use.

CRIME AND PUNISHMENT

By the late 1990s the threat of AIDS appeared to recede and the criminal justice agenda began to re-assert itself. The new Labour government gave priority to the reduction of crime and in particular stressed the importance of reducing drug-related crime. Drug users convicted of offences were to be compelled by the courts to undergo treatment, 'arrest referral schemes' were to be introduced and treatment agencies would be persuaded to give priority to offending drug users by placing them first in the queue for help. Overseeing policy as well as the development of a drug strategy was the newly appointed drug strategy co-ordinator – dubbed the 'Drug Tzar' by the media. The Drug Tzar produced Britain's first ten year anti-drug strategy 'Tackling Drugs to Build a Better Britain'. This built upon the previous government's three year strategy 'Tackling Drugs Together' and represented the first attempt to take a thorough and comprehensive view of the impact of illicit drug use on society and put forward aims and objectives designed to 'combat' drug use. Despite the strategy's acknowledgement of the health and social problems encountered by drug users, the tone of the strategy made it clear that law and order was back in the drug policy driving seat – if it had ever been out of it.

This brief overview of drug policy development gives rise to a number of observations. First, it seems that drugs policy of the last thirty years or so appears rarely to be developed with the needs of the drug user foremost. Rather it is developed with other concerns taking primacy, for instance the need to reduce crime. Even the swing towards a health agenda in the late 1980s, with the introduction of syringe exchange schemes, happened because of the perceived threat of infection to the general public rather than the protection of drug users' health.

Second, it is clear that the law and order issue has dominated drug policy development. Virtually every Act of Parliament concerned with drug use has been introduced with the aim of criminalising various aspects of the possession and sale of drugs, or latterly with the removals of assets thought to derive from drug dealing.

Last but not least, the student of drug policy will note that drug policy development is incremental and indebted to its history. History repeats itself and so does drug policy development, which in Britain is the story of attempts throughout the last century and beyond to control drug use by making the possession and or sale of certain drugs illegal.

Implementation – policy into practice.

The implementation of drug policy is fraught with difficulties. In order for any policy to be implemented effectively certain conditions have to exist. The policy should have:

- a target group or population
- sufficient funding for implementation
- a willing and able bureaucracy
- the political support of the governing party of the day (ideally more)
- feedback mechanisms so that the implementation is monitored, successes duplicated and mistakes rectified

Other factors affect implementation, some of which are outside policy makers' control. For instance, the appearance of a new drug not controlled by legislation cannot be acted against.

It is also worth bearing in mind that any policy about which there is widespread disagreement or dissension in the population – and drug policy is certainly one such – will inevitably have implementation problems simply because a proportion of those charged with implementation will dissent and refuse to implement or do so inadequately (Hill, 1995).

So how does the implementation of drug policy measure up? Space precludes a detailed analysis of drug policy implementation here, but it is possible to cite some examples of policy implementation that may be considered successes or failures.

Does drug policy impact on its target population?

Assuming that the target population is anyone with a potential to use drugs (likely to be aged between 15 and 35) the answer is a resounding no. Take cannabis as an example; controlled under the 1971 Act, the possession or sale of cannabis was liable to carry a prison sentence, but came to be routinely smoked by between two and five million people in Britain. A policy that sets out to deter people from using a drug and fails to do so is failing. It is possible to argue that if only half the population have tried a drug then the policy is working, because the other half have been deterred from experimenting. Unfortunately this argument falls down when one considers the complex set of circumstances which determine whether or not an individual experiments with a drug, or indeed with any other risk-taking behaviour, legal or not. The influence of culture, family and friends, the likelihood of discovery, the cost and availability of the drug are all of greater influence on the decision to experiment than the legal status of the substance. In 2001 the Home Office announced plans to reclassify and reduce the penalties for cannabis use, perhaps in recognition of the normalisation of cannabis use among young people.

How much does it cost?

Until recently no one really knew how much was spent on dealing with drug use in the UK. The Drug Tzar's office has attempted to discover the level of expenditure, and a figure of £1.4 billion per year is thought to be the amount spent directly on combating drug use. At least that was the figure for 1998. This does not take in to account 'invisible' spend on drug related issues. For example, Police Services argue that it is impossible to extract spend on drugs from more general spend on crime because it is impossible to calculate the amount spent on crimes cleared up, which may be related to drug use but are not direct offences under the 1971 Act. Some burglary and car crimes will fall into this category.

What is certain is that there has been an enormous rise in spending on fighting illicit drug use in the last thirty years, as drug use itself has increased. As the problem increases the spending increases, and it is reasonable to ask at what point the Treasury will look to reduce or stop spending? To cite the poll tax again – Chancellor Nigel Lawson turned off the money tap when it became clear that the policy was failing. If, despite thirty or more years of the modern war on drugs the problem continues to increase, with a similarly inexorable rise in expenditure, then the time will surely come when the Treasury will say 'enough' and refuse to give financial support without a change of policy direction? In the meantime hard-pressed frontline services clamour for more resources with which to implement the existing policy. Any policy that requires regular frequent injections of new cash with no end in sight may well be in trouble.

Summary

If the above seems a bleak assessment of the impact of drug policy then that is the reality. Modern British drug policy has evolved over the past hundred and fifty years from its foundation in attempts to control the use of opium through to today's legislation which seeks to control an ever more sophisticated global illicit drug business. It is a complex policy arena encompassing enforcement whilst attempting to deter potential users and provide treatment and other interventions for existing users. It seems that we are stuck with existing policy because any alternative appears unacceptable politically, nationally and internationally, to elements of the media and a proportion of the population. So, those of us directly concerned with drug policy delivery, those who work both in specialist or generic services such as education or health, are going to have to continue to implement current policy. No doubt this policy will evolve and indeed we are seeing such evolution today as drug treatment and testing orders come on stream alongside other initiatives. What we are unlikely to see are radical changes such as legalisation or decriminalisation of some or all illicit drugs. The unacceptability of such a step to politicians lies partly in the difficulty in answering some basic practical questions. How would the legal outlets for drugs be policed? Who would vet the quality of newly legal drugs? How much would such a change in policy cost? Despite the passion with which adherents of such changes argue their case, until questions such as this are addressed, few policy makers are likely to see legalisation or decriminalisation as serious alternatives to current policy.

Yet in a field so riven with dissension about how best to manage the use of psychoactive drugs one can only ask how committed the bureaucracies charged with drug policy implementation are likely to be to new policy developments? Any policy, no matter how well developed, is in the end reliant upon bureaucracies to undertake effective implementation. At the moment British drug policy is not so much an elephant as an elderly car with punctured tyres and an engine misfire. It is unlikely to be traded in for a better model.

READER INPUT

(1) Is it possible to create a perfect policy on drug or alcohol use? What factors lead you to this conclusion?

(2) What effect will altering the classification of cannabis have on the overall level of cannabis use in society? What costs will be saved? What costs will be incurred? What risks will individuals using cannabis reduce? What risks might individuals using cannabis face? If cannabis were to be fully legalised (like alcohol or tobacco) how much should cannabis cost? Who should sell it? Who should be allowed to buy it (how old, how identified)? How would your answers to the first five questions change?

(3) What effect would legalising heroin have on the overall level of heroin use in society? What costs would be saved? What costs would be incurred? What risks would individuals using heroin reduce? What risks might individuals using heroin face? How much should heroin cost after it is legal? Who should sell it? Who should be allowed to buy it (how old, how identified)?

(4) If there is good evidence that treatment is moderately effective and that preventive initiatives are relatively ineffective, why would you, as a politician, persist in the pursuits of control and education as the two main pillars of your policy?

(5) The United States famously prohibited alcohol during the early part of the twentieth century. What would happen if the United Kingdom took the same step in the early twenty first century?

FURTHER READING

Tackling Drugs To Build a Better Britain, (1980) London: HMSO.
P. O'Hare (ed.) (1992) *The Reduction of Drug-Related Harm*, London: Routledge.

REFERENCES

Berridge, V. (ed.) (1994) 'Aids and British drug policy: history repeats itself . . .?' in R. Coomber, *Drugs and Drug Use in Society*, Greenwich: University Press.
Berridge, V. (1999) *Opium and the People*, London: Free Association Books.
Gossop, M. (1993) *Living with Drugs*, Vermont: Ashgate.
Hill, M. (1995) *Understanding Social Policy*, Oxford: Blackwell.

CHAPTER 18

COERCION AND THE CRIMINAL JUSTICE SYSTEM

Zelda Summers

LEARNING OBJECTIVES

By the end of this chapter you will be able to:

1 Identify the various agents involved in the criminal justice system and how these may offer an opportunity for intervention in relation to substance misuse.

2 Demonstrate an understanding of the concept of coercion, how this may relate to the criminal justice system, your own role and the role of agencies outside the criminal justice system.

INTRODUCTION

This chapter provides an overview of the criminal justice system in regard to substance misuse in the UK. It also raises the issue of the nature of coercive treatment and explores the concept of coercion both inside and outside the criminal justice system.

In the UK the management of the substance misuser has long been in the domain of medicine. Funding has historically come via the Department of Health, the focus for the treatment of the individual being their health and welfare. Contemporary sources of funding also come from the Home Office. The government's concern with drug misuse is made clear in its strategy documents *Tackling Drugs to Build a Better Britain* (Home Office, 1998) and is reflected in the strategies and policies of those agencies which come into contact with offenders, such as the prison service and the police.

SUBSTANCE MISUSE AND CRIME

In the UK it is estimated that one-fifth of people serving probation orders are problem drug users whilst 11 per cent of convicted male prisoners and 23 per cent of convicted female prisoners have been assessed as drug dependent on admission to prison (Department of Health, 1996a).

A large proportion of problem drug users are reported as financing at least part of their drug misuse through acquisitive crime. A study of 738 arrestees identified that 50 per cent had committed some kind of property crime, the most common being shoplifting (28 per cent) and handling stolen goods (27 per cent). Drug supplying and car theft were reported by 12 per cent. Of this sample 69 per cent tested positive for drugs. Users of heroin and crack/cocaine were more likely to report property offences (Bennett and Sibbitt, 2000). Burglary is the second most common crime amongst sentenced prisoners (Cullen and Minchin, 2000).

The costs of drug related crime

The costs of drug related crime are high: 70,000 separate crimes were estimated to have been committed by 60 per cent of one cohort of 1,110 people in one three-month period. In the two years prior to treatment the cost of dealing with these offenders to the point of decision by courts was estimated to be £4 million (Department of Health, 1996b). The value of property stolen to buy heroin in 1995 in the UK was an estimated £1.3 billion or £55 per household. (Home Office, 1996). Arrestees in Bennett and Sibbitt's study (2000) had an average weekly expenditure on drugs of £129. For those using heroin and crack/cocaine this rose to an average of £308 a week.

The costs of non-illicit substance misuse

It is important to recognise that illegal behaviour does not exclusively relate to illegal drug misuse though it is harder to quantify the costs of non-illicit misuse of substances. For example, alcohol consumption is a major factor in driving offences and 20 per cent of drivers who die in road traffic accidents are over the legal limit for driving (Royal College of Psychiatrists, 2000). Other crimes include acts of violence carried out under the influence of alcohol or prescription drugs and alcohol.

The concept of coercion

The criminal justice system offers an essentially coercive approach. Unlike the client in the community who may (arguably) have the choice of seeking help or continuing with their current behaviour, the individual in contact with the criminal justice system does not have this option. The client may, for example, agree to volunteer for a community based treatment and testing order but their choice is not 'treatment' or 'no treatment', it is treatment or imprisonment.

Agents in the criminal justice system

There are a variety of agents within the criminal justice system well placed to influence substance-misusing offenders to take up appropriate services. A range of contact points exist which offer opportunity for referral or coercion into treatment:

At the point of arrest

1. Cautioning and advice by police.
2. Arrest referral scheme.
3. Drug worker in police station or on-call.

Once the case comes to court

4. Court liaison schemes, usually run by a general psychiatric service. This may vary from a lone CPN to a high-powered team including psychiatrists, CPNs and social workers.
5. Probation assessment and referral.
6. Psychiatric court reports.
7. Drug Treatment and Testing Orders.
8. Drug courts.

If the individual enters prison

9. Screening at point of entry.
10. Mandatory drug testing schemes in prison.
11. CARAT schemes (Care, Assessment, Rehabilitation and Through care).

Drug misusers and the police

The police may intervene early in a substance misuser's career. They can caution the offender and refer on a voluntary basis to treatment services. Individuals apprehended for possession of class B or C drugs may simply be cautioned, although this is variable across police forces.

The custody suite is not an ideal place to treat a substance misuser. Police surgeons often have no prior knowledge of arrestees and no objective confirmation of their drug history. They must rely on the custody sergeant, not trained health personnel, to monitor the detainee. Particular risks may be attached to those about to be arrested, who may swallow all the drugs they have or hide them in body cavities. If the drugs are not discovered the detainee may be at risk of intoxication, overdose and death.

Guidelines on the management of substance misusers are available for police surgeons (Department of Health, 2000). Where arrestees are already on prescribed medication, such as Methadone, it is recommended that treatment be continued. Care is necessary, unless the person has been consuming medication on the premises of the dispensing agent (clinic or pharmacist); there may be uncertainty as to compliance and the true level of tolerance for the prescribed drug in question. The police surgeon should check with existing prescribers. This is usually verifiable but is likely to be more difficult 'out of hours'.

Withdrawal symptoms in the opiate user are best managed with short-acting drugs as these will not interfere with the person's functioning on discharge from the custody suite. This does not always provide satisfactory symptomatic control of symptoms but is the best available compromise. Benzodiazepines and alcohol carry particular risks because of their potentially dangerous withdrawal syndromes.

Some detainees may engage in self-harm in order to force a prescription of psychoactive medication. Threats of self-harm must always be taken seriously. There is a need for risk assessment, close observation and maintenance of a safe environment.

In addition to assessing the immediate threats of intoxication and withdrawal the police surgeon is well placed to discuss other health related issues, e.g. transmission risks of blood-borne infections. They may be able to advise on sites of needle exchange schemes, family planning clinics, genito-urinary medicine clinics and drug treatment agencies. Time may be short however, as police surgeons are often general practitioners who have to fit their police work in around other commitments. It may not be practical or appropriate at the time of the first, and perhaps only, assessment to address all these issues with the detainee, and the role of the police as a conduit for appropriate help should also be recognised.

Arrest referral schemes

Arrest referral schemes exist in most areas, ranging from printed leaflets/cards to strong links between police and treatment services where arrest referral practitioners may be part of a wider prescribing, counselling and specialist intervention service. Some agencies have a worker placed in police stations, some work an 'on call' system. In other cases the arrest referral worker is assigned to a court.

Edmunds *et al.* (1998) evaluated arrest referral schemes across three areas. Nearly half the individuals seen had no history of previous drug services input. Follow up six to eight months later identified a reduction in drug misuse, injecting and expenditure among those referred. Such schemes offer an important early intervention.

THE PROBATION SERVICE

Probation officers are able to identify and assess drug misuse at the point of preparation of pre-sentence reports and supervision planning; delivering information to help courts make bail decisions, supervising those serving community sentences and supervision of prisoners and ex-prisoners after release. Some probation officers provide drug relevant treatment, e.g. counselling, anger management and treatment of Post Traumatic Stress Disorder. Probation officers also refer on to and liaise with treatment agencies. Liaison should take place at strategic and all other levels of service delivery.

Drug treatment and testing orders

The Home Office has made probation services responsible for commissioning services for a target group of offenders. Drug Treatment and Testing Orders (DTTOs) can be given to convicted offenders as an alternative sentence when appropriate. Turnbull *et al.* (2000) evaluated outcomes of DTTOs amongst 210 offenders. The impact was evaluated as promising but it was recognised that long-term impact requires further investigation. It is worth noting that the services evaluated were small in number and may not necessarily reflect the diversity that future schemes may demonstrate.

DTTOs present an alternative to custody and, like their predecessors – probation orders linked to treatment – represent a coercive element in getting the offender to treatment services. Offenders are assessed by the DTTO team member(s) for suitability, though the ultimate decision to proceed is taken by a court of law. The offender has a say in the decision, being offered the option of custody if preferred. The client may be returned to custody if he/she fails to comply. The shortest possible period for a DTTO is six months, the longest three years. The offender is expected to spend substantial periods in treatment although the interpretation of 'treatment' is very broad. A DTTO may include the provision of Methadone and other medication and episodes of detoxification. Naltrexone is being used post-detox in some areas to encourage continued abstention (see Chapter 11).

Although a national standard exists, services will reflect different priorities within this. Turnbull *et al.*'s evaluation focused on three schemes which demonstrated three differing approaches, not necessarily generalisable to all services. For example, one centre had a strict abstinence focus, therefore breaching many participants, whilst the other two were more focused on achieving reduced drug use. Regional variation may, in part, result from existing service provision and historical context. Some regions have skeletal services whilst others have a history of comprehensive provision prior to the introduction of DTTOs.

DRUG MISUSERS AND THE PRISON SERVICE

Prisoners receive a varied approach to their treatment. There is a standardised assessment format at inception into prison although it has been suggested that initial screening may underestimate drug misuse (Mason *et al.*, 1997). Differences exist in treatment options between the community and prison and between prisons themselves. There have been international calls for equivalent services in and out of prisons (WHO, 1993; Council of Europe, 1995). Contemporary policy advocates the development of a range of interventions more closely reflecting those found in the community (HM Prison Service, 1998).

Drug tests in prison have revealed the presence of a range of substances with 30 per cent of prisoners testing positive for one or more substance (NACRO, 1996). Prison service strategy aims to reduce the level of drug misuse in this setting. One means by which this was hoped to be achieved was via the introduction of random mandatory drug testing of prisoners. The value of this has been debated. The sensitivity for opiates in urine screens is low whilst the presence of cannabis metabolites is prolonged and easily detected. Early anecdotal evidence suggested that some individuals may switch to heroin with less risk of detection and subsequent punishment instead of cannabis (ACMD, 1996). However, more recent investigations do not support this (Farrell *et al.*, 1999). Sensitivity of tests needs to be taken into account in relation to statistics obtained.

Imprisonment is more likely to result in cessation of substance misuse, but for those who continue the risks are significant. Risk of transmission of blood-borne infection such as hepatitis and HIV through shared injecting equipment is high. This was graphically demonstrated in one outbreak of HIV infection at a Scottish prison in 1993 (Taylor *et al.*, 1995). Rates of Hepatitis C amongst substance misusing prisoners have been estimated to be between 50 per cent and 75 per cent (McBride *et al.*, 1994; Rich *et al.*, 1997). In another study, just under half of ninety-four prisoners tested positive for Hepatitis B (Nelles *et al.*, 1997). Risk is not limited to infection; the intermittent nature of misuse in prison may lead to reduced tolerance and potential overdose post-release (Zador *et al.*, 1995).

Responses to drug misuse in prison include: 'punishment' – positive tests may result in loss of privileges, including parole and home leave, treatment in the form of prescribed medication, harm reduction, detoxification and support and counselling.

The Advisory Council on the misuse of Drugs (ACMD) recommend that where a prisoner has previously been prescribed Methadone this should be continued in prison. This applies to short-term and remand prisoners only. Petersen and Stone (2001) suggest that changes in the Crime (Sentences) Act, which include a mandatory three year sentencing for third offence burglars, may increase the numbers of drug misusers entering prison, raising issues about the appropriateness of this. In some cases even this minimum recommendation is not followed. Inconsistency between prisons has been identified by both the authorities (Department of Health, 1996a) and by prisoners themselves (Hughes, 2000). Detoxification, as with prescribing, varies across institutions. Some offer only the shortest of regimes.

Harm reduction approaches include the provision of injecting equipment and bleach cleaning programmes for cleaning syringes. Prison needle exchanges are rare. A 1994 pilot study of syringe dispensers in a Swiss women's prison indicated that reduced sharing resulted (Nelles *et al.*, 1997). Bleach programmes exist in some prisons but given that it is now recognised that bleach will not necessarily destroy the Hepatitis C virus the ethics of providing these in the absence of other forms of harm reduction may be debatable.

Another harm reduction aspect which is being taken up by many prisons in response to initiatives from the government and Department of Health is the provision of Hepatitis B vaccination. Prison offers a good opportunity to commence vaccination and links may be established with external services to enhance programme retention post-release.

Throughcare and aftercare

Responsibility for through care arrangements is placed with prison and probation services. This is addressed through voluntary CARAT schemes which provide counselling, assessment, rehabilitation and through care/aftercare for drug misusing offenders. Unfortunately, the prison medical service, local GPs and community prescribing agencies have not been included as a rule, so that medical treatments are not part of the seamless delivery of services. The CARAT scheme enables the prisoner to start to address some of the issues around their substance misuse whilst they are in prison, in preparation for discharge. The aftercare component probably presents the greatest difficulty as many agencies such as housing, social services, statutory and voluntary agencies do not have additional funding to accommodate graduates of the scheme.

Other schemes related to the criminal justice system

In addition to the agencies and approaches described above there are a range of other coercive services related to, or within, the criminal justice system including:

- Youth Offending Teams (YOTs)
- drink/drive diversion schemes
- diversion schemes for people presenting with public drunkenness
- drug free wings in prison
- the forensic arm of psychiatry who deal with mentally disordered offenders which can include substance misusers

Coercion – the remit of the criminal justice agencies?

Some substance misuse practitioners would not align themselves with coercion. They argue that the service they offer is voluntary, clients choose to seek help or comply with treatment but ultimately it is 'up to them' whether they continue with their current behaviour. How true is this? Marlowe *et al.*, (1996) point out that coercion is not always linked to legal mandate and may be perceived as coming (sometimes more forcefully) from other sources such as emotional disturbance, health problems, interpersonal or social conflict or employment problems.

Hser *et al.* (1998) studied 276 assessed patients referred to treatment programmes. At six month follow up 38 per cent had not entered treatment. Investigation into influencing variables suggested that legal status, psychological distress, problems in family or social relationships, prior experience of treatment success and source of referral had significant predictive value of subsequent entry into treatment after assessment and referral.

An example of a non-criminal justice coercive scheme can be seen in the development of workplace/employee referral schemes. There is a fine balance here between the employers' right to a productive, safe workforce and employees' 'rights' to consume substances outside work time, even when this includes the right to commit an illegal act such as smoking cannabis. Random testing of employees is applied widely in the USA and is gaining support in the UK. Some studies suggest that this has resulted in lower levels of misuse and reduced accidents at work (Royal College of Psychiatrists, 2000).

In the USA coercion has become a feature of the competitive market of private health care. Advertisements placed in the media urge relatives of problem drinkers to coerce the drinker into private (often expensive) residential treatment. This raises the questions of who is being coerced, by whom and for what reason?

Conclusion

Research suggests that coercion in the criminal justice system appears to be no less effective than voluntary treatment. The system can effectively coerce people into treatment and keep them there (Hough, 1996). However, the coercive nature of treatment in the criminal justice system may create a certain amount of philosophical discomfort amongst some practitioners. Hough raises interesting questions about the type of treatment offered. Coercing a drug misuser into inappropriate treatment may, it is suggested, be arguably regarded as a miscarriage of justice. Issues also arise around confidentiality.

Coercion may be considered 'unethical' by some; a form of social control, not to be condoned by those who consider the rights of the individual to be paramount. Yet the criminal justice system offers many opportunities for intervention which may precipitate change in individuals who might otherwise not come into contact with services. Hser *et al.*'s study (1998) suggested that individuals not complying with treatment referral were seen as more dysfunctional, with higher levels of drug and alcohol misuse and more severe degrees of psychological and family problems. For these individuals legal involvement was the only enabling factor significantly related to treatment entry. It would seem that treatment services should be mindful that those in greatest distress may be the least likely to take up treatment.

Changes in government and health strategy emphasise a need for closer working relationships between traditional treatment providers and the criminal justice system. Although there is a long-established relationship between these, the nature of this has altered and needs to become established. At the very simplest practical level there is a need for practitioners to understand who does what, where and with whom. On a more complex level there are important issues to be considered, such as the role of harm reduction, how agencies can work together in different settings, the rights of the individual versus the rights of society and the ethics and meaning of coercion for all of us working in the field of substance misuse. The criminal justice system may offer opportunities to provide much needed help and this should be viewed optimistically and positively. But practitioners should also question where initiatives evolve from and be aware that there may be several agendas at play. The meaning of this in relation to practice issues, partnerships, the focus of interventions and the effect on the individual should continue to be a major focus for debate.

READER INPUT

Case scenarios

(1) The following individuals have come into contact with the criminal justice system. What type of help or intervention might they experience as a result of this?

- (a) Carla is an 18-year-old woman who has been found in possession of a small amount of cannabis, when her flat is being searched for stolen property. She has no previous criminal history.
- (b) Carl is a 23-year-old man arrested for a number of car crimes and thefts. He has served a couple of previous short sentences. He misuses a number of substances, including heroin and crack cocaine. He both injects and smokes. He has never had any contact with a treatment agency. His only service contact is through the voluntary sector needle exchange. He considers himself dependent on heroin and is worried that he will experience unpleasant withdrawals in the police station.
- (c) Colin is a 36-year-old man with a long history of property crime, mainly burglary. He has been relatively stable on a Methadone prescription for the last four months. Prior to this he was injecting heroin on a daily basis. Colin is awaiting trial in two weeks' time when he faces his third offence of burglary. He thinks it is likely that he will be imprisoned. His probation officer is not optimistic about the outcome of the case.

Discussion points

(1) To what degree do you consider your current role coercive? What about the roles of other people within your profession/area of work, or outside this? How do you feel about this? Does this affect the way you work with clients and other practitioners?

(2) A survey of 199 'expert panel' individuals explored the ethics of a range of aspects related to substance misuse. This included questions on the criminal justice system and the legal status of various substances (West, 1997). Questions included:
  (a) Should possession of cannabis be legal?
  (b) Should the supply of cannabis be legal?
  (c) Should possession of 'hard' drugs be legal?
  (d) Should assets from illegal drug dealing be seized?
  (e) Is it acceptable for countries to impose the death penalty for supplying drugs?

- What is your opinion in relation to these questions and what is the rationale behind your response? Are you, for example, able to back up any of your beliefs with appropriate literature?
- If you are in a group situation it may be interesting to debate each of these in turn with one person taking a 'pro' stance and another an 'anti' stance. The idea is not to compete, to be 'right' or 'wrong' but to provide a considered response.

FURTHER READING

Royal College of Psychiatrists (2000) *Drugs Dilemma and Choices*, London: Gaskell.

Petersen, T. and Stone, S. (2001) 'Prison injecting, methadone maintenance and the potential impact of changes in the Crime (Sentences) Act', *Journal of Substance Use* 5: 312–19.

REFERENCES

Advisory Council on the Misuse of Drugs (1996) *Drug Misusers and the Criminal Justice System. Part III: Drug Misusers and the Prison System – an integrated Approach*, London: HMSO.

Bennett, T. and Sibbitt, R. (2000) 'Drug use among arrestees', *Research Findings No. 119. Research, Development and Statistics Directorate*, London: Home Office.

Council of Europe (1995) 'Prison and criminological aspects of the control of transmissible diseases including AIDS and related health problems in prisons', *Recommendation No. R (93) and Explanatory Report*, Strasbourg: Council of Europe Press.

Cullen, C. and Minchin, M. (2000) 'The prison population in 1999: a statistical review', *Research findings No. 118. Research, Development and Statistics Directorate*, London: Home Office.

Department of Health (1996a) 'Task force to review services for drug misusers', *Report of an Independent Review of Drug Treatment Services in England*, London: HMSO.

Department of Health (1996b) *The National Treatment Outcome Research Study: Summary of the Project, the Clients and Preliminary Findings*, London: HMSO.

Department of Health (2000) *Substance Misuse Detainees in Police Custody: Guidelines for Clinical Management*, London: HMSO.

Edmunds, M., May, T. and Hearnden, I. *et al.* (1998) in Royal College of Psychiatrists (2000) *Drugs Dilemma and Choices*, Chapter 8: 182, London: Gaskell.

Farrell, M., Macauley, R. and Taylor, C. (1999) 'An analysis of the random mandatory drug testing programme', *A Report to the Prisons Directorate of Health Care. Research Findings*, London: Home Office.

HM Prison Service Tackling Drugs in Prison (1998) *The Prison Service Drug Strategy*, London: HM Prison Service.

Home Office (1996) *Breaking the Vicious Circle: Labour's Proposals to Tackle Drug Related Crime*. London: HMSO.

Home Office (1998) *Tackling Drugs to Build a Better Britain. The Government's 10 Year Strategy for Tackling Drug Misuse*. London: HMSO.

Hough, M. (1996) 'Drugs misuse and the criminal justice system: a review of the literature', *Drugs Prevention Initiative. Paper 15*, London: Home Office.

Hser, Y.I., Maglune, M., Polinsky, M. and Angun, M.D. (1998) 'Predicting drug treatment entry along treatment seeking individuals', *Journal of Substance Abuse Treatment* 15(3): 213–20.

Hughes, R. (2000) 'Its like having half a sugar when you were used to three' – drug injector's views and experiences of substitute prescribing inside English prisons, *International Journal of Drug Policy* 10: 455–66.

Marlowe, D.B., Kirby, K.C., Bonieshire, L.M., Glass, D.J., Dodds, L.D., Husband, S.D., Platt, J.J. and Festinger, D.S. (1996) 'Assessment of coercive and non-coercive pressures to attend drug abuse treatment', *Drug and Alcohol Dependence* 42: 77–84.

Mason, D., Birmingham, L., Grubin, D. (1997) 'Substance use in remand prisoners: a consecutive case study', *British Medical Journal* 315(7099): 8–21.

McBride, A.J., Ali, I.M. and Clee, W. (1994) 'Hepatitis C and injecting drug use in prisons', *British Medical Journal* 309(6958): 876.

NACRO (1996) *Drugs on the Inside*, NACRO.

Nelles, J., Bernasconi, S., Dobler-Mikola, A. and Kaufmann, B. (1997) 'Provision of syringes and prescription of heroin in prison: the Swiss experience in the prisons of Hindelbank and Oberschongrun', *The International Journal of Drug Policy* 8(1) 40–52.

Petersen, T. and Stone, S. (2001) 'Prison injecting, methadone maintenance and the potential impact of changes in the Crime (Sentences) Act, *Journal of Substance Use* 5: 312–19.

Rich, D.J., Chin Hong, P.V., Busi, K.A., Mayer, K.H. and Flanigan, T.P. (1997) 'Hepatitis C and HIV in male prisoners', *Journal of Acquired Immune Deficiency Syndrome* 16: 408–9.

Royal College of Psychiatrists (2000) *Drugs Dilemma and Choices*, London: Gaskell.

Taylor, A., Goldberg, D., Emslie, J., Wrench, J., Gruer, L., Cameron, S., Black, J., Davis, B., McGregor, J., Follett, E., Harvey, J., Basson, J. and McGavigan, J. (1995) 'Outbreak of HIV infection in a Scottish prison', *British Medical Journal* 310(6975): 289–92.

Turnbull, P.J., McSweeney, T., Webster, R., Edmunds, M. and Hough, M. (2000) 'Drug treatment and testing orders: final evaluation report', *Home Office Research Study 212*.

West, R. (1997) 'Addiction, ethics and public policy', *Addiction* 92(9): 1061–70.

World Health Organisation (1993) 'World Health Organisation guidelines on HIV infections and AIDS in prison', Geneva: WHO.

Zador, D., Sunjic, S. and Darke, S. (1995) 'Toxicological findings and circumstances of heroin caused deaths in New South Wales', National Drug and Alcohol Research Centre Monograph. Sydney: Australia.

CHAPTER 19

HEALTH PROMOTION, PUBLIC HEALTH AND SUBSTANCE MISUSE

Judy Orme and Fenella Starkey

LEARNING OBJECTIVES

By the end of this chapter you will be able to:

1. Demonstrate an understanding of the relationship between health education, health promotion and public health.
2. Discuss the contribution health promotion makes to the area of substance misuse.

INTRODUCTION

This chapter discusses the contribution of health promotion and public health to the field of substance misuse. It is important firstly to explore the relationship between health education, health promotion and public health.

HEALTH PROMOTION

The World Health Organisation defines health promotion as 'a process of enabling people to increase control over and improve their health' (WHO, 1984). The five core principles adopted in the Health for All 2000 programme (WHO, 1978) and endorsed by all subsequent World Health Organisation conferences and declarations are:

- A focus on populations rather than individuals.
- A focus on the social and environmental determinants of health.
- The use of diverse and complementary methods including communication. education, legislation and community development.
- The facilitation of effective public participation.
- Recognition of the key role of health professionals, especially those in primary healthcare settings.

The Ottawa Charter (WHO, 1986) identified five key areas for health promotion:

1 Building a **healthy public policy**.
2 Creating **supportive environments**.
3 Developing **personal skills** including information and coping strategies.
4 Strengthening **community action** including social support and networks.
5 **Reorienting health services** away from primary treatment and care towards a more proactive health promotion stance and improving access to health services (from tertiary to primary).

The Charter highlighted three ways in which health could be promoted:

- **Advocacy** on behalf of individuals and communities in order to promote public health.
- **Enablement** to support people in communities to achieve their full health potential and to reduce health inequalities.
- **Mediation** between different agencies and disciplines so that collaborative work is possible. The principle of collaborative working may be supported through inter/multiprofessional education. This is discussed later in the chapter.

HEALTH EDUCATION AND PREVENTION

The terms health education and health promotion are often used interchangeably but whilst health promotion can be seen as an umbrella term incorporating aspects of health education, the former is a much broader concept. Health education does, however, make a substantial contribution to health promotion goals and is often categorised as being concerned with primary, secondary and tertiary prevention work (Naidoo and Wills, 1998).

Primary prevention seeks to avoid the onset of ill health by the detection of high risk groups and the provision of information, advice and counselling. Secondary prevention seeks to shorten episodes of illness and prevent the progression of ill health through early diagnosis and treatment. Tertiary prevention seeks to limit disability or complications arising from an irreversible condition. In relation to substance misuse, primary prevention is usually considered to refer to activities which attempt to stop people from experimenting with drugs and alcohol in the first place. Secondary prevention work acknowledges that people may be at an experimental stage of drug and alcohol use and uses harm minimisation approaches to encourage safer drug use and avoid a shift from experimental use to problematic drug use. Tertiary prevention refers to drug treatment work with problematic substance misusers.

Drug prevention encompasses a wide variety of targets and interventions. It is important to note that drug education is not synonymous with drug prevention. The process of drug education contributes to drug prevention goals. As a form of health education, drug education is a process of teaching and learning rather than an aim or an outcome (Coggans, 1999).

Using the Ottawa Charter framework, the contribution of health promotion to the area of substance misuse is now discussed in more detail and illustrated by research findings from work involving young people.

Building healthy public policy

Public health strategy

This identifies the importance of putting health on the agenda of policy makers in all sectors and at all levels, directing them to be aware of the health consequence of their decisions and to accept their responsibilities for health. The importance of government departments working together to contribute to the public health agenda is emphasised in the current public health strategy for England, *Saving Lives – Our Healthier Nation*, which identifies two key aims (Department of Health, 1999):

1. To improve the health of the population as a whole by increasing the length of people's lives and the number of years people spend free from illness.
2. To improve the health of the worst-off in society and to narrow the health gaps.

'Our Healthier Nation' introduces the concept of three-way contracts for health, which include government responsibility, local organisations and communities, and individuals. The strategy proposes the following health promotion responsibilities across the following three levels:

- Assessing risks and communicating these risks clearly to the public (a responsibility of government and national players).
- Ensuring that the public and others have the information they need to improve their health.
- Taking responsibility for one's own health and making healthier lifestyle choices.

The public health strategy emphasises a need for partnership working and recognises the contribution a range of sectors can make to promoting health. This includes education and youth work, primary health care, social and welfare workers, police, voluntary organisations and businesses.

Drug strategy

The ten-year drug strategy *Tackling Drugs Together to Build a Better Britain* (Cabinet Office, 1998) contains a similar emphasis on partnership working and 'joined up thinking', with the following principles of the strategy endorsed by all government departments:

- **integration** of activities, recognising that drug problems are often related to other social problems and that there is therefore a need to locate substance misuse prevention work within the broader policy agenda to tackle social exclusion and health inequalities
- **evidence**, obtaining accurate information on substance misuse to underpin the strategy
- **joint action**, in recognition of the complexities of drug problems
- **consistency of action**, acknowledging that while sensitivity to local circumstances is important, substance misuse is a national issue
- **effective communication** of information to both young people and to society in general
- **accountability**, to track the government's progress in tackling substance misuse

Four main aims are identified:

1. Help young people resist drug misuse in order to achieve their full potential in society.
2. Protect our communities from drug-related anti-social and criminal behaviour.
3. Enable people with drug problems to overcome them and live healthy and crime-free lives.
4. Stifle the availability of illegal drugs on our streets.

The strategy incorporates an emphasis both on different levels of prevention activity and on responsibilities of government, agencies, local communities and individuals to work towards tackling substance misuse problems. It also recognises the many different forms which young people's drug use may take in highlighting the need for flexibility in drug prevention approaches, stating that:

> Information, skills and support need to be provided in ways which are sensitive to age and circumstances and particular efforts need to be made to reach and help those groups at high risk of developing very serious problems.
>
> (Cabinet Office, 1998: 13)

Creating supportive environments

Creating supportive environments emphasises close links between people and their environment and constitutes the basis for a socio-environmental approach to health. This approach identifies a range of factors which impact on health (Naidoo and Wills, 1998). These factors can be categorised as follows and can all be linked to issues around drug use:

- Risk *conditions*, e.g. poverty, social marginalisation and discrimination, poor housing.
- Risk *behaviours*, e.g. legal and illegal drug use, smoking, unsafe sex, poor diet.
- Risk *factors*, e.g. self-esteem, lack of social support.
- *At Risk* groups, e.g. unemployed, lone parents, travellers, homeless or inadequately housed.

Young people are seen as an 'at-risk' group in terms of their potential exposure to drugs. Current drug strategy targets young people as a particular group in society who are vulnerable to drug misuse (Cabinet Office, 1998). It could be argued that the aim of targeting young people is to create a more supportive environment for them. Department for Education and Employment (DfEE) guidelines for drug education work (DfEE, 1998) raise the issue of 'targeting' young people, stating that:

> Schools and youth services have the responsibility for devising (drug education) programmes that answer the needs of young people, appropriate to their knowledge, experience, race and gender. Careful targeting is needed. Not all young people need the same thing at the same time.
>
> (DfEE, 1998: 14)

Attention in the drugs field has turned towards the use of early drug education interventions for groups of young people identified as being 'at risk'. The concentration on this area has resulted in part from research evidence suggesting that young people may be vulnerable to drug misuse due to physiological factors, such as disability; family factors, such as family conflict and parental substance use; psychological and behavioural factors, including mental health problems, early behaviour problems, early peer rejection and academic problems; and economic factors, such as neighbourhood deprivation. Young people with complex problems (i.e young offenders, school excluded, homeless, those in care and those with mental health problems) are identified as potentially more vulnerable to drug misuse (SCODA, 1997).

Strengthening community action

The participation and empowerment of communities is central. This emphasises involving people in decisions about their own health at every level and every stage of policy making and service development. Community action is identified as one form of community development work, within the following typologies:

- Community *development* approaches, which promote self-help and involve collaboration between statutory and voluntary organisations.

- Community *action* approaches, which emphasise action and campaigning by community groups.
- Community *services* approaches, which focus on improving service provision by reflecting community needs and harnessing existing skills within the community (Henderson, 1995; Duke *et al.*, 1996).

Duke *et al.* (1996) note that prevention work can be aimed at both individual and community levels, working to increase both individual and collective confidence, power and resources. Prevention work using a community development approach has tended to emphasise self-help (Henderson, 1995). Community development work highlights the importance of knowing and understanding complex local conditions and problems. Five areas are identified as having particular relevance to drug prevention work (Henderson 1995).

- **Education**, e.g. informal adult and community education.
- **Youth work**, particularly detached and outreach youth work, which meet young people 'on their own "territory"' (Henderson, 1995: 8).
- **Neighbourhood family centres**, which work as community resources.
- **Approaches targeted at specific groups or specific issues**, e.g. HIV/AIDS.
- **Crime prevention** community development strategies.

Developing personal skills

The importance of health promotion in supporting personal and social development through providing information, education for health and enhancing life skills is underscored. Individually focused education designed to empower and facilitate decision making delivered in a school and youth work setting has been a feature of government strategy (DfEE, 1997).

The government's aims relating to drug education are elaborated upon by the DfEE drug education guidance documents (DfEE, 1995, 1998) and SCODA's quality standards in drug education (SCODA, 1999). These documents outline key aspects found to underpin effective drug education including;

- A progressive curriculum which builds throughout a school career and forms part of an integrated health education programme.
- Skills-based approaches.
- An emphasis on meeting the particular needs and circumstances of pupils in each class, including those with special educational needs.
- Interactive teaching methods.
- Comprehensive teacher training.

Approaches to drug education

With regard to translating government drug education policy guidance into practice, a range of approaches to drug education have been used, including information-based, life skills, resistance training and peer education (Coggans and Watson, 1995) delivered via schools, the youth service and the media.

Life skills and social influences approaches

Social influence approaches to drug education encourage young people to develop a range of life skills, e.g. increasing self-esteem, decision-making skills and moral values on the basis that these will act as resistance factors against developing substance misuse problems. On the research evidence available to date, such approaches are relatively the most effective. The most favourably evaluated life skills approaches are those based on developmental theories of problem behaviour (i.e. not specifically focused on drug use), targeting risk factors such as personal and social competencies, attitudes and values (O'Connor *et al.*, 1999).

Such approaches assume that young people have personal and social deficits which make them more vulnerable to engaging in delinquent behaviours including drug misuse. This is not necessarily supported by the research evidence. It appears that life skills approaches have a limited impact, if any, as primary prevention, but they may inhibit escalation and/or develop skills (Coggans and Watson, 1995).

Tobler and Stratton (1997) carried out a meta-analysis of 120 school-based life skills programmes, and found that interactive life skills programmes had a small positive impact on knowledge, attitudes and drug use but that many young people remain unaffected by these programmes.

Resistance training approaches

Resistance training approaches include life skills elements but include a particular focus on social skills, e.g. peer resistance, 'say no' techniques and refusal skills required to resist drug offers. These programmes are very popular in the USA and have a serious foothold in the UK. The main resistance training programme used is DARE – Drug Abuse Resistance Education – which 50 per cent of US children go through at school and which is police-led.

Even though this approach is widespread, there is no evidence in the literature to support the effectiveness of DARE in affecting drug taking behaviour: evaluations tend to show a 'feel good' factor amongst parents and teachers for these programmes, but little more. A large-scale US Congress mandated study published in 1998 by the National Institute of Justice (O'Connor *et al.*, 1999) concluded that DARE does not work.

Peer education

Although there are varying definitions of 'peer' (e.g. people of the same age, people with similar experiences) and a range of activities encompassed by the label of 'peer drug education', all such initiatives appear to share the common characteristic of the communication of information around drugs and drug use by peers (of equal age and/or similar experiences) to others with the aim of educating.

Evaluations of peer drug education approaches have tended to focus on process issues and benefits of involvement for the peer educators themselves rather than outcome measures in relation to substance misuse (e.g. Orme and Starkey,

1997) although Coggans and Watson (1995) report research findings of positive effects of peer education on knowledge and attitudes relating to drug use.

Key issues for the development of drug education can be identified from consideration of the range of drug education approaches currently being used with young people in the UK. Orme and Starkey (1999) pose and discuss central questions that need to be addressed. These are:

- Who is the programme targeting?
- What is the programme trying to achieve?
- How do we judge the effectiveness of drug education?
- Can any approach be effective on its own?

The issues raised by these questions include the need for programmes to be tailored to meet the needs of a clear target audience which will involve considering the appropriateness of primary and secondary prevention approaches. The complexity of drug taking behaviour shows the importance of both qualitative and quantitative approaches to programme evaluation. The issues of the appropriateness and relevance of drug education for the vastly heterogeneous section of society that is 'young people' are important. These are likely to be enhanced by the adoption of a multi-agency and multi-method approach to evaluation.

Reorienting health services

Pelosi (2000) claims that Britain spends almost as much on drug education as on treatment. The need for approaches to drug prevention to be better integrated nationally and locally is well documented (Cabinet Office, 1998). The main responsibility for ensuring action is taken on drug prevention lies centrally with the Department of Education and Employment, the Department of Health, the Home Office and locally with the education service, youth and community services and health promotion services.

Individuals, community groups, health professionals and government all have a part to play in reorienting health services. The emphasis on the Primary Care Group and Trust structure encourages innovative partnership working as the Board includes the Health Authority, Social Services, primary care professionals and a lay member. The need for the health sector to move increasingly in a health promotion direction is identified, beyond its responsibility for providing clinical and curative services.

Conclusion

Understanding the breadth of health promotion is an important prerequisite to recognising its potential impact on substance misuse. The aforementioned literature on young people provides examples of this potential in terms of primary and secondary prevention. The need to address inequalities in health span both youth and adult fields. The concepts of health promotion and health education in relation to adults and existing substance misusers require consideration.

READER INPUT

Discussion points

- This chapter focuses on health promotion and health education primarily with young people. Referring to the five key areas (healthy public policy, creating supportive environments, developing personal skills, strengthening community action and re-orientating health services) to what extent does your role accommodate the principles of health promotion and health education? How does this transcribe to 'adult' situations?
- How could your place of work develop in relation to health promotion either in its own primary function or in relation to other agencies? What partnerships currently exist, what potential partnerships might be possible. Can you identify any tensions that may emerge and how could these be dealt with?

FURTHER READING

Cabinet Office (1998) *Tackling Drugs to Build a Better Britain: The Government's 10-Year Strategy for Tackling Drug Misuse*, London: Stationery Office.

Coggans, N. and Watson, J. (1995) 'Drug education: approaches, effectiveness and delivery', *Drugs: Education, Prevention and Policy* 2(3): 211–24.

Orme, J. and Starkey, F. (1999) 'Young people's views on drug education in schools: implications for health promotion and health education', *Health Education* 99(4): 142–52.

Orme, J. and Starkey, F. (1999) 'Peer drug education: the way forward? *Health Education* 99(1): 8–16.

SCODA (1999) *The Right Approach: Quality Standards in Drug Education*, London: Standing Conference on Drug Abuse.

REFERENCES

Cabinet Office (1998) *Tackling Drugs Together to Build a Better Britain: The Government's 10-Year Strategy for Tackling Drug Misuse*, London: Stationery Office.

Coggans, N. (1999) 'What's in a word?', *Drug Education Matters* 5:4.

Coggans, N. and Watson, J. (1995) 'Drug education: approaches, effectiveness and delivery', *Drugs: Education, Prevention and Policy* 2(3): 211–24.

Department for Education and Employment (1995) *Drug Prevention and Schools*, London: DfEE.

Department for Education and Employment (1997) *Excellence in Schools*, London: Stationery Office.

Department for Education and Employment (1998) *Protecting Young People: Good Practice in Drug Education in Schools and the Youth Service*, London: DfEE.

Department of Health (1999) *Saving Lives – Our Healthier Nation*, London: Stationery Office.

Duke, K., MacGregor, S. and Smith, L. (1996) *'Activating Local Networks: A Comparison of Two Community Development Approaches to Drug Prevention'*, London: Home Office.

Henderson, P. (1995) *Drugs Prevention and Community Development: Principles of Good Practice*, London: Home Office.

Naidoo, J. and Wills, J. (1998) *Practising Health Promotion. Dilemmas and Challenges*, London: Bailliere Tindall.

Naidoo, J. and Wills, J. (2000) *Health Promotion. Foundations for Practice*, London: Bailliere Tindall.

O'Connor, L., Evans, R. and Coggans, N. (1999) *Drug Education in Schools: Identifying the Added Value of the Police Service within a Model of Best Practice*, London: Roehampton Institute.

Orme, J. and Starkey, F. (1997) *Evaluation of Somerset Peer Education (Drugs Prevention) Project 1996/97*, Bristol: UWE Bristol.

Orme, J. and Starkey, F. (1999) 'Peer drug education: the way forward? *Health Education* 99(1): 8–16.

Pelosi, A. (2000) 'Dilemmas and choices in facing the drugs problem', *British Medical Journal* 30: 885–6.

SCODA (1997) *Drug Related Early Intervention: Developing Services for Young People and Families*, London: Standing Conference on Drug Abuse.

SCODA (1999) *The Right Approach: Quality Standards in Drug Education*, London: Standing Conference on Drug Abuse.

Tobler and Stratton (1997) 'Effectiveness of school-based drug prevention programmes: a meta-analysis of the research', *Journal of Primary Prevention* 18(1): 71–128.

WHO (1978) *Alma Ata 1978 Primary Health Care*, Copenhagen: World Health Organisation.

WHO (1984) *Health Promotion: A Discussion Document*, Copenhagen: World Health Organisation.

WHO (1986) *Ottawa Charter for Health Promotion: An International Conference on Health Promotion*, Geneva, World Health Organisation.

CHAPTER 20

ORGANISATION OF SERVICES – PUTTING IT ALL TOGETHER

Gillian Tober and Duncan Raistrick

LEARNING OBJECTIVES

After you have read this chapter you will be able to demonstrate an understanding of:

1 How alcohol and other drug services have developed in the UK, and how a typical district service might be configured.

2 The elements that are important to the structure of a specialist agency.

3 How different treatment philosophies and treatment modalities should and should not be combined within an agency.

INTRODUCTION

One of the fascinations of the addiction field is that the problems related to substance misuse come up in almost every aspect of life. This means that agencies dealing with healthcare, housing or social care, agencies within the criminal justice system, and all manner of leisure industries, are tied into alcohol and other drug policies. The UK has a ten-year national drugs strategy (Central Drugs Coordinating Unit, 1998), which has four clear objectives addressing: (1) help to young people; (2) community safety; (3) improved treatment services; and (4) reducing the availability of illicit drugs. The strategy assumes that there is general support for minimising illicit drug use, and, while this may have some truth, there are many who would argue for legalising drugs such as cannabis and ecstasy. Nonetheless the strength of the strategy is that it sets out clear objectives and the means to measure whether or not these objectives have been achieved. Setting alcohol policy is a much more difficult task. The majority of people in the UK drink alcohol and many do so regularly (Office for National Statistics, 2000). While it is the case that there is a consensus in the general population in favour of some alcohol controls, for example to minimise drinking and driving, there is also much ambivalence; for example proposals to extend licensing hours have been welcomed. So it is likely that agencies will need to define their role against a backdrop of sometimes conflicting government policies. For example, increasing the opening times of public houses may well achieve the objective of reducing violent incidents but is also likely to increase alcohol related health problems. Similarly in the illicit drugs field, a policy aimed at reducing criminal activity might lead to an increase in high dose substitute prescribing with less effort put into helping people to become drug free and rehabilitate.

GOVERNMENT INITIATIVES MAKE THINGS HAPPEN

It would be nice if services were planned on the basis of a needs analysis matched by the commissioning of service providers. Historically this has not been the case; rather, the provision of substance misuse services has been reactive either to pressure from local clinicians or politicians, or to some perceived national crisis.

The UK approach to illicit drug use is usually said to have been set in 1926 by the report of the Rolleston Committee. The so-called 'British System' defined by Rolleston saw addiction as a medical rather than a legal problem and acknowledged the prescription of substitute drugs as a legitimate treatment for addiction. The establishment of services as we know them today began in the 1960s when there was a marked increase in the use of illicit drugs, particularly amphetamines and opiates. Regional Drug Dependency Units (DDUs), were set up with the good intentions of providing detoxification, substitute prescribing, psycho-social therapies, and social rehabilitation. These clinics were quickly overwhelmed by demand and before too long were unable to deliver much more than a substitute prescribing service. In a landmark report called Treatment and Rehabilitation (Department of Health and Social Security, 1982), the Advisory Council on the Misuse of Drugs recommended a broadening of the base of treatment agencies and professionals involved in delivering treatment. Central funding ensured a rapid expansion of drug services on locally based community drug services and away from DDUs and rehabs. The growth of drug misuse services continued in response to the AIDS threat which brought with it a resurgence of harm reduction as a treatment goal. The National Drug Strategy, first published in 1998 and implemented locally by Drug Action Teams, is now driving the pattern and range of services through a process of commissioning. See *Heroin Addiction and Drug Policy – the British System* (Strang and Gossop, 1994) for a detailed historical review.

Alcohol services have developed in a remarkably similar way to drug services, albeit driven by a health rather than criminal justice agenda. In the 1960s Regional Alcohol Treatment Units were set up with similar ambitions to drug dependency units. In contrast to drug services there was a stronger tradition of providing information and counselling to people with alcohol problems through local Councils on Alcohol. It was perhaps this tradition that influenced the landmark Pattern and Range of Services Report, published in 1978, to recommend a shift towards community based services for alcohol problems as happened four years later for drug misuse services. There has, however, been no AIDS threat, no criminal justice agenda and no national policy to fund and drive alcohol services forward; and so, at the turn of the century, alcohol services find themselves the poor relation to drug services. In some districts Drug Action Teams have become Drug and Alcohol Action Teams, but local interest in alcohol policy and service development is uneven across the country. *Tackling Alcohol Together* (Raistrick *et al.*, 1999) describes the historical context of UK alcohol policy and includes an appendix of alcohol policy landmarks 1950–1998.

The terminology used to describe treatment services is confusing. One way of getting around this problem is to use treatment programmes as a means of bridging the gap between the broadly defined objectives of commissioner, tiers of treatment, and specific service agreements needed by providers.

- Tier 1 – generic and direct access services providing information, identification, and first line interventions.
- Tier 2 – addiction focused treatments provided by practitioners with some specialist knowledge.
- Tier 3 – specialist services working with complex cases where multidisciplinary teamwork and cross-agency working is common.
- Tier 4 – very specialised and usually intensive forms of intervention.

Within these four tiers of service delivery it is easy to think of specific programmes. For example, minimal interventions, usually in primary care, would belong to Tier 1; addictions counselling and advice would belong to Tier 2; a pregnant user's programme or a structured methadone programme would belong to Tier 3; and a dual diagnosis programme would belong to Tier 4.

What services are available?

Much of the change that people make in their drinking or drug use occurs without formal treatment, and so services need to be understood within the context of a dynamic social system (Holder, 1998). The social networks that people move in will have a strong influence on their substance misuse. It follows that family, friends, mutual aids groups and others are all worthy of support. At a more formal level community action has been shown to be an effective way of changing local media messages, local attitudes, and local action by professionals. Drug Misuse and the Environment (Advisory Council on the Misuse of Drugs, 1998) gives examples of how community action might work.

There are a huge number of professionals who encounter people with substance misuse problems as part of their work: included in this list would be general practitioners, social workers, hospital staff, probation officers, workplace counsellors and others. There are others who encounter people with addiction problems through their work but not with any direct service delivery role: these include magistrates, bar staff, drug dealers, police and others. What is important here is to recognise that all of these people can be trained to influence positively people wishing to change their substance use. Health promotion units have a special role within a district. The distinction between prevention and treatment is somewhat arbitrary and health promotion forms a bridge between generic and specialist services. Substance misuse education messages are commonly built into more general healthy lifestyles advice which may be carried out in schools, workplaces and other community settings, as well as being targeted at special groups such high risk users.

One way of further enhancing the skills of the people listed here is to encourage multiagency working. Multiagency sometimes means people attending more than one specialist service at the same time. This seems illogical, at best inefficient, and at worst likely to confuse clients. Multiagency working is appropriate where the multiple needs of clients are best met, for example by bringing together a specialist addiction service and a housing agency.

Shared care is a particular example of multiagency working where general practitioners provide general medical and prescribing services and work with a specialist addiction service (Gerada and Tighe, 1999). Ideally the specialist service should be led by a consultant level doctor qualified to provide advice and back-up to the general practitioner. The idea of shared care has been developed with opiate users in mind but in principle could be applied to any kind of addiction problem. For the purpose of dealing with agreed clients it is as if the general practice and the specialist agency are one service and for this to work well there needs to be training which ensures that lines and means of communication are clearly understood, protocols are agreed and adhered to, and there is monitoring of the service.

Providing an addiction service – service delivery at the agency level

Specialist services means those services that are staffed by people who have been trained to have specialist knowledge and skills rather than agencies that are specialist in the sense of seeing clients selected on the basis of having an alcohol or other drug problems. The role of the specialist agency is:

- The treatment of more complex addiction problems with the goals of reducing dependence and improving physical, psychological and social health.
- A focus for research and development.
- Provision of training to generic workers.
- Provision of accredited specialist training.
- To provide information and advice to the public and professionals.

Addiction is a field about which everyone has a view, a view about the nature of the problem and about the optimal responses to the problem. The consequence is a high political profile and political involvement which in turn demand continual change: the setting of new targets, standards and methods for service provision. Change has also been a feature of the political landscape for health and social services over the last decade of the twentieth century and is likely to continue. Thus an organising principle of service provision is the need to accommodate change. As changes in patterns of substance misuse and changes of direction at the political level are difficult to anticipate, much of the way in which change is accommodated will be reactive rather than proactive. The extent to which the ability to manage change is built into the organisation of an agency and its service provision may well dictate the health of that agency and its ability to provide for its client group.

Clinical governance can be seen as a set of principles which provide a framework for addressing the need for continual change: giving direction for the updating of practice through routine training in evidence based treatments, demonstration of competence by audit, review and supervision of practice in an atmosphere which supports clinical excellence (Scally and Donaldson, 1998). Grand words and laudable intentions can be translated into everyday practice which is achievable. In the following paragraphs, some suggestions of how this can be achieved are made.

Clients, therapists and treatments – three way interaction

Some agencies have chosen to select clients on the basis of primary drug of misuse, stage of change, age, gender or social circumstances. Narrowing down the client group in this way creates minority groups who are disadvantaged in terms of access to a full range of treatment options. Thus, for example, it may be expedient to offer harm reduction interventions where individuals are continuing in their use, at a different site from that at which the cessation of use and dependence are addressed; but it may not be so useful to have a separate harm reduction service.

A programme of stepped care as illustrated in Figure 20.1 enables an agency to build up to the intensity of treatment a client needs (Sobell and Sobell, 1998). Commencing with a motivational intervention at or after assessment ensures that an attempt to effect a change in motivation precedes the decision to pursue either a harm reduction goal or a cessation of use goal. Thereafter, decisional criteria take account of the age, gender and social circumstances of the client to choose the context for treatment which is planned on the grounds of the severity of the dependence and related problems.

Much has been made of the need for multidisciplinary staff teams in the addiction field. The choice of a multidisciplinary mix of the staff is informed by the resources required to provide the treatments listed in a comprehensive programme of stepped care: medicine, nursing, social work, clinical psychology and occupational therapy are disciplines whose training enables staff to fulfil relevant roles, including the delivery of psycho-social treatments (see Institute of Medicine, 1990). Therapist characteristics are associated with good outcomes. Identification of these at the point of staff selection is followed by in-service training and supervision which focus on those skills and attributes which are modifiable.

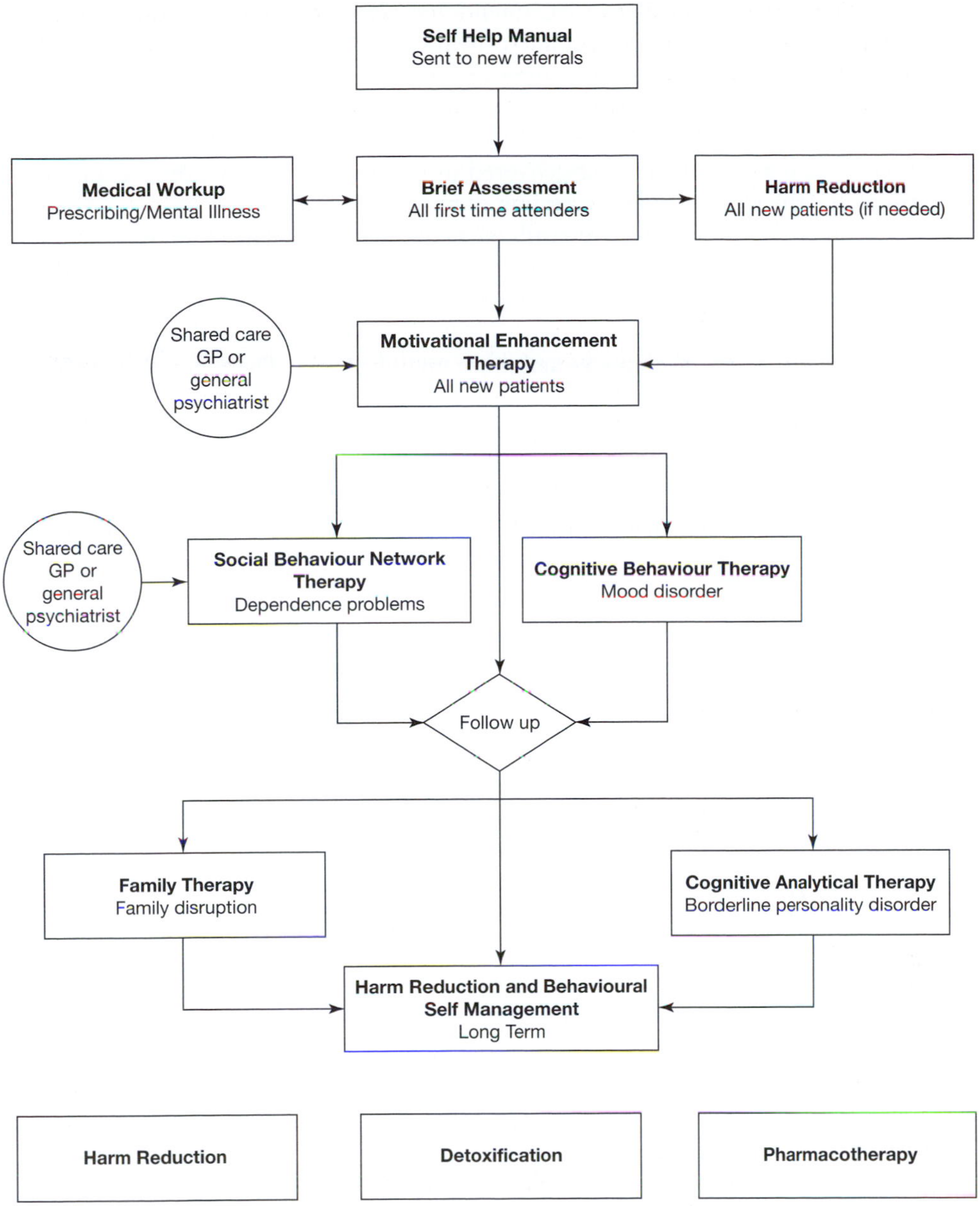

There is the possibility of 'emergency' harm reduction sessions at any stage. Pharmacotherapies can be used to enhance any psycho-social intervention. Planned or urgent detoxification may take place at any stage.

Figure 20.1 Programme of stepped care

Evidence for a number of treatments for detoxification from the various substances, for motivational, cognitive-behavioural and social network based treatments, is described in the foregoing chapters. Increasingly, treatment protocols for psycho-social treatments are described in the same way as those for pharmacological treatments (see UKATT, 2001). Two methods are essential for ensuring that treatments are delivered in line with protocols: the treatment manual and the routine video recording of practice.

Protocol led treatments are available in manual form. The manual provides the structure and the content of the treatment or intervention. It does not replace experience or training and does not compensate for a lack of these. Experienced practitioners adhere to manuals with greater consistency than inexperienced practitioners and also use the manual more imaginatively. The manual provides the basis of standardised treatment, the course text, an essential tool for supervision and for audit of practice. Practitioners have described the ways in which manuals have helped to keep them on course with difficult clients, complex cases and have provided the agreed common ground for the purpose of supervision. Project MATCH found that building a therapeutic alliance made an important contribution to outcome and is itself probably facilitated by the use of therapy manuals (Connors *et al.*, 1997).

In order to be supervised and monitored, practice must be seen. A retrospective verbal account of practice is, by definition unable to address the points that the therapist missed, indeed is unlikely to be able to produce an accurate and objective account of the content of the session. The use of one-way mirrors means that the supervisor must be available for the duration of the practice and this is often unrealistic. It is also a less efficient method for identifying problems and changing practice. The routine video recording of practice is a cost-effective method of supervision which enables the therapist and the supervisor to watch and discuss practice simultaneously. It provides the focus of peer supervision, demonstration of good practice and opportunities for identifying departures from treatment protocols.

The video recording of practice provides the material for audit of the delivery of a treatment and for independent rating of the extent and quality of adherence to the treatment protocol. Furthermore it may be used for demonstration in teaching practice.

Management serves the needs of service delivery

When managers are practitioners, their ability to manage derives from knowledge of the field and the client group; management procedures are designed to serve and support the tasks of meeting client need rather than organisational need. The requirement of continually updating practice to keep abreast of new evidence and a rapidly changing field places high demands upon the staff group, and managers who are clinicians are able to lead by example rather than decree. Moreover where the routine of video recorded practice is adopted, the performance of senior staff is as transparent as that of junior staff, and an atmosphere of mutual support and problem solving is more readily established and maintained.

An important management function is to know what is happening in an agency. For example, where an agency has not designed and implemented its own evaluation procedures, these are likely to be imposed by commissioners with various political agendas. It is preferable that the criteria for and practice of goal setting, audit of treatments and the evaluation of outcome be set on the basis of clinical need and utility while subsuming external political requirements. Agency goals are set by the prevailing problems relating to drug and alcohol use in the community served by the agency. Where audit instruments assist the staff in carrying out their job, they will be welcomed for their utility rather than neglected for their irrelevance (Alcohol Concern and SCODA, 1999). Treatment protocols specified in manual form provide this sort of instrument. The same principle applies to the collection of data for outcome evaluation; measures chosen for the purpose of outcome evaluation are more likely to be completed where they are clinically meaningful. Job satisfaction is enhanced by knowledge that the task is well done, that the client derived benefit from attending the agency. Outcome evaluation instruments that serve both clinical and political needs can be chosen (Tober *et al.*, 2000). Outcome measures should be capable of assessing the extent to which the organisation has met its goals both with the entire client group and in individual cases.

Conclusion

Large centres of population are able to support 'one stop' centres that are able to provide practice which is supported by training, information and clinical research. Indeed, having centres of a 'critical mass' were central recommendations of both the Kessel and Treatment and Rehabilitation reports, discussed earlier. A district should:

- Encourage community action groups, and, support mutual aid groups and other 'helpers' and 'carers'.
- Identify the role of different agencies in delivering Tier 1–4 services.
- Provide evidence based therapies and train therapists to deliver these therapies.
- Ensure agencies have a transparent system of clinical supervision and audits.

READER INPUT

Activity

Find out what services are available for substance misusers in your locality. Which category do they fit into? How does this compare to neighbouring areas, rural or urban? Where does your agency sit in relation to other services? What is the multidisciplinary/multiagency mix of services? What is the service structure from the top down and how do services relate or communicate with each other? Are there any formal means of doing this?

Questions

(1) How does your agency monitor the quality and type of service it provides?
(2) What dilemmas or difficulties may exist in relation to video recording of practice and how might these be overcome?

REFERENCES

Advisory Council on the Misuse of Drugs (1998) *Drug Misuse and the Environment*, London: The Stationery Office.

Alcohol Concern and SCODA (1999) *Quality in Alcohol and Drug Services (QuADS) Organisational Standards for Alcohol and Drug Treatment Services*, London: Alcohol Concern and SCODA.

Central Drugs Coordination Unit (1998) *Tackling Drugs to Build a Better Britain: The Government's 10-year Strategy for Tackling Drug Misuse*, London: The Stationery Office.

Connors, G.J., Carroll, K.M., DiClemente, C.C., Longabaugh, R. and Donovan, D.M. (1997) 'The therapeutic alliance and its relationship to alcoholism treatment participation and outcome', *Journal of Consulting and Clinical Psychology* 65: 588–98.

Department of Health and Social Security and the Welsh Office (1978) *The Pattern and Range of Services for Problem Drinkers*, London: HMSO.

Department of Health and Social Security (1982) *Treatment and Rehabilitation: Report of the Advisory Council on the Misuse of Drugs*, London: HMSO.

Gerada, C. and Tighe, J. (1999) 'A review of shared care protocols for the treatment of problem drug users in England, Scotland and Wales', *British Journal of General Practice* 49: 125–6.

Holder, H.D. (1998) *Alcohol and the Community: A Systems Approach to Prevention, International Research Monographs in the Addictions (IRMA)*, Cambridge: Cambridge University Press.

Institute of Medicine (1990) *Broadening the Base of Treatment for Alcohol Problems*, Washington, National Academy Press.

Office for National Statistics (2000) *Living in Britain: Results from the 1998 General Household Survey*, Norwich: The Stationery Office.

Raistrick, D., Hodgson, R. and Ritson, B. (eds) (1999) *Tackling Alcohol Together*, London: Free Association Books.

Scally, G. and Donaldson, L.J. (1998) 'Clinical governance and the drive for quality improvement in the new NHS in England', *British Medical Journal* 317: 61–5.

Sobell, M.B. and Sobell, L.C. (1998) 'Stepped care for alcohol problems: an efficient method for planning and delivering clinical services', in J.A. Tucker, D.A. Donovan and G.A. Marlatt (eds) *Changing Addictive Behavior*, New York: Guilford Press.

Strang, J. and Gossop, M. (eds) (1994) *Heroin Addiction and Drug Police – the British System*, Oxford: Oxford University Press.

Tober, G., Brearley, R., Kenyon, R., Raistrick, D. and Morley, S. (2000) 'Measuring outcomes in a health service addiction clinic', *Addiction Research* 8: 169–82.

UKATT Research Team (2001) 'United Kingdom alcohol treatment trial (UKATT): hypotheses, design and methods', *Alcohol and Alcoholism* 36: 11–21.

CHAPTER 21

EVALUATING TREATMENT SERVICES

Kim Hager

LEARNING OBJECTIVES

After studying this chapter, you will be able to:

1 Describe different types of evaluation.

2 Distinguish between evaluation, audit, monitoring and quality assurance.

3 Understand some of the pleasures and dilemmas that can be involved in evaluating substance services.

INTRODUCTION

This chapter seeks to describe what evaluation is, the focus of evaluation historically and the current preoccupations. Because the term has been applied to almost anything that looks at monitoring or researching services, the chapter will also briefly distinguish evaluation from monitoring and quality assurance. Additionally, we will look at some of the debates, issues and appeals of evaluating substance services.

WHAT IS EVALUATION?

In the early days of its development, evaluation was applied mainly to assessing the impact of interventions. Did they have the planned results? What was the most effective means of achieving the desired outcomes? Through attempting to evaluate outcomes, it became apparent that greater clarity was often needed as to what our aims and objectives are and how best to measure them.

> Evaluation aims to assess the *feasibility*, *effectiveness* and *efficiency* of an intervention in achieving stated aims and objectives.
>
> (Rhodes *et al.*, 1991)

In other words, is it possible? Is it the best way of doing it? Were the intended results achieved? And is it the best use of the resources available? All too often our clients are not seen to be of sufficient worth to merit the allocation of resources, nor is it often believed that they will benefit from them.

What are we evaluating?

Evaluation can be applied to any of the three strands of Substance Strategies: Prevention, Control, and what gets grouped together as 'Treatment'. A term with its basis in medicine, it has not always been commonly acceptable across the field. It is now used to cover the full range of services and interventions from open access services such as drop-in and advice and information through to in-patient and residential services.

Why do evaluation?

We are all motivated to work with people experiencing problems with substances for different reasons. We have in common wanting to have a positive impact on their lives. How do we know that we have had that positive impact? How then do we prove it to others? Our subjective experience and assessment is a natural place to start.

We all work in services with stated aims and objectives about the positive benefit these services exist to convey. Our agencies usually receive public funds to undertake this work, funds that are given with a view to achieving a positive benefit to society. How do we demonstrate to what extent we are meeting our aims and objectives and that we are making the best use of these resources?

Similarly, those responsible for allocating public funds are accountable for their use. How do they know that they are giving those funds to services that will achieve the best results? Can they demonstrate that they are doing so? Do they have a choice amongst alternatives of service provision?

To articulate our successes and develop tools for evaluating our work together, there has to be some common agreement between commissioners, providers and other stakeholders upon the most important things to evaluate, how we define them and how we measure them. These have to be acceptable to all the relevant parties. Therein lies the art of evaluation.

Social scientists have worked for the last three decades developing methods to articulate, measure, demonstrate, prove and improve the impact our work is having, just as practitioners have done in working with those experiencing substance-related problems. Both groups are still at the very early stages of their respective crafts. Thus, there is still much work to be done before we can successfully evaluate our work. There remains some confusion as to what does and doesn't constitute evaluation at any given time, and what the current evaluation fads are.

Most reasons for undertaking evaluation fall into one or more of three categories:

1 Increasing our knowledge about what works (and what doesn't).
2 Improving the quality and effectiveness of what we do.
3 Demonstrating accountability – showing that we are achieving what we are set up and funded to do.

Evaluation addresses three broad categories of questions (Clarke and Dawson, 1999):

1 Descriptive. Who is using the service? How many of them? What are their characteristics? What aspects of the service do they use? Most evaluation until the 1990s was of this type.
2 Normative. To what extent is an intervention, aspect of a service or whole organisation operating as intended? (Scriven, 1991)
3 Cause-and-effect questions. Has it worked or not? What changes that the client has achieved can be directly attributed to the service? (Patton, 1982; Chen, 1996)

Evaluation is often perceived by practitioners to be anything from threatening, to uninteresting or irrelevant. This can be for a number of reasons:

- Social science research, with its own language and methods can seem mysterious to those who aren't professional evaluators.
- Practitioners have little faith in those doing the evaluating to understand the work they do and thus do them justice. The cliché is that someone (an evaluator) from outside an organisation comes and evaluates your work.
- Those commissioning the evaluation have not chosen topics of interest or relevance to practitioners (or clients).
- If the topics are interesting, the time delay between undertaking evaluation and having access to the results renders the exercise useless because people have moved on, lost motivation or the study has dated (Nizzoli, 1996).

If the reasons for evaluating are of interest and value to practitioners, then the process becomes a vehicle for discussion and agreement between all parties and a training and development tool for service teams. Many researchers write about developing a 'culture' of evaluation, by which they mean creating a climate in which everyone in a team, organisation or locale routinely and actively participates in the design and development of evaluation. This creates a rewarding culture of curiosity, innovation, enthusiasm and learning, as evaluation is a systematic means of obtaining feedback about our work.

Lincoln and Guba (1985) describe evaluation as a collaborative and participative activity between practitioners and researchers. Patton (1986) identified a number of additional 'stakeholders' who have a vested interest in evaluation studies, including commissioners, planners and those for whom the service has been developed. If evaluation means to judge the merit or worth of a service, who better to do this than those who utilise it, their families and their local communities?

Good evaluation is a vital and rewarding process that encourages our professional confidence, provides a means of communicating about our work with each other, and demonstrates good practice. It should be an integral part of all service provision and funding.

Types of evaluation

Different people have categorised types of evaluation in different ways. What follows is a range of commonly used terms that you may come across:

1. Formative – done to provide feedback to people who are trying to improve something. The primary objective is to support the improvement. The emphasis is on identifying the strengths and weaknesses of a service or intervention and whether changes are needed.
2. Summative – aims to determine the overall effectiveness or impact of a programme or project, sometimes with a view to recommending whether or not it should continue. Primarily concerned with determining the effectiveness of a treatment or intervention (Scriven, 1967).
3. Knowledge generating – helps to clarify our thinking and to develop concepts. This may not result in changes, but helps to get a clearer understanding of the aims and objectives of a service or an element of a service (Patton, 1986).

These are not mutually exclusive categories, so that in practice many evaluations will embrace all of these aspects.

Evaluation can be applied to different stages in the development and delivery of services:

1. Front-end analysis (Patton, 1982) or Conceptualisation and Design (Dale, 1993). Studies undertaken to look at what needs there are for services and what sort of services or specific interventions should be set up or revised. Included under this heading are situation assessments, feasibility studies and needs assessments.
2. Process Evaluation, also called Implementation Studies (Chambers *et al.*, 1992). This seeks to establish whether a programme, treatment or intervention has been set up and is working as planned, the quality of the service and who uses it.

3 Outcome Evaluation. Ascertaining the extent to which a planned intervention actually works and whether it has the desired impact. This also includes economic evaluation, such as cost-effectiveness studies and cost–benefit analysis. It may also include consumer satisfaction, although this is usually separated out into a category of its own.

Historically substance misuse services conducted predominantly descriptive and, at best, process evaluations. The focus is now very much more on economic, health and social outcomes.

Economic evaluation

Economic evaluation identifies, measures, values and compares costs and consequences of alternative uses of public funds (Drummond *et al.*, 1987). The three broad questions addressed in economic evaluation are:

- Is it worthwhile allocating scarce resources to this health procedure, service, or intervention?
- Should investment (or further investment) be made in treatment A or treatment B?
- Could the resources allocated be spent more productively?

Services can be evaluated on a number of levels:

- Treatment activity – evaluating the impact of a particular treatment activity or component, such as one-to-one counselling *or* pharmacotherapy for an individual or group of service users.
- Treatment service – evaluating the impact of a range of treatment activities provided through a single service (e.g. counselling *and* pharmacotherapy *and* relapse prevention in a community service) for individuals and groups.
- Treatment system – evaluating the impact of the full range of services (e.g. a combination of community, in-patient, and residential) available in a community or area or a community partnership system.

Or to put it another way, it is possible for everybody to evaluate their work.

- Small groups or teams within an organisation can evaluate their work in a specialised area.
- The organisation can evaluate its work.
- Groups of organisations can evaluate their work and interworking.
- Planners, policy-makers, commissioners/investors and other stakeholders can evaluate the strategies they follow and the work of those that they fund.

To evaluate adequately a treatment system we must consider:

- its aims and objectives
- the needs and wants of clients
- the stated aims and objectives of all the relevant organisations

- the objectives of specific pieces of work within an organisation, such as methadone prescribing, outreach work, work with young people

Stages of evaluation – doing it

According to Babbie (1995) the main stages of evaluation are:

- measurement
- study design
- execution.

Measurement

Evaluation involves articulating what we value, including what we define as success. This is one of the greatest challenges, but if we can't define success we can't evaluate it. To take a seemingly simple example: if 'success' is taken to mean abstinence, then abstinence from what and for how long? All drugs, including legal and prescribed drugs? Forever? Our intentions are usually more complex, covering a range of health and social needs. Debating the priorities is one of the more interesting and challenging aspects of evaluation. It highlights our value systems and can challenge the beliefs and theories upon which our services have been developed.

Within any agency or area of work, there will be a number of things which the staff and clients might consider to be a 'success'. The challenge is to define these in ways which can be measured. This isn't always as easy as it sounds. It takes a while to develop the knack and some people in teams are 'naturals' in this role.

For many possible outcomes, other researchers will already have developed valid and reliable instruments, which can be employed for measuring change. For example, The Task Force to Review Services for Drugs Misusers (1996), as part of its early deliberations, established a set of measures against which outcomes of different drug services could be assessed. This questionnaire, the Maudsley Addiction Profile (MAP) is now commonly used. Other similar instruments are available, such as the Christo Inventory in the UK.

Study design

In any evaluation the following must be specified in the design:

- The reasons for the evaluation.
- The components of the service to be evaluated.
- The questions to be addressed.
- The measures to be used (what data is to be collected).
- The data-collection strategies (who will collect the data, where and when).
- The analysis to be used.

This is where those with research skills come in.

Execution

Evaluation uses social science methods and procedures. There is no one research method that is 'evaluation'. Because social sciences are the most recent addition to the sciences, they have had to prove that they really are science and the methods they use have to some extent been adopted or adapted from the physical sciences.

The randomised control trial

In the past fifty years the randomised control trial has come to be seen as the 'gold standard' for evaluating medical treatments. It is useful to understand the basics of this method of doing research because it increasingly determines whether or not a new or innovative treatment will be purchased. Readily applicable to relatively simple interventions such as drug treatment, such a methodology is rarely achievable in service evaluation. You can probably work out why.

After the treatment to be evaluated has been defined, the next task is to identify a group of people for whom the treatment is thought to be relevant. You randomly allocate half the people to the treatment, and the other half to a control group who may get either no active intervention or the best current treatment. Before and after measurements are taken by somebody outside the treatment process and ideally blind to who is in which group. You then compare results. For example, if you want to test the effectiveness of prescribed dexamphetamine, you might take all new amphetamine users to the service who have been using daily for the past eighteen months. You randomly assign half of them to the existing best available treatment (such as advice and information, and cognitive-behavioural therapy) and the other half to the best available treatment plus a substitute prescribing regime. The measures of effectiveness of treatment, which are defined beforehand, might include stopping injecting, stopping use of illicit amphetamines, improved physical and mental health and reduced crime. If the treatment other than the substitute prescribing is similar but those prescribed dexamphetamine do better, then you have some evidence for the effectiveness of the treatment.

You can probably already see some of the problems in this type of study. Is it right to withhold 'treatment' from anyone who needs it (ethics)? How many of those who don't receive help would stay in touch for you to study (drop-out rate)? How do you know it was the treatment that did it (causality) and not some other factor? What is the impact of being part of a research project?

However desirable, such a purist approach is usually too costly, time-consuming and resource-intensive to be applied to every intervention in the field of substance treatment. It is also practically impossible for many of the complex problems that confront the clients of such services. So, we have to do other things.

Quasi-experimental design

The next group of methods is called quasi-experimental design. It means trying to get as close as possible to the experimental design described above. Usually this means that instead of randomly allocating clients, they are chosen in some systematic way. The experimental designs described above come from a background of natural science which believes that there are universal laws of cause and effect which we can measure and that there is such a thing as objectivity. The world is made up of objectively defined facts and all we have to do is find the means to standardise, measure and quantify.

Qualitative methodology

The alternative is known as qualitative methodology. This approach accepts the inevitability of being subjective – that the world looks different according to whose eyes it is seen through. Examples of qualitative methods include questionnaires, interviewing clients, looking at documents, observation and action research.

Nowadays, quantitative and qualitative methods are usually used together, understanding the shortcomings and values of both. Criticism of either approach can signify the hidden agendas of opinion leaders, rather than scientific discussion, and this can be a way for ordinary mortals to be sidelined. Beware!

What evaluation isn't

Audit

Evaluation is more of a research activity which should address questions of what works, how and why? Audit is a process of *checking* what happens against previously agreed standards of practice, with a view to improving practice. In the audit process, auditors (peers) identify where actual practice does and does not meet the standards set. Where it doesn't, auditors make recommendations for improvement. Those audited implement the recommended action to improve and then the topic is re-audited to establish whether improvements have taken place.

Monitoring

In monitoring, we are usually collecting information in a standardised and routine manner about the procedures and processes that have been agreed to deliver the intervention concerned. The purpose is to provide feedback about levels of compliance, rather than why or how it works. Monitoring can be a source of information for evaluation.

Performance monitoring

Performance monitoring is monitoring of pre-set targets often called Key Performance Indicators (KPIs). These can be set for whole organisations or individual staff. All the main public sector services publish annual performance figures. The same distinctions apply here between monitoring and evaluation as above.

Outcome monitoring

It is hard to talk about evaluation in the twenty-first century without talking about outcomes and outcome monitoring. This is the current preoccupation and looks like being so for some time. It may even be a milestone on the way to higher quality evaluation; but this is monitoring, not evaluation in the strictest sense. It may be as far as we can get without putting more resources into evaluating services than providing them. Outcome monitoring and milestone management is the compromise that has been struck to fill the evaluation gap.

Lavoie (1999), writing in *Findings*, says that the way to show treatment works is by answering three main questions:

1 Who uses the service (client demography)?
2 What does the service do to/with them (activity)?
3 Who benefits from the service, how many, and in what ways (outcomes)?

He argues that this is sufficient information for contract monitoring purposes and represents a sufficient challenge to services to answer. For many it is, but to argue that this is how to show that treatment 'works' misses some important steps along the way. How do we know that anything we did had any effect on the outcome?

Milestone management is a way of monitoring what we believe to be the important steps a person must take on the way to achieving the desired outcomes, as little has been done to unpack what happens in the so-called 'black box' of treatment. This is an American initiative, which has caught on as it is easily achievable.

One of the greatest developments in treatment evaluation has been the joint project between the World Health Organisation (WHO), the United Nations Drug Control Programme (UNDCP) and the European Monitoring Centre for Drugs and Drug Addiction (EMCDDA). They have produced an international framework for the evaluation of treatment services (WHO, 2000b) and workbooks in each of the following five areas:

- needs assessment
- process
- client satisfaction
- outcomes
- economic evaluation

The project is also developing standardised international measures, instruments and training in these areas, with the aim of facilitating greater international communication and comparison of our work.

Conclusion

- Evaluation is a systematic means of obtaining feedback about our work, demonstrating and improving effectiveness.
- It is routine in some countries, for example in the United States, but rare elsewhere.

- We are in the process of developing a 'culture' of evaluation.
- Key to this is the involvement of all stakeholders, such as service users, their families (if they have them) and communities.
- Evaluation can be applied at every stage of service development.
- Evaluation is not always resource-intensive or highly specialised. We can all undertake some level of evaluation of our work.
- Some areas of evaluation are becoming standardised and prescribed, such as outcome domains, measures and instruments.

READER INPUT

(1) Find out what types of evaluation (audit, monitoring and quality assurance) are currently being undertaken in the:
  (a) academic institution in which you are studying
  (b) alcohol/drug service in which you are working

(2) Consider, or better, discuss with colleagues/managers/educators, the reasons for evaluating those things that are being evaluated and the methods used. Ask and reflect on whether the methods used are theoretically the most appropriate?

(3) What are the three most important things that should be evaluated? Speak to a user of the service (or more if possible) and ask them what they think is of value and should be checked out.

(4) How does evaluation, as described in this chapter, line up with Evidence Based Practice? Why might conflict arise between service users, service providers and service commissioners? You might consider Chapter 16, which critically reviews the largely negative findings for 'Alternative Therapies', which are popular with service users and many service providers.

FURTHER READING

World Health Organisation (2000a) *International Guidelines for the Evaluation of Treatment Services and Systems for Psychoactive Substance Use Disorders*, www.who.int/substance_abuse/pubs_psychoactive_drugs.htm

World Health Organisation (2000b) *Framework*, Evaluation of Psychoactive Substance Use Disorder Treatment Workbook Series, www.who.int/substance_abuse/pubs_psychoactive_drugs.htm

Clarke, A. and Dawson, R. (1999) *Evaluation Research*, London: Sage.

European Monitoring Centre for Drugs and Drug Addiction (1999) *Evaluating the Treatment of Drug Abuse in the European Union*, Luxembourg: Office for Official Publications of the European Communities.

REFERENCES

Babbie, E. (1995) *The Practice of Social Research* (7th edn), Belmont, USA: Wadsworth.

Chambers, D.E., Wedel, K.R. and Rodwell, M.K. (1992) *Evaluating Social Programs*, Boston: Allyn & Baker, 1992.

Chen, H.T. (1996) 'A comprehensive typology for program evaluation', *Evaluation Practice* 17(2): 121–30.

Dale, A. (1993) 'Evaluation methodology: an overview', Executive Summary, *The Centre for Research on Drugs and Health Behaviour*.

Drummond, M.F., Stoddart, G.L. and Torrance, G.W. (1987) *Methods for the Economic Evaluation of Health Care Programmes*, Oxford: Oxford University Press.

Lincoln, Y.S. and Guba, E.G. (1985) *Naturalistic Enquiry*, Newbury Park, CA: Sage.

Lavoie, D. (1999) 'How to show treatment works', *Drug and Alcohol Findings*, 1.

Nizzoli, U. (ed.) (1996) *The Way Things Are, The Evaluation of Medical, Psychological, Socio-Educational Interventions with Drug Users in Europe*, Italy: Mucchi Editore.

Patton, M.Q. (1986) *Practical Evaluation*, Beverly Hills, CA: Sage.

Rhodes, T., Holland, J. and Hartnoll, R. (1991) *Hard to Reach or Out of Reach: An Evaluation of an Innovative Model of HIV Outreach Health Education*, London: Tufnell.

Scriven, M. (1991) *Evaluation Thesaurus* (4th edn), Newbury Park, CA: Sage.

The Task Force to Review Services for Drug Misusers (1996) *Report of an Independent Review of Drug Treatment Services in England*, London: Department of Health.

PART IV

SOME SPECIFIC POPULATIONS

CHAPTER 22

DUAL DIAGNOSIS

Jeff Champney-Smith

LEARNING OBJECTIVES

After you have studied this chapter you will be able to demonstrate:

1 An understanding of the nature and prevalence of co-existent substance use and mental health problems.

2 An awareness of current literature relating to effective interventions for such problems.

INTRODUCTION

Practitioners in the fields of substance misuse and mental health are increasingly coming into contact with individuals who have both drug/alcohol problems and mental health problems. Such clients usually have poorer outcomes in relation to cessation or reduction of substance use and in regard to their mental health.

The use of diagnostic labels such as dual diagnosis and comorbidity is the subject of some controversy. Manley (1998) points out that in practice individuals rarely receive a formal diagnosis of both mental illness and substance misuse, so that the term 'dual diagnosis' can properly be considered a 'misnomer'. The literature on the subject of dual diagnosis is usually written from the point of view of either substance misuse or mental health, and little research into dual diagnosis as a specific diagnostic category has been undertaken. Petersen (1998) argues that if the term is applied carefully and with forethought, closer working relationships between substance use services and general mental health services may be fostered.

Zimberg (1999) defines the term by splitting dual diagnosis into three types of co-existing mental health and substance misuse problems:

- Type 1 – Primary mental health problem with a substance use disorder which becomes apparent only when the person is experiencing mental ill-health symptoms, i.e. the substance is used as self-medication by the client to enable them to cope with or obliterate symptoms.
- Type 2 – Primary substance misuse with substance induced mental health problems. For example the amphetamine user who develops 'amphetamine psychosis'.
- Type 3 – Mental health and substance misuse problems co-existing in the same individual over a long period of time (considered 'true' dual diagnosis).

PREVALENCE AND INCIDENCE

The literature suggests that the prevalence of dual diagnosis has increased over time. The increase may be due to two factors. First, the increased exposure of individuals with psychiatric illnesses to illicit drug and alcohol use, as a consequence of community care programmes. Second, the general increase in alcohol use and experimentation with illicit drugs in the population as a whole (Smith and Hucker, 1993). Changing diagnostic criteria, doctors' awareness, knowledge and competence in assessment of both substance misuse and mental health disorders and patients' increased willingness to disclose drug use may also impact on statistics.

Evidence from the Epidemiological Catchment Area Study (ECAS) (Regier *et al.*, 1990) shows an 83 per cent prevalence of substance misuse in individuals with personality disorder and a 47 per cent prevalence of substance misuse in those diagnosed with schizophrenia. The overall rate of substance misuse in those with a mental illness was 29 per cent, estimated to be 2.7 times higher than the general population. Rates of mental illness in individuals with substance misuse were found to be similarly high: 53 per cent in drug users and 37 per cent in problem drinkers, 4.7 and 7 times the rate for the rest of the sample. From these figures it was estimated that substance misusers with a comorbid mental illness made 62 per cent of 56.3 million visits to walk-in psychiatric services.

Up to 53 per cent of psychiatric service users with a diagnosis of schizophrenia have been identified as also having an alcohol related problem (Drake *et al.*, 1990). Nearly half (44 per cent) of amphetamine users in another study showed significant psychological problems (Hall *et al.*, 1996). Such problems correlated highly with transitions from the oral route to the intravenous injection of amphetamine.

UK STUDIES

There are currently few published British studies. One cohort of 171 individuals with a psychotic illness in South London revealed a prevalence rate of 36.3 per cent for drug and alcohol problems (Menezes *et al.*, 1996). Young males were identified as being the most likely to have substance misuse problems. Clients with substance misuse problems were also found to have spent almost twice as long in hospital as those without such problems in the two-year period preceding the study. Significant mental health problems were identified in opiate dependent and amphetamine dependent attendees at one South Wales substance misuse clinic (Barrowcliff *et al.*, 1999).

Statistics need to be considered in relation to geography and sample type. Urban studies centred on areas of deprivation where social drift and transience is high may show different results to rural or affluent areas and more stable populations.

Subject to the type of assessments used and the nature of the research samples, up to two-thirds of individuals with alcohol dependence have been identified as having co-existent psychopathology (Davidson and Ritson, 1993), the most common disorders being antisocial personality disorder and affective disorder, with women being more affected by both conditions than men.

Forensic importance

The role of substance misuse in violent crime is an important one and often overlooked. An examination of seventeen reports into murders committed by mentally ill individuals in the UK found that thirteen involved significant substance misuse. But only one report mentioned this as a contributory factor to murder. The failure to recognise the role of substance misuse in these cases demonstrates a failure to give sufficient credence to the existence and the potentially dangerous sequelae of dual diagnoses (Ward and Applin, 1998).

SUBSTANCES OF MISUSE

Studies of the prevalence of comorbidity show that the substances used most commonly by people with mental health problems are alcohol and cannabis. Two distinct patterns of substance misuse were identified in individuals diagnosed as suffering from schizophrenia; one being the use of high levels of alcohol and cannabis, with little or no other drug use; the other, the use of a number of substances (sometimes including alcohol and cannabis) (Cuffel *et al.*, 1993). Although, as Gournay *et al.*, (1997) point out:

> There is clearly a great deal of heterogeneity in this area and the types of substances used are obviously determined by availability and cultural variations. Furthermore, there is a need to investigate the

similarities and differences between populations who use single drugs, such as alcohol or cannabis, and populations that show multiple use.

Cannabis ingestion, often not considered 'problematic' by drug services, can have significant effects on mental health and treatment outcomes, including an increase in negative symptoms, more severe symptoms and more likely relapse (Martinez-Arevalo *et al.*, 1994).

The chicken and egg 'which comes first' question needs consideration. Allan (1995) found convincing evidence that alcohol use is likely to be a causative factor in the development of anxiety disorders. However, Davidson and Ritson (1993) suggest caution when interpreting their findings that affective disorders remit after detoxification from alcohol, arguing that confusion over what constitutes a dual diagnosis and a failure to differentiate between current and lifetime diagnosis of depression has led to an 'overstatement' of the relationship between alcoholism and affective disorder.

Siegfried (1998) notes that dual diagnosis is also associated with increased uptake of services, violence, non-compliance with treatment, involvement with criminal justice system and social deprivation. Despite the high prevalence and increased morbidity associated with dual diagnosis, detection remains low and both specialist and generic services have failed to adopt flexible responses to the problem:

> Our concern as mental health workers should not be to debate whether certain people suffer a certain syndrome known as 'dual diagnosis', but rather how we can ensure that individuals with these intensive and complex problems are able to access a service which understands and responds appropriately to their multiple needs.
>
> (Leahy and Hawker, 1998: 275)

Treatment

In the United States it has been suggested that the co-existence of mental illness and substance misuse problems is best approached in an integrated manner (Gournay *et al.*, 1997). The development of a service specifically designed for individuals with co-existent mental health and substance use problems based in seven Community Mental Health Centres (CMHC) in New Hampshire is described by Drake and Noordsy (1994). The authors suggest a model of care (Assertive Community Outreach, ACO) in which caseworkers have 24-hour responsibility for around twelve clients. The smaller caseloads allow workers time to engage individuals more frequently and for longer periods. Interventions include helping with finances, taking people to work and encouraging access to community facilities. Individual and group methods are employed, which are non-confrontational and do not require immediate abstinence. The programme is stepped, comprising:

- engagement
- persuasion

- treatment
- relapse prevention.

Drake *et al.* (1998) conducted a study in which 114 individuals received standard case management (SCM) treatment and 109 ACO. Validated substance use and quality of life measures showed little difference in outcome between the groups, but the researchers noted a reduction in the severity of substance use and a reduction in the necessity for hospitalisation in the ACO group. Similar models of assertive outreach are currently favoured by many mental health services and some UK dual diagnosis projects are similarly constituted (Dodd, 2001).

Minkoff (1989) proposes a combined model in which traditional bio-psycho-social and rehabilitation mental health treatments are run alongside the recovery model favoured by some substance misuse services. Four treatment stages are suggested:

- acute stabilisation
- engagement
- prolonged stabilisation
- rehabilitation.

During each of the four stages, psychiatric and addiction treatments are offered alongside each other. Education of clinical staff in the particular philosophies of each treatment model, continuous validation of treatment methods and practical demonstration of treatment efficacy are seen as central to success of the model.

It has been suggested that individuals with schizophrenia and co-existent substance misuse who have low motivation be treated using a harm minimisation approach, whereas those with high motivation should be steered towards abstinence (Ziedonis and Trudeau, 1997).

In one approach (Clenaghan *et al.*, 1996), the principles of integrated services, intensive case management and assertive outreach are supplemented by an innovative residential treatment programme for dually diagnosed clients.

Gournay *et al.* (1997) believe that the training in case management and psychosocial interventions provided by such training programmes as the Thorn initiative (Butterworth, 1994) could be supplemented with specific training in assessment, group methods and motivation enhancement techniques required for the treatment of substance misusers.

It should be remembered that of all these integrated treatment approaches, only the New Hampshire model (Teague *et al.*, 1995) has been evaluated.

Effectiveness

A recent Cochrane review of effective interventions for dual diagnosis (Ley *et al.*, 2000) found little evidence to support the effectiveness of any particular treatment, or to recommend one approach over any other. However, Siegfried (1998) suggests that there is a growing consensus that integrated mental health and substance misuse services offering tolerant, non-confrontational approaches are the best and most appropriate way forward for those people with a dual diagnosis.

In summary, although evidence of effectiveness in managing this client group is limited there are a number of steps services should consider:

- Comprehensive assessment of both mental health and substance use problems.
- Training for mental health workers in the recognition and management of substance use problems.
- Training for substance misuse workers in the recognition and management of mental health problems.
- Services that are non-judgemental, flexible and take account of the principles of harm minimisation.
- Assertive outreach teams with appropriate case loads.
- Clear understanding of roles and responsibilities.
- Good liaison between agencies, clearly identifying who has the lead.
- Development of care pathways.
- Evaluation of new services using a range of outcome measures.

Conclusion

It is clear that the increasing co-existence of substance misuse and mental illness presents a challenge to both substance misuse services and generic mental health services. Evidence for effective interventions is limited, but a consensus suggests that integrated services offer the best prospect for effective assessment and treatment. Treatment programmes should recognise the relapsing and chronic nature of substance dependence and embrace the principles of harm minimisation.

For those involved with this client group face-to-face, the challenge is to provide appropriate interventions tailored to the needs of the individual. This may not always be possible because of constraints imposed by service philosophies and practical barriers such as waiting lists, caseload size and complexion, working hours, geography and discharge criteria.

Each client should be considered individually. There may be a need to re-consider service and treatment boundaries if the client is unable to comply, but discharge is thought potentially unhelpful or damaging. Services need to develop closer liaison to ensure a cohesive and gap-free approach.

The importance of early risk assessment and effective risk management cannot be over-emphasised. All practitioners need to recognise the vulnerability of this client group which has increased risks for deliberate self-harm, suicide and aggressive behaviour. Mental health assessment from a suitably qualified doctor should be sought whenever appropriate and referral mechanisms in place for this to be available to all relevant agencies.

Change can come from both the ground up and the top down. Practitioners in both mental health and substance misuse services need to increase their knowledge base. Increased knowledge levels should enhance practitioners confidence in dealing with dual diagnosis clients and allow further work towards improved attitudes. Practitioners should be prepared to question and challenge established practice. Contemporary developments such as GP and psychiatric liaison services, closer links with the criminal justice system and the current emphasis on partnership working may help pave the way for future change. Evaluation of newly developing services and service models is essential if future services for this challenging group are to be firmly based on good evidence.

READER INPUT

Case scenario

Melanie is a 24-year-old woman with a history of psychotic episodes going back to her early teens. She has a three-year history of heroin misuse and is currently on a Methadone prescription. Her last psychotic episode was nearly a year ago. She has a CPN in the mental health team who she sees monthly for a depot injection. She has self-harmed during these periods, cutting her arms and hands in response to orders from hallucinatory 'voices'.

You normally see Melanie once a fortnight. She missed her last appointment because her flat had been burgled. In an emergency situation like this her father would call in for her prescription but he had recently been admitted to hospital with a suspected tumour so you sent the prescription to the chemist.

At this visit she is quiet and withdrawn, sitting with her head down much of the time and picking at a scab on the back of her arm. She seems to hear little of what you say and several times you hear her muttering under her breath. It sounds like she's saying 'go away, get away'. You ask her what she said but she replies that she hasn't said anything. At one point she spotted a police car out of the clinic window and hurriedly pulled her chair back out of sight. She looks uncomfortable and sweaty. Her nose is running. She sits hunched up, gripping her stomach with both arms.

(1) What might make you suspect that Melanie is experiencing symptoms of psychiatric distress?
(2) What symptoms is Melanie demonstrating that might make you suspect that she may have significantly increased her heroin use on top of her prescription?
(3) Why might she have increased her use? Could she, for instance, be self-medicating? What may have triggered this off?
(4) Melanie's last urine test showed evidence of cocaine metabolites. How might this account for her behaviour?
(5) How might you respond to this situation?

FURTHER READING

Ley, A., Jeffrey, D.P., McLaren, S. and Siegfried, N. (2000) 'Treatment programmes for people with both severe mental illness and substance misuse' (Cochrane Review), in *The Cochrane Library* 1, Oxford: Update Software.

Rorstad, P., Checinski, K., McGeachy, O. and Ward, M. (eds) (1996) *Dual Diagnosis: Facing the Challenge*, Kenley: Wynne Howard Publishing.

REFERENCES

Allan, C. (1995) 'Alcohol problems and anxiety disorders – a critical review', *Alcohol and Alcoholism* 30(2): 145–51.

Barrowcliff, A., Champney-Smith, J. and McBride, A. (1999) 'The opiate treatment index (OTI): treatment assessment with Welsh samples of opiate prescribed or amphetamine prescribed clients', *Journal of Substance Use* 4(4): 98–103.

Butterworth, T. (1994) 'Developing research ideas from theory to practice: psychosocial interventions as a case example', *Nurse Researcher* 1: 78–87.

Cleneghan, P.S., Rosen, A. and Colechin, A. (1966) 'Serious mental illness and problematic substance use', *Journal of Substance Misuse* 1: 199–204.

Cuffel, B., Heithoff, K. and Lawson, W. (1993) 'Correlates of patterns of sustance abuse among patients with schizophrenia', *Hospital and Community Psychiatry* 44(3): 247–51.

Davidson, K. and Ritson, B. (1993) 'The relationship between alcohol dependence and depression', *Alcohol and Alcoholism* 28: 147–55.

Dodd, T. (2001) 'Clues about evidence for mental health care in community settings: assertive outreach', *Mental Health Practice* 41(7): 10–14.

Drake, R., McHugo, G., Clark, R.,Teague, G., Xie, H., Miles, K. and Ackerson, T. (1998) 'Assertive community outreach for patients with co-occurring severe mental illness and substance use disorder: a clinical trial', *American Journal of Orthopsychiatry* 68(2): 201–15.

Drake, R., Osher, F. and Noordsy, D. (1994) 'Diagnosis of alcohol use disorders in schizophrenia', *Schizophrenia Bulletin* 16(1): 57–67.

Gournay, K., Sandford, T., Johnson, S. and Thornicroft, G. (1997) 'Dual diagnosis of severe mental health problems and substance abuse/misuse: a major priority for mental health nursing', *Journal of Psychiatric and Mental Health Nursing* 4: 89–95.

Hall, W., Hando, J., Darke, S. and Ross, J. (1996) 'Psychological morbidity and route of administration among amphetamine users in Sydney, Australia'. *Addiction* 91(1): 81–7.

Leahy, N. and Hawker, R. (1998) 'Re-inventing the wheel', *Mental Health Care* 1(8): 275.

Ley, A., Jeffrey, D.P., McLaren, S. and Siegfried, N. (2000) 'Treatment programmes for people with both severe mental illness and substance misuse' (Cochrane Review), in *The Cochrane Library* 1, Oxford: Update Software.

Manley, D. (1998) 'Dual Diagnosis: approaches to the treatment of people with dual mental health and drug abuse problems', *Mental Health Care* 11(6): 190–92.

Martinez-Arevalo, M., Calcedo-Ordoñez, A. and Varo-Prieto, J. (1994) 'Cannabis consumption as a prognostic factor in schizophrenia', *British Journal of Psychiatry* 164: 679–81.

Menezes, P., Johnson, S., Thornicroft, G., Marshall, J., Prosser, D., Bebbington, P. and Kuipers, E. (1996) 'Drug and alcohol problems among individuals with severe mental illness in South London', *British Journal of Psychiatry* 168: 612–19.

Minkoff, K. (1989) 'An integrated treatment model for dual diagnosis of psychosis and addiction', *Hospital and Community Psychiatry* 40(10): 1031–36.

Petersen, T. (1998) 'Is "Dual Diagnosis" a useful term?' *Nursing Times* 94(37): 56–7.

Regier, D.S., Farmer, N. and Rae, D. (1990) 'Co-morbidity of mental disorders with alcohol and other drugs of abuse: results from the epidemiological catchment area (ECA)', *Journal of American Medical Association* 264: 2511–18.

Siegfried, N. (1998) 'A review of comorbidity: major mental illness and problematic substance use', *Australian and New Zealand Journal of Psychiatry* 32: 707–17.

Smith, J. and Hucker, S. (1993) 'Dual diagnosis patients: sustance abuse by the severely mentally ill', *British Journal of Hospital Medicine* 50(11): 650–4.

Teague, G., Drake, R. and Ackerson, T. (1995) 'Evaluating use of continuous treatment teams for persons with mental illness and substance abuses', *Psychiatric Services* 46(7): 689–95.

Ward, M. and Applin, C. (1998) *The Unlearned Lesson: The Role of Alcohol and Drug Misuse in Inquiries into Homicides by People with Mental Health Problems*, Ware, Herts: Wynne Howard Books.

Ziedonis, D.M. and Trudeau, K. (1997) 'Motivation to quit using substances among individuals with schizophrenia: implications for a motivation-based treatment model', *Schizophrenia Bulletin* 23(2): 229–38.

Zimberg, S. (1999) 'A dual diagnosis typology to improve diagnosis and treatment of dual disorder patients', *Journal of Psychoactive Drugs* 31(1): 47–51.

CHAPTER 23

WOMEN AND ALCOHOL

Moira Plant

LEARNING OBJECTIVES

After you have read this chapter you will:

1 Have an understanding of alcohol-related issues, specifically related to women.

2 Have an understanding of physical and psychological problems due to heavy consumption specifically related to women.

3 Have an understanding of some of the problems encountered in treatment, specifically related to women.

INTRODUCTION

There are some areas in the wider field of substance misuse which are important to examine. One of these is gender. Originally the majority of work carried out on this topic related to men. It was assumed that women would have similar problems and similar predictors of developing problems. More recent work has shown some of these assumptions to be incorrect.

ALCOHOL CONSUMPTION: LEVELS AND PATTERNS

The pattern of alcohol consumption in the UK is what is known as a 'Northern European' pattern. That is, little drinking typically takes place during the week while quite a lot occurs during the weekend. This holds true for both genders and all age groups. The level of consumption in this country has changed over the years. It nearly doubled between 1945 and 1979 but has remained fairly static since then. For many years any changes in drinking levels of women and men tended to follow a similar pattern. If men's drinking increased, remained stable, or decreased then so did women's. Over the past fifteen years or so, men's drinking in the UK has stayed reasonably stable but women's drinking has been steadily increasing.

UK health professionals still use the guidelines for 'low risk' or 'sensible' drinking of 14 units a week for women and 21 units a week for men. The mean weekly consumption for women in the UK in the year 1996 was 9.5 units for the age group 16–24, reducing over the age ranges, to 3.5 units in the 65 years and over group (Office for National Statistics (ONS) 1998).

Self-image

In relation to 'risk drinking' and alcohol consumption, in 1984 9 per cent of women in the UK were drinking over the 14 units a week level. By 1996 this had increased to 14 per cent. This was in comparison to men: in 1984 25 per cent of men were drinking over the 21 units level, in 1996 the percentage was 27 per cent. This issue of self-image is an interesting and important one. The General Household Survey (ONS, 1998) measured the amounts people reportedly consumed with the aid of the information on drinking history. Respondents were also asked how they would describe themselves in relation to their drinking. In the survey, 65 per cent of women who had drunk between 26 and 35 units in the past week (defined as high consumption in the survey) described themselves as 'moderate drinkers'. Furthermore 43 per cent of women who had drunk 36 units or more in the past week (defined as very high consumption in the survey) still defined themselves as drinking a 'moderate amount'. Obviously there will be many reasons for this, for example a lack of awareness and understanding about alcohol measures and health education messages. It may also be a wish to be seen by self or others as not drinking too heavily. It is a good example of the importance of being specific when asking questions about a woman's drinking. Generalisations such as 'light, social or moderate' are of little use and may hinder the identification of a problem. This may be a particular problem for women.

Psychological aspects

There are many reasons why people drink, and people drink for different reasons at different times in their lives. Women in the 18 to 25 age range have been drinking more. This may simply be due to more disposable income and fewer responsibilities. It may also be due to work pressure where they will drink alcohol for the same reasons as their male colleagues do. Women with young families are more likely to continue working than in the past, or to return to work earlier. The pressure of working all day then returning home to look after the children means increased tiredness and the need for a quick way to unwind. One of the most powerful aspects of alcohol is the expectation of how it will affect the individual. If a person thinks a drink will help them unwind it probably will. Women who are older, who may be at the time in their lives when the children have left home, may drink to cope with the feelings of loss, both loss of children but also loss of one of the most important roles they see themselves as having, that of carer. This is known as the 'empty nest' syndrome. Reduction of anxiety is often given as a reason for drinking by both women and men. However, in problem drinkers the aspect of panic disorder is not uncommon, and this often becomes a vicious cycle with each reinforcing the other (Cowley, 1992).

Alcohol and sexuality

As noted earlier in this chapter, expectation influences alcohol's effects. This not only relates to an individual's expectation of their own behaviour but also their expectation of the behaviour of others. It has long been the case that women who drink are perceived by others as more sexually available. An interesting study by George *et al.* (1988) explored how others perceived women when they were drinking and particularly when someone else paid for the drink. As reported by George *et al.* (1988: 1295) the women who drank alcohol compared to a non-alcoholic drink were:

> significantly more aggressive, impaired, sexually available and, as significantly more likely to engage in foreplay and intercourse. Perceptions of her sexual disinhibition and likelihood of sex play were significantly enhanced if the man brought the drinks.

It is now well established that people who take sexual risks will be no more or less likely to do so when they have been drinking. Alcohol does not 'make' you behave in a way that is alien. However, it is certainly the case that alcohol is often used as an excuse for inappropriate behaviour. This is true for both women and men.

Dual diagnosis

In relation to problem drinking the issue of dual disorders has recently become recognised. Women in general are more likely to experience bouts of depression than their male counterparts. The majority of depressions linked to alcohol problems develop after the drinking problem. For this reason it is recommended that 'detox' be completed before assessment for depression takes place.

PHYSICAL ASPECTS

Gastro-intestinal system

For many years it has been the accepted wisdom that women are more 'sensitive' to alcohol than their male counterparts. This was based on a mixture of science and sexism. More recently studies on enzymes and tissue saturation have suggested that women do break down alcohol slightly differently from men. This is mainly due to the lower levels of alcohol dehydrogenase (ADH) in the stomach (Di Padova *et al.*, 1988). Alcohol begins to be broken down in the stomach, known as the 'first pass' metabolic process. This breakdown continues in the small intestine and the liver. In women with drinking problems the level of ADH is even lower or non-existent. For this reason problem-drinking women who have been abstinent for a while and then return to problem drinking may become severely ill more quickly than their male counterparts (Frezza *et al.*, 1990). This reduction in ADH may also be related to age, with pre-menopausal women having lower levels of this gastric enzyme than do older women (Lucey *et al.*, 1993).

There is now a well-established causal relationship between problem drinking and liver disease (Lieber, 1991, 1992). However, there are factors which exacerbate this harm due to heavy drinking. The major factors associated with liver disease at this time appear to be viral. Hepatitis B and particularly hepatitis C are highly correlated with the development of liver cancer in those with established liver disease.

Cardiovascular disease

Current evidence suggests that small amounts of alcohol are protective in relation to coronary heart disease (for review see Grobbee *et al.*, 1999). The issue of age is relevant here. The protective effects of low to moderate alcohol consumption, (1–2 units a day), appear to be present at all ages (Fuchs, 1995). However, the risks of coronary heart disease in women do not really come in to play until after the menopause. Therefore any beneficial effects for women come post-menopausally.

In relation to problem drinking women the picture is very different. The risk of cardiac damage is increased both with 'binge' drinking (Kauhanen *et al.*, 1997) and with prolonged problem drinking (USDHHS, 1994; Rehm *et al.*, 1997). This relates to hypertension (Witteman *et al.*, 1989; Marmot *et al.*, 1994; Seppä *et al.*, 1996; Keil *et al.*, 1998), coronary heart disease (Rehm *et al.*, 1997), and stroke (van Gijn *et al.*, 1993). There is a clear causal link between high blood pressure and alcohol consumption at higher levels (Seppä *et al.*, 1996).

An added factor in relation to women and heart disease is the worrying evidence from some studies which suggests that women are less likely than men to be diagnosed early and referred appropriately (Steingart *et al.*, 1991; Petticrew *et al.*, 1993). Given the acknowledged unpopularity of women with drinking problems combined with this delay in diagnosis the issue becomes potentially life threatening.

Breast cancer

One of the most frightening diseases for women is breast cancer. It brings fear of death, disfigurement and possible negative changes in the relationship with their partner. Although past evidence has suggested an association between moderate amounts of alcohol and increased risk of breast cancer, more recent work has not shown evidence of a causal mechanism (McPherson *et al.*, 1999)

Gynaecological problems

Many women with drinking problems will describe self-medicating with alcohol for pre-menstrual tension. This may be relevant to know in relation to relapse prevention. It may be that the woman's risks of drinking are increased immediately before her period. Enabling her to recognise 'at risk' times like these can be very useful (Allen, 1996). Other examples of gynaecological problems include sub-fertility, and sexual difficulties. The topic of drinking in pregnancy is addressed in Chapter 24. It has been shown that problem-drinking women who initially report sexual difficulties such as reduced libido or pain on intercourse may find their sexual function improved after a period of abstinence (Gavaler *et al.*, 1993, 1994). It must be noted that women with past experiences of abuse do not fit into these groups (see treatment section).

Osteoporosis

The risk of osteoporosis in menopausal women has long been established. There does appear to be some initial protective effect of moderate alcohol consumption. Alcohol changes testosterone into oestrogen (one of the reasons for breast enlargement and testicular atrophy in men). This added oestrogen, at a time when oestrogen levels are falling, helps protect against bone loss. However, as with all these physical aspects of drinking, increased consumption brings increased risk of harm. Furthermore, as women are living longer and, in this country, continuing to drink into their seventies and older, the risk of fractures due to falls and slow healing will become an increasing burden on an already overburdened health service (Hingson and Howland, 1987; Charles *et al.*, 1999).

TREATMENT

There is now a growing literature on treatment aspects for problem drinking women (for review see Plant, 1997). Work by Thom has usefully divided the problems experienced by women seeking help into two groups. These are internal and external problems. Examples of internal problems include shame and guilt. An example of the external problems that hinder a woman seeking help sadly is failure on the part of the professional to recognise the problem (Thom, 1986, 1987).

There are many myths about treating women with drinking problems. These myths include, women are more difficult to treat than men, have a poorer prognosis, and are not as truthful as men. The most recent large-scale treatment study was carried out in the USA. Called 'Project Match', it randomly assigned problem drinkers to three treatment groups:

1 Cognitive behavioural coping skills.
2 Motivational enhancement therapy.
3 Twelve-Step facilitation.

The patients were then monitored over a three-year period. By the end of that time the major factors in how successful patients were in the treatment programmes related to their readiness to change and self-efficacy, that is, whether they believed they would be able to make the changes in their lives. The other interesting aspect was that women did slightly better than men in relation to number of days abstinence.

There are particular issues relevant to women in relation to treatment. Those are the treatment of pregnant problem drinkers and women who have a past history of physical or sexual abuse. For pregnant women, detox needs to be carried out carefully and testing for such things as HIV, Hepatitis B and C should be routinely offered. In the future, testing for tuberculosis may also become necessary. Clear role division among staff needs to be observed due to the possibility of the frightened pregnant problem drinker trying to manipulate professionals into helping her in an unhealthy way. This manipulation needs to be seen for what it is, a desperate behaviour of a frightened woman. This is one group who should not be discharged from treatment even if they continue to relapse: the risk to the child is too high. The other group who need special recognition are women who have been abused. The treatment for these women is long-term and complex. Detox means that the 'cotton wool' which they have used to keep the nightmares away has been removed and they often have terrifying 'flash-backs' to the abuse situations. They need help to contain the terror: cognitive behavioural therapy helps with this. Then slow, gentle hard work, with a dependable skilled therapist.

READER INPUT

Questions

(1) What is ADH, how do ADH levels differ in women and how might this impact on the consequences of women drinking?
(2) How do the protective effects of small amounts of alcohol differ in women compared to men?
(3) Why is pregnancy an important issue for women problem drinkers?

(4) How could a woman who is 'self medicating' with alcohol during times of premenstrual tension be helped to recognise this and what strategies might she employ to help deal with this?

Discussion point

What impact do you think the mass media (television, newspapers, film, etc.) have on current images of women drinking? It may help to monitor one day's newspapers or a range of television programmes for implicit and explicit messages about alcohol and women.

Activity

Who produces information for the general public about alcohol? Find out what health messages have been disseminated in relation to alcohol during the past ten years? How do these apply to women? What kinds of material might be most useful in developing contemporary health messages for women drinkers?

FURTHER READING

Macdonald, I. (ed.) (1999) *Health Issues Related to Alcohol Consumption*, Oxford: Blackwell Science.

Plant, M.A., Single, E., Stockwell, T. (eds) (1997) *Alcohol: Minimising the Harm: What Works?* London: Free Association Books.

Plant, M.A. and Cameron, D. (in press) *The Alcohol Report*, London: Free Association Books.

Plant, M.L. (1997) *Women and Alcohol: Contemporary and Historical Perspectives*, London: Free Association Books.

Wilsnack, R.W. and Wilsnack, S.C. (eds) (1997) *Gender and Alcohol: Individual and Social Perspectives*, New Jersey: Rutgers Center of Alcohol Studies.

BIBLIOGRAPHY

Allen, D. (1996) 'Are alcoholic women more likely to drink premenstrually?' *Alcohol and Alcoholism* 31: 145–7.

Charles, P., Laitinen, K. and Kardinaal, A. (1999) 'Alcohol and bone', in I. Macdonald (ed.) *Health Issues Related to Alcohol Consumption* (2nd edn) Oxford: Blackwell Science.

Cowley, D.S. (1992) 'Alcohol abuse, substance abuse and panic disorder', *American Journal of Medicine* 92: 41S–47S.

Di Padova, C., Frezza, M. and Lieber, C.S. (1988) 'Gastric metabolism of ethanol:

implications for its bioavailiability in men and women', in K. Kuriyama, A. Takada and H. Ishii (eds) *Biomedical and Social Aspects of Alcohol and Alcoholism*, Barking: Elsevier.

Frezza, M., di Padova, C., Pozzato, G. *et al.* (1990) 'High blood alcohol levels in women. The role of decreased gastric alcohol dehydrogenase activity and first pass metabolism', *New England Journal of Medicine* 322: 95–9.

Friedman, G.D. and Kimball, A. (1986) 'Coronary heart disease mortality and alcohol consumption in Framingham', *American Journal of Epidemiology* 124: 481–9.

Fuchs, C.S., Stampfer, M.J., Colditz, G.A. *et al.* (1995) 'Alcohol consumption and mortality among women', *New England Journal of Medicine* 332: 1245–50.

Gavaler, J.S., Rizzo, A., Rossaro, L., Van Thiel, D.H., Brezza, E. and Deal, S.R. (1993) 'Sexuality of alcoholic women with menstrual cycle function: Effects of duration of alcohol abstinence', *Alcoholism: Clinical and Experimental Research* 17: 778–81.

Gavaler, J.S., Rizzo, A., Rossaro, L., Van Thiel, D.H., Brezza, E. and Deal, S.R. (1994) 'Sexuality of alcoholic postmenopausal women: Effects of duration of alcohol abstinence', *Alcoholism: Clinical and Experimental Research* 18: 269–71.

George, W.H., Gournic, S.J. and McAffe, M.P. (1988) 'Perceptions of post-drinking female sexuality: Effects of gender, beverage choice, and drink payment', *Journal of Applied Social Psychology* 18: 1295–317.

Grønbæk, M., Deis, A. Sørensen, T.I.A. *et al.* (1995) 'Morality associated with moderate intakes of wine, beer or spirits', *British Medical Journal* 310: 1165–69.

Grobbee, D.E., Rimm, E.B., Keil, U. *et al.* (1999) 'Alcohol and the cardiovascular system', in I. Macdonald (ed.) *Health Issues Related to Alcohol Consumption* (2nd edn), Oxford: Blackwell Science.

Hingson, R. and Howland, J. (1987) 'Alcohol as a risk factor for injury or death resulting from accidental falls: A review of the literature', *Journal of Studies of Alcohol* 48: 212–19.

Kauhanen, J., Kaplan, G.A., Goldberg, D.E. *et al.* (1997) 'Beer binging and mortality: Results from the Kuopio ischemic heart disease risk factor study, a prospective population based study', *British Medical Journal* 315: 846–51.

Keil, U., Liese, A., Filipiak, B. *et al.* (1998) *Alcohol, Blood Pressure and Hypertension in Alcohol and Cardiovascular Diseases*, Chichester: Wiley.

Klatsky, A. and Armstrong, M.A. (1993) 'Alcohol use, other traits and risk of unnatural death: A prospective study', *Alcoholism: Clinical and Experimental Research* 17: 1156–62.

Lieber, C.S. (1991) 'Hepatic, metabolic and toxic effects of ethanol', *Alcoholism: Clinical and Experimental Research* 15: 573–92.

Lieber, C.S. (1992) 'Alcoholic liver injury', *Current Opinions in Gastroenterology* 8: 449–57.

Lucey, M.R., Egerer, G., Young, J. *et al.* (1993) 'The interplay of age, sex and gastric function on ethanol metabolism', *Gastroenterology* 104: A945.

McPherson, K., Cavallo, F. and Rubin, E. (1999) 'Alcohol and breast cancer', in I. Macdonald (ed.) *Health Issues Related to Alcohol Consumption*, Oxford: Blackwell Science.

Marmot, M.G., Elliot, P., Shipley, M.J. *et al.* (1994) 'Alcohol and blood pressure: The Intersalt study', *British Medical Journal* 308: 1263–7.

Office for National Statistics (1998) *Living in Britain: Results from the 1996 General Household Survey*, London: The Stationery Office.

Petticrew, M., McKee, M. and Jones, J. (1993) 'Coronary heart disease: Are women discriminated against?' *British Medical Journal* 306: 1164–6.

Plant, M.L. (1997) '*Women and Alcohol: Contemporary and Historical Perspectives*', London: Free Association Books.

Rimm, E.B., Klatsky, A., Grobbee, D. and Stampfer, M.J. (1996) 'Review of moderate alcohol consumption and reduced risk of coronary heart disease: Is the effect due to beer, wine or spirits?', *British Medical Journal* 312: 731–6.

Rehm, J.T., Bondy, S.J., Sempos, C.T. *et al.* (1997) 'Alcohol consumption and coronary heart disease morbidity and mortality', *American Journal of Epidemiology* 146: 495–501.

Seppä, K., Laippala, T. and Sillanaukee, P. (1996) 'High diastolic blood pressure: Common among women who are heavy drinkers', *Alcoholism: Clinical and Experimental Research* 20: 47–51.

Stampfer, M.J., Colditz, G.A., Willet, W.C. *et al.* (1988) 'A prospective study of moderate alcohol consumption and the risk of coronary disease and stroke in women', *New England Journal of Medicine* 319: 267–73.

Steingart, R.M., Packer, M., Ham, P. *et al.* (1991) 'Sex differences in the management of coronary disease', *New England Journal of Medicine* 325: 226–30.

Thom, B. (1991) *Dealing with Drink: Alcohol and Social Policy: From Treatment to Management*, London: Free Association Books.

Thom, B. (1986) 'Sex differences in help seeking for alcohol problems, 1: The barriers to help seeking', *British Journal of Addiction* 81: 777–8.

Thom, B. (1987) 'Sex differences in help seeking for alcohol problems, 2: Entry into treatment', *British Journal of Addiction* 82: 989–97.

Van Gijn, J., Stampfer, M.J., Wolfe, C. and Algra, A. (1993) 'The association between alcohol and stroke', in P.M. Verschuren (ed.) *Health Issues Related to Alcohol* (1st edn) Brussels: ILSI Europe.

US Department of Health and Human Services (1994) *Eighth Special Report to the US Congress on Alcohol and Health*, (NIH Pub No 94–3699), Washington DC: UD Government Printing Office.

Wilsnack, R.W. and Wilsnack, S.C. (eds) (1997) *Gender and Alcohol: Individual and Social Perspectives*, New Jersey, USA: Rutgers Center of Alcohol Studies.

Witteman, J.C.M., Willett, W.C., Stampfer, M.J. *et al.* (1989) 'A prospective study of nutritional factors and hypertension among US women', *Circulation* 80: 1320–7.

CHAPTER 24

DRUG USE AND WOMEN'S REPRODUCTIVE HEALTH

Mary Hepburn

LEARNING OBJECTIVES

After you have studied this chapter you will be able to demonstrate an awareness of:

1. The specific service needs of women, including pregnant women, who use drugs.
2. The medical and social effects of drug use on women's health, the limitations of scientific research in this area, and the consequent need for a pragmatic approach to management.

INTRODUCTION

An estimated one-third of drug users are female and virtually all are in the reproductive age range. They may have been pregnant already, want to become pregnant in the future, not want to become pregnant, or have no interest in the question. Drug use can directly affect women's reproductive functions including pregnancy, while pregnancy can affect their drug use. Consequently women who use drugs have specific service requirements. The relevance of reproductive functions and role is not confined to pregnancy and should always be borne in mind by those who work with women who use drugs.

REPRODUCTIVE HEALTH ISSUES FOR NON-PREGNANT WOMEN

Planning of pregnancy and pre-pregnancy care

Ideally, all pregnancies should be planned; the medical and social problems associated with drug use make it especially important that drug using women do not become pregnant unless they want to. An unplanned pregnancy may be welcome but may also be destabilising and can cause distressing dilemmas if the timing is medically or socially inappropriate.

It is especially important for drug using women to maximise their health before becoming pregnant. Improving lifestyle and diet are helpful. Control of drug use and elimination or reduction in risky practices is extremely important. Screening for sexually transmitted infections may be relevant while women over 20 years of age should have regular cervical smears. If drug use is financed by prostitution it is also important to ensure conception can only occur with the chosen partner.

Fertility

Use of heroin and/or poor diet may cause women to stop menstruating. However, ovulation may not cease and adequate contraception is essential for those who do not want to become pregnant. Ovulation may restart with control of drug use or treatment with methadone and can restart (with restoration of fertility) before menstruation recommences. Adequate contraceptive advice should therefore always accompany provision of substitution therapy. Conversely, for those trying unsuccessfully to become pregnant control of drug use or substitution therapy may restore fertility in the absence of other problems.

Choice of contraception

Contraception and protection against sexually transmitted infections should always be addressed separately since both cannot be reliably provided by the same method. It is therefore important to raise both issues.

Contraceptive advice should be medically, socially and individually appropriate. For example, the contraceptive pill may be unusable if the woman is highly mobile, chaotic, loses the pill or can't take it correctly, and it may be ineffective if she has frequent vomiting. Longer-acting progestogen by injection may be more appropriate but needs an effective three monthly recall system, independent of an unreliable memory. Mobility may also be a problem if the woman cannot be contacted at the appropriate time. The intrauterine contraceptive device is effective for several years, but is associated with an increased risk of pelvic infection. However, this does not apply to the progestogen releasing coil. Like progestogen by injection, this coil causes lighter and less frequent (though often irregular) periods, or even cessation of menstruation. Since it provides protection for five years, this can be an excellent method for drug using women.

In the care of drug using women there is an important role for reproductive health services, which should provide regular input to addiction services. It is also helpful if at least some input is provided by the reproductive health service which would care for the woman if she became pregnant, since continuity of care with prior establishment of a positive relationship promotes earlier attendance for maternity care.

DRUG USE AND PREGNANCY

Attendance for care

Pregnant drug using women are often reported to attend late if at all for antenatal care. This is frequently attributed to lack of awareness of the pregnancy due to absence of menstruation. In fact it is usually due to competition from other pressures in their lives, together with feelings of guilt about their drug use and consequent fear of negative responses from health care professionals. In Glasgow, where there is a specialist service, drug using women book just as early as other women and if confused by their lack of menstruation tend to overdiagnose rather than underdiagnose pregnancy (Hepburn and Elliot, 1997).

Service design and delivery

The effect, if any, of drug use on pregnancy will depend on the drug(s) used, the level, pattern and route of use and the presence or absence of other medical and/or social problems. Significant problematic drug use, particularly if accompanied by a chaotic lifestyle, is associated with poorer maternal health and increased rates of perinatal morbidity and mortality. Drug using women thus have potentially high risk pregnancies and their maternity care must be obstetrically led. Although unsuitable for midwife-only care much of the care of the pregnant drug user can nevertheless be delivered by midwives in the community.

Ideally all women should have access to information and discussion about reproductive choices before they become pregnant to ensure optimum timing and optimum health at conception. While universal prepregnancy counselling has not been achieved it is especially important that it is provided for women with health problems that could affect pregnancy. Thus, in the same way that it is considered essential for women with conditions such as diabetes and epilepsy, it is also essential for women with drug and/or alcohol problems and is best provided by reproductive health care nurses (not necessarily midwives but linked to maternity services). Similarly, input from addiction services to maternity care of pregnant drug using women is also desirable. Close collaboration between addiction and reproductive health care services is necessary, with reciprocal contributions to each service from both specialist teams. Professionals from both teams therefore need training to develop the knowledge and skills to care for drug using women before, during and after pregnancy.

Pregnant drug using women should be regarded as pregnant women who have a drug problem rather than drug users who happen to be pregnant. Since drug using women have potentially high risk pregnancies (as do women with problems such as diabetes and epilepsy that carry comparable maternal and child health risks) they need specialised maternity care that can meet the needs of both the mother and her baby before, during and after delivery. Such care can only be effectively provided by maternity teams with adequate experience of the problem. While in remote settings care in a small or general unit may be necessary, elsewhere it will be preferable to provide a specialist service in one centre. Some forms of care, for example home or domino deliveries, would also be inappropriate. Consequently, as in the care of all pregnant women choice of care should be available from the range of options that are medically and socially appropriate; however it must be recognised that problem drug use by virtue of its effects on pregnancy will impose some limitations on choice of management.

Since social problems can also adversely affect health, pregnant drug using women require comprehensive multidisciplinary care which addresses both medical and social problems. Like all pregnant women they should be provided with good professional care which meets their specific needs; this care should be health care based with contributions from other services as necessary. There may also be benefit from midwifery input for pregnant women within addiction services, but this should not be the main focus of maternity care. If pregnant women are unwilling to attend health services for maternity care then these services should be modified to make them acceptable; total delivery of care within addiction services should be regarded as a short-term compromise which is obstetrically unacceptable as well as stigmatising. Moreover it is important for pregnant drug using women to attend maternity services to access the range of other educational and support services available to and necessary for all pregnant women.

General effects of drug use on pregnancy

There is a dearth of reliable scientific data on effects of specific drugs on pregnancy and pregnancy outcome. This is because illicit drugs are not used under controlled circumstances and there are often other factors which affect outcome. The main adverse outcomes are an increase in low birthweight and/or preterm delivery and an increase in Sudden Infant Death (Cot Death). However, such outcomes are multifactorial and are also increased by, for example, cigarette smoking and by socio-economic deprivation and associated problems. Opiates/opioids and benzodiazepines can also cause withdrawal symptoms in the new-born.

Opiates/opioids

In Britain opioid (including heroin, dihydrocodeine and methadone) misuse is widespread (Department of Health, 1996). Heroin is short acting and many of the problems associated with its use result from the effects of withdrawal. Withdrawal causes contraction of smooth muscle; this can lead to spasm of the placental blood vessels, reduced placental blood flow and consequently reduced birthweight, while contraction of the uterine muscle can increase the risk of preterm labour.

Substitute prescribing of methadone has social and medical benefits. Legal prescription removes the need to procure and finance illicit drugs and brings drug users in contact with services. It therefore promotes stability of drug use and lifestyle and reduces drug related harm (Ward *et al.*, 1999). Maintenance methadone has additional benefits in pregnancy since its longer half life minimises fluctuations in body drug levels. It therefore does not increase the risk of preterm labour although, despite reports to the contrary (Newman *et al.*, 1974), in the series of >1,000 babies born to drug using women in Glasgow an increased rate of low birthweight and small for gestational age babies has been observed (unpublished data). Such contradictory findings no doubt reflect the variable effects of the many other social and lifestyle factors that affect pregnancy outcome and frequently accompany problem drug use. Methadone, like heroin, causes withdrawal symptoms in the neonate. There has been considerable experience of use of methadone in pregnancy and it remains the substitute drug of choice.

Dihydrocodeine is commonly abused and since oral dihydrocodeine is not a controlled drug it is sometimes prescribed as an opiate substitute instead of methadone. However, whether in standard or slow release forms it affects birthweight and can produce severe withdrawal symptoms in the neonate. Methadone substitution for dihydrocodeine users is therefore justifiable during pregnancy.

Benzodiazepines

Benzodiazepines are commonly misused in the UK and their use, especially in combination with opioids, has been a particular feature of problem drug use in Scotland (Forsyth *et al.*, 1993; Robertson and Treasure, 1996). Their use is particularly associated with social instability. However there is no good evidence of benefit from and therefore no indication for substitution therapy in pregnancy. Exposure to benzodiazepines in early pregnancy increases the risk of major malformation and oral cleft in the fetus. Accompanying medical and social problems are often associated with poorer outcomes (especially low birthweight and prematurity) of multifactorial aetiology. Maternal benzodiazepine use also causes withdrawal symptoms in the neonate.

Amphetamines and ecstasy

Amphetamines are very commonly used in England and Wales (Department of Health, 1996). Their use is more problematic when injected or as a component of polydrug use, especially together with benzodiazepines. Such patterns may be associated with a chaotic lifestyle. While harm reduction measures such as needle exchange will be beneficial, and theoretically substitute prescribing could increase contact with services, there is no evidence of benefit from substitute prescribing in pregnancy. Also there is no evidence that amphetamines *per se* directly affect pregnancy outcome although there may be indirect effects due to associated problems. Amphetamines do not cause withdrawal symptoms in the neonate.

There has been no substantial published evidence of any effect on pregnancy outcome, or of withdrawals in the neonate following ecstasy use in pregnancy, and no such effects have been observed among ecstasy using women in the Glasgow cohort.

Cocaine

Cocaine use is increasingly common in the UK but not on a scale comparable to its use in North America. As with all drugs it is more problematic when injected and heavy use can lead to social instability. Use of 'crack' cocaine is particularly associated with instability and consequent problems. Cocaine is a powerful vasoconstrictor and this effect on blood vessels is reported to increase the risk of adverse pregnancy outcomes including placental separation, reduced brain growth, underdevelopment of organs and limbs, and of fetal death in utero. However, there is evidence of a publication bias in favour of data showing adverse outcomes (Koren *et al.*, 1989) and such outcomes seem to be largely associated with heavy, problematic use rather than with recreational use. Cocaine does not cause withdrawal symptoms in the neonate, and problems in the baby, if they occur, are attributable to antenatal complications.

Cannabis

Cannabis is widely used both by those who do and do not use other drugs. Cannabis is frequently used together with tobacco which itself causes problems (see below). There is no evidence of a direct effect on pregnancy outcome for cannabis itself (Fried, 1986) although very heavy use may cause jitteriness in the baby (Fried, 1989).

Tobacco and alcohol

It is important to remember that maternal use of the legal drugs tobacco and alcohol can affect the pregnancy. Smoking during pregnancy is associated with increased perinatal mortality and morbidity (Butler and Bonham, 1963), a reduction in birthweight and is a major risk factor for cot deaths (King and Fabro, 1983). Babies of women who smoke heavily during pregnancy may also exhibit jitteriness in the neonatal period.

Low levels of alcohol consumption during pregnancy seem harmless, but safe levels cannot be precisely identified. At higher levels alcohol causes reduction in birthweight while amongst women who drink heavily in pregnancy (especially binge drinkers) a small number deliver babies with the combination of effects known as 'fetal alcohol syndrome' (Jones and Smith, 1973). These features include low birthweight with reduction in all parameters of growth (including head circumference and brain size), central nervous dysfunction including learning difficulties and characteristic facial abnormalities. The correlation with dosage is not exact, suggesting that other factors may contribute to the aetiology.

Maintenance v. detoxification

Opioid maintenance and detoxification each have advantages and disadvantages. Methadone maintenance improves stability, but methadone has effects in common with the drugs it replaces including withdrawal symptoms in the baby. Detoxification improves fetal growth and reduces the likelihood of neonatal withdrawals, but carries the risk of failure and consequent loss of stability. There is an observable increase in liquor catecholamines following acute detoxification which suggests that antenatal opioid detoxification could be stressful for the fetus (Zuspan *et al.*, 1975) but in practice it is not unacceptably risky for women to undergo detoxification at any responsible speed or at any stage of pregnancy (Hepburn, 1997). Nevertheless opioid withdrawal is not always a realistic objective and stability is more important than abstinence. Opioid maintenance and detoxification are often wrongly viewed as mutually exclusive. A compromise is often best, reducing the dose of methadone gradually to the lowest compatible with stability by the time of delivery.

Sudden withdrawal of large doses of benzodiazepines can lead to maternal convulsions so that detoxification should be covered with reducing doses of a longer-acting benzodiazepine such as diazepam. Regardless of the level of use, complete withdrawal can be safely achieved within a week, but should be carried out on an inpatient basis with obstetric supervision both for medical safety and to increase the chance of success. Post-detoxification problems, especially sleep disturbance (which is common among drug users), can persist for much longer. Relapse is therefore a very real possibility (but is not necessarily prevented by a slower regime). Repeated admissions for detoxification or reduction may be necessary. Since benzodiazepine misuse is both medically and socially problematic, maximum overall reduction in maternal consumption is the objective. Repeated detoxification is therefore acceptable and does not indicate that the original attempt was misguided.

There are no problems for mother or baby with detoxification from any of the other commonly used drugs all of which can be withdrawn immediately, or as quickly as the mother will tolerate.

Care of the baby

Withdrawal symptoms and their treatment do not require the babies of drug using women to be routinely admitted to the Special Care Nursery and whenever feasible babies should remain with their mothers.

Neonatal withdrawal symptoms and breastfeeding

Heroin, dihydrocodeine and methadone all cause withdrawal symptoms in the neonate. While these are broadly dose related, other factors which affect the baby's condition at birth will influence severity. The severity of withdrawal symptoms therefore cannot be predicted simply on the basis of maternal drug use.

Breast feeding, by providing drug replacement, will reduce the severity of neonatal withdrawal symptoms. It will also have other benefits for these vulnerable babies and should be encouraged for all mothers whose drug use is stable and for whom breastfeeding is not absolutely contraindicated. Successful establishment of breastfeeding is in itself a sufficient measure of stability.

Women should be advised that sudden cessation of breastfeeding may precipitate or exacerbate withdrawal symptoms; with breastfeeding established few women would do so voluntarily, but the risk should be borne in mind if breastfeeding women are involuntarily separated from their babies. Current evidence indicates that breastfeeding increases the risk of vertical transmission of HIV (Dunn *et al.*, 1992; Nduati *et al.*, 2000) so at present women known to be HIV positive should not be encouraged to breastfeed. Although Hepatitis C might theoretically be transmissible by breastfeeding the evidence suggests this does not happen (Thomas *et al.*, 1998), so that infection with Hepatitis C (including PCR+ve status) is not a contraindication to breastfeeding.

Other drug related health problems in pregnancy

In addition to their poor general health, drug using women may also have specific health problems directly or indirectly due to their drug use. Genital tract infections which may be transmitted to the baby or affect the pregnancy in other ways have already been mentioned. Dental caries can be a significant focus of infection for women with previous endocarditis and damage to heart valves, while detoxification from pain killing drugs may precipitate toothache. Women with a history of venous thrombosis due to injecting may require anticoagulant therapy during and after pregnancy. Injecting can cause infection locally, with development of abscesses, or systemically with organisms including Hepatitis B (HBV), Hepatitis C (HCV) and Human Immunodeficiency virus (HIV) which can be transmitted to the baby (vertical transmission). Vertical transmission of Hepatitis B can be prevented by immunisation of the baby, so that antenatal screening of pregnant women for HBV carrier status is now required of all maternity units in the UK. The risk of vertical transmission of HIV can be reduced by interventions including antiretroviral therapy for mother and baby, delivery by caesarian section and avoidance of breastfeeding. The offer of antenatal screening of mothers for HIV is recommended but not universally provided. Vertical transmission rates for HCV appear to be much lower than for HIV, although as with HIV individual risk will depend on a number of factors, especially the mother's viral load. Co-infection with HIV increases the risk of transmission of HCV. There is as yet no proof that any interventions reduce the risk of vertical transmission of HCV. Consequently women infected with HCV should be managed as obstetrically indicated and the

WHO recommendation is that women with HCV infection be encouraged to breastfeed. Women should receive appropriate specialist care for all these health problems and increased fetal monitoring during pregnancy may be necessary.

Social effects of drug use in pregnancy

Most drug using women are adequate parents. However, heavy drug use and a chaotic lifestyle can compromise a mother's ability to care for her child, while women from dysfunctional backgrounds may have poorly developed parenting skills independent of their drug use. Caring for a baby that is sick and/or has withdrawals will be especially demanding. Women with a history of significant drug use should be assessed early in pregnancy to determine what type of support will be needed to ensure they can adequately care for their child(ren). This requires effective interagency collaboration.

A multidisciplinary meeting held at thirty-two weeks gestation will allow identification of problems, planning of support and setting of goals. Such meetings should not be restricted to women with current major problems; the potentially relapsing nature of drug use should be recognised and contingency plans made for such an eventuality.

During pregnancy the main focus of care will be with specialist maternity services (including paediatric services) with contributions from primary care, social work, addiction services and other agencies as required. After delivery care will be centred in and mainly provided by community medical and social services. Consequently, regardless of whether there are major concerns, good professional practice demands that a similar multidisciplinary meeting be held after delivery, preferably before postnatal discharge, to allow effective transfer of care.

Drug use by the mother is not necessarily a child protection issue but each individual situation should be assessed in this respect and where there are such concerns they should be separately addressed under the relevant legislation – the Children's Act or the Children's Act (Scotland). Pregnant women may be afraid that involvement of social services will result in their children being removed from their care, but the social services contribution should take the form of family support rather than child protection unless the latter is specifically indicated. Women should be encouraged to view the involvement of social services as supportive and preventive rather than punitive, and professionals from all agencies involved should work together with the women to promote this approach. Women should know that all agencies, not just social services, will contribute to assessments and should be reassured that they too will be involved in all decision making. Sharing of relevant information is essential for effective multidisciplinary management. Agencies should discuss their confidentiality policies with women at the outset and whenever possible women's permission to share information should be sought. This will enable women to feel they have some control over the process and even though it may occasionally take a little longer, is more likely to be successful. Experience in Glasgow using this approach has been that women almost invariably agree to involvement of all relevant services and to sharing of information where this can be justified. Individual agencies should all have policies to ensure that services provided are appropriate to women's needs and reflect their social, cultural and religious circumstances; it is important that this approach is also adopted by the multidisciplinary team.

Long-term outcomes

The presence of confounding factors makes it difficult to study long-term developmental outcomes for these babies. While there is no doubt that their physical, emotional, intellectual and social development can be compromised, this is often attributable to their disadvantaged circumstances and there is no evidence that such compromise is a direct effect of drug use *per se*.

Conclusions

Problem drug use can have long-term adverse consequences for mother and baby. The wide range of medical and social problems associated with such drug use makes multidisciplinary management essential. Punitive measures aimed simply at trying to eradicate drug use are unlikely to be effective in either the short or the long term. Instead there should be recognition that the problem is inextricably linked with poverty and inequality with introduction of policies to effectively deal with these issues while providing support to those suffering the consequences.

READER INPUT

Questions

(1) What are the major risks of heroin withdrawal in pregnancy?
(2) Which is best used as a substitute: dihydrocodeine or methadone and why?
(3) What are the potential effects of cocaine on the foetus?
(4) Should women on substitute prescriptions be encouraged to breastfeed or dissuaded from doing so?

Case scenario

Sandra, a single 25-year-old injecting heroin user, has not experienced a period for over a year. She recently started on a methadone prescription. She does not want to become pregnant but admits that she has had unprotected sex on several occasions in the last year. She did not think that she could become pregnant if she did not menstruate. Sandra is currently in unstable housing, moving between hostels and friends' houses.

(1) Was Sandra correct in her assumption that she could not become pregnant whilst not menstruating?
(2) What contraceptive advice and forms of contraception may be best suited to Sandra's situation?
(3) What other information and advice might be helpful in this situation?
(4) What risk factors, other than pregnancy, exist for Sandra and how might these be addressed?

REFERENCES

Butler, N.R. and Bonham, D.G. (1963) *Perinatal Mortality: The First Report of the 1958 British Perinatal Mortality Survey*, Edinburgh: E. and S. Livingstone.

Department of Health (1996) 'Drug misuse statistics 1996/24', *Statistical Bulletin Dec 1996*, London: Department of Health.

Dunn, D.T., Newell, M.-L., Ades, A.E. and Peckham, C. (1992) 'Estimates of the risk of HIV-1 transmission through breastfeeding' *Lancet* 340: 585–8.

Forsyth, A.J.M., Farquhar, D. and Gemmell, M. *et al.* (1993) 'The dual use of opioids and temazepam by drug injectors in Glasgow (Scotland)', *Drug and Alcohol Dependence* 32: 277–80.

Fried, P. (1986) 'Marijuana and human pregnancy', in I.J. Chasnoff (ed.) *Drug use in pregnancy: mother and child*, Norwell, MA: MTP Press.

Fried, P. (1989) 'Postnatal consequences of maternal marijuana use in humans', *Annals of the New York Academy of Science* 562: 123–32.

Hepburn, M. (1997) 'Drugs of addiction', in F. Cockburn (ed.) *Advances in Perinatal Medicine*, Carnforth: Parthenon Publishing Group.

Hepburn, M. and Elliott, L. (1997) 'A community obstetric service for women with special needs', *British Journal of Midwifery* 5(8): 485–8.

Jones, K.L., Smith, D.W. (1973) 'Recognition of the fetal alcohol syndrome in early infancy', *Lancet* 2: 999–1001.

King, J.C. and Fabro, S. (1983) Alcohol consumption and cigarette smoking. Effect on pregnancy', *Clin Obstet and Gynecol* 26: 437–48.

Koren, G., Graham, K., Shear, H. and Einarson, T. (1989) 'Bias against the null hypothesis: the reproductive hazards of cocaine', *Lancet* 2: 1440–2.

Newman, R.G., Bashkow, S. and Calko, D. (1974) 'Results of 313 consecutive live births of infants delivered to patients in the New York City Methadone Maintenance Treatment Program', *Am J Obstet Gynecol* 121(2): 233–7.

Nduati, R., John, G. and Mbori-Ngacha, D. *et al.* (2000) 'Effect of breastfeeding and formula feeding on transmission of HIV-1: a randomised clinical trial', *JAMA* 283: 1167–74.

Robertson, R., Treasure, W. (1996) 'Benzodiazepine abuse. Nature and extent of the problem', *CNS Drugs* 5(2): 137–46.

Thomas, S.L., Newell, M.-L. and Peckham, C.S. *et al.* (1998) 'A review of hepatitis C (HCV) vertical transmission: risks of transmission to infants born to mothers with and without HCV viraemia or human immunodeficiency virus infection', *Int J Epidemiol* 27: 108–17.

Ward, A., Hall, W. and Mahick, R. (1999) 'Role of maintenance treatment in opioid dependence', *Lancet* 353: 221–26.

Zuspan, F.P., Gumpel, J.A., Mejia-Zelaya, A. *et al.* (1975) 'Fetal stress from methadone withdrawal', *Am J Obstet and Gynecol* 122: 43–6.

CHAPTER 25

YOUNG PEOPLE

Jane Christian and Eilish Gilvarry

LEARNING OBJECTIVES

After you have studied this chapter:

1 You should be aware of the principles of good practice that guide children's services.

2 You should be aware of the need for comprehensive assessments.

3 You should be aware of the importance of early and targeted interventions.

INTRODUCTION

Substance misuse amongst young people has been a matter for increasing concern among politicians, policy makers, service providers and the general public throughout the 1990s. This concern is justifiable. Successive prevalence studies in the UK confirm an upward trend in the availability and use of controlled drugs, particularly cannabis and 'dance drugs' (amphetamines, LSD, ecstasy), with a minority using heroin and crack cocaine (Gilvarry, 2000). This increased use is associated with early experimentation, poly-drug use and a high degree of acceptance of drug use by young people (Measham *et al.*, 1998). Cigarette smoking is commonplace, especially among girls, with greater alcohol consumption and higher rates of drunkenness and binge drinking found more amongst teenagers in the UK, Denmark and Ireland than other European countries (Hibell *et al.*, 1997).

There is a substantial literature on the aetiological and risk factors associated with substance misuse, arising from a combination of environmental, legal, individual and family risk factors. These risks are thought to be multiple in more vulnerable young people, such as the young homeless, young offenders, school truants or excluded students, those in the 'looked after' system, those with learning difficulties and those with mental health problems. Identification of these 'at risk' groups, has received greater emphasis recently. These special populations present with multiple and more complex problems that may demand more intense interventions and specific expertise. This increased interest reflects a focus on secondary and targeted prevention.

It is therefore of great concern that there is a paucity of services and developmentally appropriate interventions for young drug users under the age of 18. In 1996, the Health Advisory Service (HAS) Thematic Review of Substance Misuse Services for Children and Young People reported that services were generally scarce and operated without a strategic framework or effective co-ordination. Some progress in the development of specific youth services has been achieved latterly with modest central government funding, as well as an emphasis on the needs of young drug users within government strategy documents. While there is cause for some optimism, evaluations of models of service delivery and specific interventions are much needed. Young people's services 'tagged on' to adult services, usually by the provision of one dedicated young people's worker, fall substantially short of what is required.

PRINCIPLES OF YOUNG PEOPLE'S SUBSTANCE MISUSE SERVICES

The first and over-riding principle when planning responses to young people's substance use is that children are not adults. Service models and interventions must adopt a developmental approach that reflects the differences in age and developmental maturity of the young person, the need to involve those with parental responsibility (balanced against the young person's need and desire for confidentiality), and the legislative framework for children (Christian and Gilvarry, 1999).

The legal position can be daunting, particularly in the delivery of some interventions, such as needle exchange and substitute prescribing. Advice has been formulated which reviews case law which deals with possibly comparable circumstances (HAS, 1996). In England and Wales young people of 16 or 17 years can legally consent to medical treatment. Generally, children under 16 cannot give consent to treatment, but a child who has sufficient intelligence and understanding to fully comprehend the proposed treatment may be deemed legally competent to give consent. In this situation, the child may be described as 'Gillick competent' (Gillick *v.* West Norfolk Health Authority 1985), but this ruling has not been applied in substance misuse cases. The Children Act 1989 emphasises a 'duty to consult', with the involvement of the family accepted as good practice. Given the significant degree of uncertainty, it is of importance that all those working with young people know the legal framework, understand the principles of good practice, and have supervision available as well as legal advice. A full assessment of maturity and understanding, ability to consent, as well as detailed information of the risks of the intervention, or of no intervention, are essential.

Services need to be attractive and accessible, appropriate to the needs of children and their families, and capable of responding to the varied and often complex needs of young people. The young person's own views must be taken into account, so far as this is compatible with their maturity and competence to make their own decisions and choices. Agencies must be able to co-ordinate and communicate with a number of organisations and individuals that might be involved in providing care, hence the need for policies on confidentiality and information exchange. For all the varied professionals involved there is a need for training in substance misuse, as well as awareness and confidence in dealing with associated mental health problems, both from a developmental perspective.

To address these complexities, and to promote best practice, the HAS review detailed the key issues for commissioning and provision of services for this client group. A manual of guidance, designed to assist professionals working with children and young people, has been produced by the Standing Conference on Drug Abuse (now DrugScope), which draws on the HAS review and other sources (SCODA, 1999). This guidance helpfully summarises principles for policy and practice (Figure 25.1).

1. A child or young person is not an adult.
2. The overall welfare of the individual child or young person is of paramount importance.
3. The views of the young person are of central importance, and should always be sought and considered.
4. Services need to respect parental responsibility when working with a young person.
5. Services should recognise and co-operate with the local authority in carrying out its responsibilities towards children and young people.
6. A holistic approach is vital at all levels, as young people's problems do not respect professional boundaries.
7. Services must be child-centred.
8. A comprehensive range of services needs to be provided.
9. Services must be competent.
10. Services should aim to operate, in all cases, according to the principles of good practice.

Figure 25.1 Ten key policy principles

Assessment

Assessing drug misuse in children and young people is unfamiliar territory for many practitioners, both in children's services and substance misuse services. In response to this, and in light of the development of treatment services for young people, SCODA (2000) has produced a manual of practical guidance for practitioners on assessing young people's drug use, which recommends a child-centred, child-protecting and comprehensive approach to assessment and care planning.

Comprehensive guidance was produced for clinicians in the assessment of adolescent substance abuse, based on clinical consensus and critical reviews of the scientific evidence by Buckstein with a working party (1997). They provide guidance on assessing the substance misuse itself; physical, social, emotional, and mental health functioning; scholastic and lifestyle attainments; peer relationships; parental and family history; appropriate other informants (e.g. school and juvenile justice); and treatment history.

Comprehensive assessment forms the basis for any treatment intervention. It is especially important in young drug users who may present with a complex array of needs. Antecedent risks, current use and consequences of use need to be assessed. For example, alcohol and drug misuse are important risk factors for suicide and self-harm, with conduct and mood disorders frequently reported as antecedents or in association with substance misuse (Gilvarry, 1998).

A comprehensive assessment should take account of the quantity, frequency, and the context of use, as well as any potential harmful practices that may increase the risk of infection or other adverse consequences. In addition, attention should be paid to the social context including school attendance and performance, training or employment issues, friendship networks and family relationships, peer involvement in substance misuse, use of leisure time, and any criminal behaviour. A physical health assessment should be undertaken to identify any illnesses or infections (e.g. Hepatitis C), overdoses or accidents, as well as assessing any lifestyle consequences of substance misuse such as pregnancy, poor nutrition and so on. The presence or otherwise of depression, suicidal thoughts, conduct problems and current or past abuse should be identified as part of a comprehensive assessment of the mental health of the young person (Gilvarry, 1998).

In adult treatment services there are some specific validated assessment tools and questionnaires to aid screening and diagnosis. Any attempt to adapt these for children and young people should be approached with caution. There are some instruments validated for adolescents; the interested reader is referred to the Bukstein article (1997). Unfortunately there is little evidence on the relative importance of individual instruments for specific populations in particular settings.

TREATMENT INTERVENTIONS

Treatment interventions for young substance misusers are rapidly being developed, often with little theoretical basis and against a background of a dearth of research on what constitutes effective treatment. There is also confusion on the acceptable goals of treatment. It has been stated that abstinence is the only defensible treatment goal for minors (Fulkerson *et al.*, 1999); others argue that harm reduction is an acceptable approach but should not be the ultimate aim of treatment (Buckstein *et al.*, 1997). Retention in treatment may affect outcome, to the extent that those who remain in treatment do better than those who drop out, irrespective of the degree of difficulties faced by the individual. Therefore treatment philosophies which over-emphasise the importance of abstinence may prove counter-productive if this approach fails to attract and engage young people.

Recommended treatment models put significant emphasis on multi-disciplinary working. The range of skills and expertise required could be achieved with collaboration between drug and alcohol services, child and adolescent mental health services, child health services, social and educational services and non-statutory sector services. A small number of specialist young people's drug services have been created in the United Kingdom in this way. In one such model, an addiction psychiatrist worked with a core team of project workers, who had prior experience of working with young people in nursing, youth work and social work settings (Crome *et al.*, 2000). An art therapist, a community paediatrician and a child and adolescent psychiatrist provided sessional input. Extensive links were made with educational services, criminal justice agencies and other medical specialists. In this way a comprehensive package of treatment and care could be delivered. Almost 40 per cent complied with or completed their agreed treatment plan, and demonstrated improved psychosocial functioning.

To date there has been little systematic evaluation of service models or treatment modalities in this country. In the United States, the strongest conclusion of effectiveness was that any treatment was better than none, but no one treatment modality was shown to be superior to others and post-treatment relapse was found to be high (Catalano *et al.*, 1990–1991). There is evidence for the effectiveness of cognitive and behavioural therapies, brief interventions, motivational enhancement and relapse prevention in adults, but whilst these approaches have been adapted for adolescents, there has not as yet been any research into their effectiveness with this age group (Buckstein and van Hasselt, 1993). There is evolving evidence on family therapy techniques, with improved engagement and retention of families in treatment, a reduction in criminal rates and improved family relationships. Multisystemic therapy shows interesting early results (Henggeler, 1999).

Pharmacotherapy in the adolescent, as part of a comprehensive care plan, may be directed at a number of areas: detoxification, treatment of overdose emergencies, substitution or maintenance therapy, adjuncts to relapse prevention and treatment of comorbid disorders. The prescription of substitute medication is not generally recommended for adolescents, and methadone maintenance in particular is controversial. Nevertheless, there may be a role for medication for young people who are dependent substance misusers. The Guidelines on Clinical Management (Department of Health, 1999) recommend that controlled drugs should only be prescribed to young people following a full assessment and with guidance from a substance misuse treatment specialist. Attention is drawn to the importance of informed consent which, in the case of young people under 16 years, should be sought from a person with parental responsibility for the young person.

Working within a harm minimisation framework, easy access to needles and syringes might be regarded as good practice in services for adults. The same is not necessarily so where young people are concerned, owing to the different statutory and legal requirements for minors. Full assessment and informed consent are essential, and where young people under 16 are involved, needle exchange should only be provided in the context of a regularly reviewed care plan.

Prevention/Early intervention

Discussion of young people and substance misuse rightly highlights the importance of prevention. Universal education programmes, delivered in a school setting, are often cited as a central plank of prevention activity. Evidence for the effectiveness of these programmes in influencing behaviour is limited, even though they may impact on levels of knowledge and attitudes to drugs and alcohol (HAS, 1996). While primary prevention is clearly important, there is a growing awareness of the need to target specific interventions to different groups of young people. 'Indicated' and 'selective' programmes aim to reduce both drug and alcohol use and also intervene to improve scholastic achievement, family functioning, self-esteem and mental health. Unlike their adult counterparts, young substance users are often not a hidden population. They are likely to be known to, if unrecognised by, the staff of a range of agencies already involved in their lives. Since many will be excluded from school, struggling academically, known to the police or social services, they present numerous opportunities for intervention.

In addition to targeting, interventions are more likely to succeed if they are timely and relevant to the experience of the young people involved. The substance misuse histories of young people referred to a treatment service illustrate the importance of reaching young people early. The average age of first use of alcohol and nicotine was 11 years; for LSD, cannabis, benzodiazepines, amphetamines and ecstasy it was 13 years; and, for heroin 15 years (Crome *et al.*, 2000).

Effective early intervention programmes are likely to be multifaceted in nature, including elements of universal, targeted and clinical interventions (Offord *et al.*, 1998). Prevention strategies that combat social exclusion, address the complex needs of vulnerable young people, support family management skills, and maintain young people's involvement in education or training appear most likely to achieve positive outcomes. The interested reader is referred to the National Institute on Drug Abuse website-www.nida.nih.gov.

Conclusion

The level of public and professional concern about the growth of substance misuse in young people has not been matched by a corresponding development of age appropriate interventions. Much has been written that describes prevention and treatment programmes in the UK and elsewhere, but there is little empirical research on treatment outcome and less on evaluation of specific treatments (Gilvarry, 2000). This may in part be due to the lack of service provision, though the development of a few models of good practice could provide a robust basis for much needed longitudinal research (Crome *et al.*, 2000).

Summary

- There is an increase in substance misuse amongst young people, with frequent poly-drug use and early age of initiation.
- Risk factors that increase the risk of substance misuse have been identified, as have factors which may have some protective effect.
- Socially excluded young people are at particular risk of developing substance use problems.
- Interventions for young people need to be child-centred, competent and comprehensive.
- Those with parental responsibility have an important part to play in treatment and care plans for young people.
- Individual assessments should be comprehensive and within a developmental framework.
- Treatment interventions should be capable of meeting a complex array of needs and are therefore likely to involve a multi-agency partnership approach.
- An important goal for young people's services is engagement and retention in treatment and other interventions.
- There is a lack of specific, targeted services providing prevention and treatment.
- Effective prevention and early intervention approaches should be timely, targeted and multifaceted.
- Research concentrating on evaluations of service delivery, interventions and longitudinal studies are particularly required.

READER INPUT

Questions

(1) What is meant by the term 'Gillick competent?'

(2) What recommendations/guidelines apply in relation to under 16s regarding:

  (a) substitute prescribing?

  (b) needle exchange provision?

Discussion point

How do you feel about treatment aims for under 16s? Should treatment be abstention orientated only or is there a defensible place for harm reduction?

Activity

Find out what services exist for under 16s in your locality. How are these services organised and how can they be accessed. Include statutory, non-statutory and self-help agencies and services.

FURTHER READING

Bukstein, O. and the Working Group on Quality Issues (1997) 'Practice parameters for the assessment and treatment of children and adolescents with substance use disorders', *Journal of the American Academy of Child and Adolescent Psychiatry* 36 Supplement: 140S–156S.

Crome, I.B., Christian, J. and Green, C. (2000) 'The development of a unique designated community drugs service for adolescents: policy, prevention and education implications', *Drugs: Education, Prevention and Policy* 7(1): 87–108.

Gilvarry, E. (1998) Young Drug Users: early intervention, *Drugs: education, prevention and policy* 5(3): 281–92.

Health Advisory Service (1996) *Children and Young People, Substance Misuse Services – The Substance of Young Needs*, London: HMSO.

Standing Conference on Drug Abuse (1999) *Young People and Drugs. Policy Guidance for Drug Interventions*, London, SCODA.

REFERENCES

Bukstein, O. and Van Hasselt, V. (1993) 'Alcohol and drug abuse', in A.S. Bellack and M. Herseu (eds) *Handbook of Behaviour Therapy in the Psychiatric Setting*, New York: Plenum Press.

Catalano, R.F., Hawkins, J.D., Wells, E., Miller, J. and Brewer, D. (1990–1991) 'Evaluation of the effectiveness of adolescent drug abuse treatment, assessment of risk of relapse, and promising approaches to relapse prevention', *International Journal of the Addictions* 25: 1085–140.

Christian, J. and Gilvarry, E. (1999) 'Specialist Services: the need for multi-agency partnership', *Drug and Alcohol Dependence* 55: 265–74.

Department of Health (1999) *Drug Misuse and Dependence – Guidelines on Clinical Management*, London: The Stationery Office.

Fulkerson, J., Harrison, P. and Beebe, T. (1999) 'DSM-IV substance use and dependence: are there really two dimensions of substance use disorders in adolescents?' *Addiction* 94: 495–506.

Gilvarry, E. (2000) 'Substance abuse in young people', *Journal of Child Psychology and Psychiatry* 41(1): 55–80.

Henggeler, S. (1999) 'Multisystemic therapy', *Child Psychology and Psychiatry Review* 4: 2–10.

Hibell, B., Andersson, B., Bjarnason, T., Kokkevi, A., Morgan, M. and Narusk, A. (1997) *The 1995 ESPAD Report: Alcohol and other drug use among students in 26 European countries*, Sweden: The Swedish Council for Information on Alcohol and other drugs. (CAN)/The Pompidou Group at the Council of Europe.

Measham, F., Parker, H. and Aldridge, J. (1998) 'The teenage transition: from adolescent recreational drug use to the young adult dance culture in Britain in the mid-1990s', *Journal of Drug Issues* 28: 9–32.

Miller, P. and Plant, M. (1996) 'Drinking, smoking and illicit drug use among 15 and 16 year olds in the United Kingdom', *British Medical Journal* 313: 394–7.

Offord, D., Kraemer, H., Kazdin, A., Jensen, P. and Harrington, H. (1998) 'Lowering the burden of suffering from child psychiatric disorder: trade-offs among clinical, targeted and universal intervention', *Journal of the American Academy of Child and Adolescent Psychiatry* 37: 686–94.

Standing Conference on Drug Abuse (2000) *Assessing Young People's Drug Taking. Guidance for Drug Services*, London: SCODA.

CHAPTER 26

ANTI-DISCRIMINATORY PRACTICE IN SUBSTANCE MISUSE WORK

Suzanne Midgley and Trudi Petersen

LEARNING OBJECTIVES

By the end of this chapter you should be able to demonstrate an awareness of:

1. Discrimination, anti-discrimination and the potential for change within your own work setting.
2. Government and national policy responses to issues around discrimination and diversity and how these may translate into practice.

INTRODUCTION

The field of substance misuse is not homogeneous in relation to substance misusers or service providers. Some people have issues that may be addressed inadequately. Practitioners need to develop an awareness of their own and others' beliefs and behaviours in relation to ethnicity, culture, gender, age and sexuality. An anti-discriminatory approach should be an essential component of good practice. It should be promoted and developed to permeate all aspects of substance misuse work, from overall policy and strategy to individual client contacts.

DISCRIMINATION AND PREJUDICE

Discriminatory behaviour stems from beliefs about certain groups of people, which are based on assumptions rather than facts – prejudice. Discrimination and prejudice are often seen to be related to skin colour or other visible characteristics, but this is only one aspect. Discrimination may occur in relation to a variety of factors – the country someone comes from, religious and cultural difference, gender, sexuality, physical impairment, mental ill health and age.

Substance misusers face marginalisation within society. Newcombe (1993) highlights some of the repercussions of being identified as a drug user and points out how drug users and their families may be discriminated against by both society and professionals. Alongside this general discrimination, certain groups may experience more specific difficulties.

Black individuals and communities

The complexion of the majority of UK substance misuse services reflects a preponderance of young, white male service users. The Black Drug Workers Forum in an analysis of drug service delivery to Black communities in Manchester found low levels of uptake by Black people, confirmed by both qualitative and quantitative data, the lowest take up being amongst Chinese and South Asian groups (Aslam *et al.*, 1998). Many agencies were identified as not seeing the potential value of monitoring uptake of services whilst lack of evaluation was also highlighted. Nearly half (40 per cent) of managers felt that monitoring was not a priority issue as the numbers of Black people living locally were low. The report points out that 'One has to challenge the notion that drug services only need to start caring when there are lots of Black service users' (Aslam *et al.*, 1998: 10).

Women

Women substance misusers have been perceived as more deviant, promiscuous and passive than their male counterparts, though male drug users significantly outnumber female. One area where this is excepted is in relation to prescribed medication, notably benzodiazepines. Women are twice as likely as men to be prescribed benzodiazepines (Tyler, 1995), (see also Chapter 23).

Age

Helping services are usually established for the 18–65 age group. Substance misuse problems are perhaps most common amongst younger adults. Young people are increasingly targeted for services because they are seen as a problem, whilst older substance misusers remain largely ignored. Older people are discussed in Chapter 27 and young people in Chapter 25.

Sexuality

Cabaj (1989) suggests that in order to address the barriers gay and bi-sexual people experience in seeking treatment, this group should be seen as another minority group. The experience of internalised homophobia needs to be explored and understood and health care providers' resistance, and anxiety, in working with this client group needs to be addressed. An increase in lesbian and gay drug workers has been identified as a potential strategy to encourage the gay community into services (Skingle, 1997). Covert homophobia may be present amongst professional groups. Rose's small-scale study of homophobia amongst doctors (Rose, 1994) found that despite initial denials of homophobic prejudice, comments made during the course of interviews suggested that an underlying, albeit probably unconscious, prejudice was demonstrated.

Mental illness

Mental illness is another area where discrimination is often encountered. This can be compounded where substance misuse is also part of the picture. One large UK survey of public opinion, focusing on seven mental disorders, found that schizophrenia, alcoholism and drug dependency elicited the most negative responses and the highest perceived rates of dangerousness and unpredictability (Crisp *et al.*, 2000). Black people have fared badly in psychiatric settings, being alienated from mainstream service provision (McGovern and Hemmings, 1994) and over-diagnosed with serious mental illness (Fernando, 1991).

Employee discrimination

Discrimination is not confined to service users. Professionals too can experience this. Ethnic minority doctors are concentrated in sub-consultant grades in 'unpopular' specialities such as psychiatry (including Addiction Psychiatry). Differences in recruitment, examinations, short-listing and merit awards have all been seen to be tarnished by racial discrimination (Esmail and Carnall, 1997; Esmail *et al.*, 1998). The health service has been identified as at real risk of lagging behind other sectors in offering equality of opportunity (Commission for Racial Equality, 2000).

Specific substances and particular groups

Certain substances, modes of use and patterns of misuse can be linked with certain ethnic groups. For example, Khat use is most commonly found amongst Somali men, but practitioners need to take care that acknowledgement of this does not lead to a stereotypical belief structure, such as that 'all Rastafarians smoke cannabis because of their religious and cultural beliefs'. Awareness is also needed of when research was carried out, the context in which it took place, the population sampled, the methodologies used and who was involved in the research team.

Substance misuse patterns are dynamic. Social roles, the meaning of certain substances within cultures, availability, environment, norms and sanctions all change over time and impact on patterns of use. An example of this may be seen in the rise of crack cocaine. Traditionally cocaine has been seen as a wealthy white drug and crack cocaine a poor, black, male drug, but changes have made both types of cocaine more accessible and affordable across groups. One Bristol based study of crack cocaine has found a male/female ratio of 2:1 compared to notification of 'any drug' use of 4:1 (Bristol Drugs Project, 2000). DrugScope's UK drug report for 2000 points out that 'both versions of the drug are used across the whole of the drug using community' (DrugScope, 2000: 1).

RECOGNITION OF DISCRIMINATION

The language of prejudice

How is discrimination recognised? It may be overt or covert. Language is probably the most obvious way that this is demonstrated. There are a multitude of nationalistic or racist 'jokes'. Physical and/or social characteristics are used as insults and collective labels may be used offensively. Discriminatory language serves a function in providing a defence against anxieties engendered by others perceived as 'different'. The creation of scapegoats promotes exploitation, legitimising and reinforcing power and privilege for the discriminator.

Language may not be so blunt yet may still show evidence of discrimination. The speaker may not be aware of the roots of the language they use or its potential connotations. Negative language stereotypes abound in everyday speech. There are phrases still in common use such as 'take it like a man' or 'he's like an old woman', which are variously discriminatory.

It is not unusual to hear 'immigrant' used as a description of someone who is not white, irrespective of their country of origin. Sometimes the term 'ethnic minorities' is used as if it meant immigrants. The use of such terms requires careful consideration. None of us knows who our earliest ancestors were other than that if we go back far enough they came from somewhere else. With such a history of diversity we could all be described as immigrants (someone who comes to this country with the intention of settling for over a year, or a descendant of immigrants). Unfortunately an awareness of such commonality does not prevent discrimination.

White people usually describe minority ethnic groups in terms of people who share certain cultural characteristics such as language, family values, religious beliefs or cuisine, which distinguish them from the majority of the population. To describe someone as belonging to an 'ethnic minority' is often seen as more socially acceptable than 'Black' or 'coloured'. Yet Pfeffer (1998) points out that 'ethnicity is as much a characteristic of white as black people and that because it has been set up as the standard against which all others are measured, white ethnicity is invisible'.

Institutional discrimination

Covert discrimination may be harder to recognise. The report of the Lawrence inquiry highlighted the concept of institutional racism in the police (Macpherson, 1999). The inquiry found no deliberately discriminatory policies but did find that the way that policies were put into practice resulted in discrimination. McKenzie (1999) explores the similarities between the police and the NHS, suggesting that racist attitudes may not be held by those working in such a setting, indeed individuals may consider themselves as acting in 'good faith', yet discriminatory practices may be perpetuated due to institutional systems. There is a need to focus on the actions of institutions. McKenzie goes on to suggest a further six points for consideration:

- The results of practice rather than the intent should be targeted.
- The interaction between medicine and a discriminatory social world needs to be acknowledged.
- The way the history of NHS treatment affects patients' perceptions and help seeking behaviour needs to be taken into account.
- Interactions between social stratification (gender, class, sexual orientation) and race need to be recognised when looking at disparities.
- There needs to be a recognition that racism changes with time and with the type of institution. Overt racism may be replaced by more subtle racism.
- The problems need to be seen as ideological with disparities being produced and perpetuated by sources both external to medicine (such as culture, class and socio-political factors) and internal, through medical ideology. This includes a lack of medical education about racism and an over-emphasis on the biomedical model at the expense of more anthropological research.

Treating the individual

Sometimes practitioners consider that if they concentrate on treating each person as a unique human being then they will deliver a quality service. Much of the emphasis of substance misuse work is based on the individual and caring for their needs. These are undoubtedly important goals but a focus on the individual ignores the mistreatment many people have experienced, not simply as individuals but as members of a group. Failure to recognise the ways in which groups of people have been oppressed in the past adds to the misrepresentations that surround us in everyday life and increases the risk of our failure to see and/or care for members of that group. Any staff group adopting a 'colour-blind' 'genderless' approach to service provision is at considerable risk of simply maintaining the status quo. Denial of access to effective treatment remains a denial of treatment however 'unintentional'.

Anti-discriminatory working

Discriminatory behaviour is learned and endures because of the functions it serves for individuals, cultures and institutions. Anti-discriminatory practice therefore requires strategies and action on all three levels.

Working with others

A good starting point is for practitioners to familiarise themselves with the local picture. What groups exist in the local area and what services are there? Who are the community leaders and who are the key people who could be communicated with? Moving on from there is a need to explore the organisation's complexion. Who does the service see? Does this reflect the wider community picture? What is the make up of the staff? Are there areas of disparity or gaps in provision and how could these be addressed? What other groups or agencies exist? Do you work with these? Are there ways that working partnerships could be developed? How are decisions made in regard to service policy? Who is involved? Could this be altered to include representatives from various groups (including service users and carers?). The importance of user involvement is highlighted in contemporary government policy: http://www.doh.gov.uk/involvingpatients

How does the service make itself accessible? What kind of literature is available and in what format is this presented to service users? The importance of working with voluntary sector groups, especially in relation to Black and minority ethnic groups, cannot be overstated and has been highlighted in recent Government reports (Home Office, 1999).

Employment practice in substance misuse services

Knowledge of employment law in regard to discrimination is necessary for employers. It is also important for employees to be aware of their rights.

Employment and race

Positive action with regard to recruitment can be taken under the provision of Section 5 (2) (d) of the Race Relations Act 1976 (Home Office, 1976). This allows the appointment of a member of a particular ethnic group where the holder of the post provides services that promote the welfare of that ethnic group and where such services can be provided most effectively by someone from that group. Section 37 and 38 of the Race Relations Act provide opportunity for training to be given to members of ethnic groups who may be under-represented at all levels within services. Employment schemes such as the Modern Apprenticeship Project can assist with training potential staff members from a minority ethnic group. Recruitment can be enhanced by advertising posts in the Black and Asian press and by forging of links between services and community organisations. A recent amendment to the Race Relations Act (Home Office, 2000) extends protection against racial discrimination by public authorities and places a new, enforceable duty on them.

Employment and gender

Sections 47 and 48 of the Sexual Discrimination Act (Home Office, 1975, 1986) permit positive measures to be taken for the recruitment and training of women, to address female under-representation at any level within the workforce. Services can recognise the additional role of female employees as principal or sole carers for dependants within the home through appropriate human resource policies that make provision for paid absence in the event of child minder sickness, and other difficulties. Organisations also need to develop and implement policies that decrease threats to the personal safety of female staff.

Employment and disability

The Disability Discrimination Act (Home Office, 1995) requires employers to look at changes that might be made to working practices and environments to accommodate disabled employees. Disability refers to conditions of physical or sensory impairment, learning difficulty or psychological distress.

Organisational responses

Government policy

Government drug strategy states a commitment to ensuring that all problem drug misusers have proper access to services, specifically citing people from ethnic minorities and women (Home Office, 1998). To support this the United Kingdom Drugs Co-ordination Unit (UKADCU) has commissioned a review of current service provision. UKADCU have funded the Federation of Black Drug and Alcohol Workers to carry out a variety of tasks including the development of benchmarking and investigation into recruitment and retention of Black drug workers. An Anti-Drugs Race Issues Group has been set up. Results and recommendations will follow in 2001/2 (Home Office, 2001).

Race equality is also highlighted in the NHS Plan (Department of Health, 1999). The Plan requires the NHS to address local inequalities, to be measured and managed through the NHS Performance Assessment Framework. The importance of voluntary sector input specifically in relation to Black and minority ethnic groups has been highlighted (Home Office, 1999) and a commitment to new funding has been made. The Government proposes a code of good practice in relation to minority ethnic sectors, which should emphasise the realities of institutional racism, recognise the diversity of minority ethnic groups themselves, highlight the difficulties faced by newer minority ethnic communities, such as asylum seekers, avoid tokenism and incorporate the voices of women.

Policy development at service level

All services should develop and implement specific policies around anti-discriminatory practice, employment and training which reflect contemporary Government aims and best practice. Recognition is needed of the interplay of race, gender, ethnicity, age and sexuality on social inequalities.

The parameters of acceptable and unacceptable behaviour need to extend to all aspects of a service. This includes the behaviour of service users. Clients need to be informed of acceptable behaviour and told that discriminatory behaviour will not be tolerated.

Policies are ineffective without monitoring. Agencies need to have in place systems to monitor recruitment, career progression and termination of employment with regards to vulnerable populations. Standards exist for racial equality in Local Government (Commission for Racial Equality, 1995). These standards can be adapted to apply to the wider diversity agenda and the addiction services. An equality audit with specific levels of attainment allows the agency to:

1. Identify existing best practice and become an example of best practice in the way services are provided and monitored.
2. Highlight shortfalls in areas for the development of improvement and use monitoring and consultations to demonstrate clear improvements.
3. Determine short- and long-term priorities.
4. Establish staff development needs in relation to diversity and anti-discriminatory practice.
5. Embark on a planned programme of action and continuous improvement.
6. Produce a written diversity policy statement and ensure that policy is communicated to staff and service users.

Training and awareness

The focus of training needs to be contextual and broad, encompassing all aspects of discrimination. For institutional change to take place, real commitment on behalf of those who manage the system is vital. It is important that all employees participate. Sadly, the people who might benefit most from attending training are often those who consider themselves to be too well educated and 'open minded' to need to attend. It is these people who are most at risk of remaining unaware of their own hidden prejudices.

The type of training offered is important. Cultural awareness training highlights the differences between cultures, then uses an educational package to promote tolerance of those differences. Any assumption that this will lead to anti-discriminatory practice needs to be treated with caution. This approach tends to minimise the difficulties of defining culture and presents ethnicity and race as fixed categories rather than social constructs. Unless such training is placed in the context of racism it carries the risk that 'foreign' cultures are seen as exotic or less developed.

Training needs to go beyond simple definitions. It needs to be meaningful to those involved, encouraging participants to explore their own day-to-day experiences in a positive way.

Roles and responsibilities

Taking responsibility

Staff are employed at different levels within an organisation and therefore have different responsibilities in ensuring the provision of equitable, effective treatment to the communities they serve. This does not mean that leadership in anti-discriminatory practice is the remit only of senior staff. Addressing discriminatory practice requires courage and persistence at all levels. Institutional change cannot be achieved on an individual basis, but by raising discussion and working with similarly motivated staff, progress is achievable. It is important that practitioners are able to obtain support as the issues raised may be sensitive and have far-ranging consequences. If support is not available inside the organisation then external support should be offered. Practitioner responsibilities and organisation responsibilities may be summarised by the use of two acronyms, QUEST and PLOT (Figure 26.1).

Conclusion

Clear communication needs to exist between practitioners, service managers and higher level policy makers. A commitment to anti-discriminatory practice must mean more than lip service, or providing training or making statements of intent. True anti-discriminatory practice is proactive, dynamic and involves everyone. A fostering of political awareness amongst practitioners is vitally important, as it is they, not politicians, who translate national policy into day to day practice.

Practitioner responsibilities – QUEST

- Question existing practices and challenge discrimination.
- Understand and explore your own beliefs.
- Educate others.
- Seek support.
- Transfer of policy into action.

Organisational responsibilities – PLOT

- Policy development and evaluation.
- Lead by example.
- Offer support.
- Training should be made available for all staff.

Figure 26.1 Practitioner and organisation responsibilities

Notes

The use of the term 'Black' in this document refers to African-Caribbean, African, Asian, Chinese and other minority ethnic people who share a common experience of discrimination in Britain as a result of their colour or race/origin.

The authors would like to thank the Nilaari agency in Bristol for inspiring this chapter.

READER INPUT

(1) Assumptions and stereotypes. Consider the following statements:

- Crack is a Black drug.
- Asians don't have drug / alcohol problems
- Rastafarians have dreadlocks and smoke cannabis.
- Black drug users don't use available services because they don't inject heroin.

- How accurate do you think these statements are?
- Why do you think assumptions such as these develop?
- What are the dangers of maintaining such beliefs?
- Can you think of other assumptive statements in relation to gender, sexuality and age?

(None of the above are facts, they are opinions which re-enforce negative images and stereotypes.)

(2) Use of language

- Think about the words and phrases you use in everyday communication. Do you use language that could be perceived as discriminatory, either overtly or covertly? What can you do to change this? What alternatives could you use?
- Could you challenge discriminatory language used by another person? How could you do this and what issues might arise?
- How do you deal with discriminatory language if it is used by a client? How does it make you feel? Do you challenge this or accept it? If you don't challenge it, why not?

(3) Exploring diversity

- What information is available for service users? How is this made available (leaflets, posters, etc.)? Consider both the language and the images used. Do these reflect diversity in relation to ethnicity, gender, age, etc.?
- Is there any written material informing service users of the agency's approach towards anti-discriminatory practice?

- Is there any information on other community services or groups such as support groups for gay people, telephone helplines or information on educational courses?

(4) Putting policy into practice

- What policies exist in your workplace in regard to anti-discriminatory practice and diversity?
- What is your own and your colleagues' level of awareness of such policies?
- If policies exist, how are they put into action, monitored and evaluated?
- What support mechanisms exist in your work environment for challenging discrimination?

REFERENCES

Aslam, H., Bashir, C., Darrell, J., Patel, K. and Steele, C. (1998) *An Analysis of Present Drug Service Delivery to Black Communities in Greater Manchester*. Project Report March 1998.

Bristol Drugs Project (2000) *The Crack Report. A Picture of Crack Cocaine Use in Bristol in the 1990s*. Bristol Drugs Project, July.

Cabaj, R.P. (1989) 'Aids and chemical dependency: Special issues and treatment barriers for gay and bisexual men', *Journal of Psychoactive Drug* 21(4): 387–93.

Commission for Racial Equality (1995) *Racial Equality Means Quality*, London: CRE.

Commission for Racial Equality (2000) *Racial Equality and NHS Trusts. A Survey by the Commission for Racial Equality*. London: CRE.

Crisp, A.H., Gelder, M.G., Rix, S., Meltzer, H.I. and Rowlands, O.J. (2000) 'Stigmatisation of people with mental illnesses', *The British Journal of Psychiatry* 177(1): 4–7.

Department of Health (1999) *The Modernisation Plan for the NHS in London 1999–2002. NHS Executive*. London: HMSO.

Drugscope – *UK drug report (2000)*, London: Drugscope.

Esmail, A. and Carnall, D. (1997) 'Tackling racism in the NHS', *British Medical Journal* 314: 618.

Esmail, A., Everington, S. and Doyle, H. (1998) 'Racial discrimination in the allocation of distinction awards? Analysis of list of award holders by type of award, speciality and region', *British Medical Journal* 316: 193–5.

Fernando, S. (1991) *Mental Health, Race and Culture*, London: MIND.

Home Office (1975/1986) *Sexual Discrimination Act*, London: HMSO.

Home Office (1976) *Race Relations Act 1976*, London: HMSO.

Home Office (1995) *Disability Discrimination Act 1995*, London: HMSO.

Home Office (1998) *Tackling Drugs to Build a Better Britain: The Government's 10 year strategy for tackling drug misuse*, London: HMSO.

Home Office (1999) *Strengthening the Black and Minority Ethnic Voluntary Sector Infrastructure*, Home Office Active Community Unit. London: HMSO.

Home Office (2000) *Race Relations (Amendment) Act 2000*, London: HMSO.

Home Office (2001) *Race Equality in Public Services*. London: HMSO.

Macpherson, W. (1999) *The Steven Lawrence Inquiry. Report of an Inquiry by Sir William Macpherson of Cluny*, London: HMSO.

McGovern, D. and Hemmings, P. (1994) 'A follow-up of second generation Afro-Caribbeans and white British with a first admission diagnosis of schizophrenia:attitudes to mental illness and psychiatric services of patients and relatives', *Social Science and Medicine* 38: 117–27.

McKenzie, K. (1999) 'Something borrowed from the blues?' Editorial, *British Medical Journal* 318 (7184): 616–17.

Newcombe, R. (1993) 'Second class citizens – how drug users are disadvantaged and discriminated against', *Druglink* 8(2): 10–13.

Pfeffer, N. (1998) 'Theories of race, ethnicity and culture', *British Medical Journal* 317 (7169): 1381–4.

Rose, L. (1994) 'Homophobia among doctors', *British Medical Journal* 308: 586–7.

Skingle, T. (1997) 'Lesbian and gay injecting drug users: Discrimination within a discriminated community', *Mainliners Ltd. Newsletter*, October: 6.

Tyler, A. (1995) *Street Drugs* (3rd edn) London: Hodder and Stoughton.

CHAPTER 27

SUBSTANCE MISUSE AND OLDER PEOPLE

Kathryn Williamson

LEARNING OBJECTIVES

By the end of this chapter you should be able to identify:

1 Three physiological changes that may occur in the elderly which could impact on vulnerability to substance related problems.

2 Five possible clinical presentations that may occur with elderly substance misusers.

3 Some of the important factors in the screening and treatment of elderly substance misusers.

INTRODUCTION

The elderly are an often overlooked population in the field of substance misuse. This chapter examines the impact of substance misuse on the elderly, exploring issues which arise in relation to this including: reporting and diagnosis, screening, substances liable to misuse and the treatment of two of the most common substances of misuse – alcohol and benzodiazepines. The elderly should be considered a separate and specific group within the field of substance misuse for several reasons.

An increasing population

The effects of improved medical care, technology, living conditions, and the post-war 'baby boom' indicate a continued increase in the elderly cohort over time (Stoddard and Thompson, 1996). This is likely to lead to an increase in the absolute numbers of problem drinkers even if the prevalence of problem drinking remains constant.

Changing social norms

Women and alcohol

Changing social conventions making women drinkers more acceptable may lead to an increase in problems in this group; thus the female predominance in the elderly may no longer serve to limit the extent of the problem (Adams and Smith-Cox, 1995).

Illicit drug use

The prevalence rate of illicit drug use in the 'baby boomers', now reaching elderly status, remains higher than age matched cohorts in previous generations. Larger numbers of current drug users are expected to continue their habit as they reach 65 years (Patterson and Jeste, 1999). A significant increase in demand on the health service from the elderly group can be anticipated.

Physiological changes

Age related physiological changes make the elderly vulnerable to drug related problems.

- The volume of distribution may change as lean body mass falls and body fat increases. Water-soluble drugs, e.g. ethanol, thus have a smaller volume of distribution and fat-soluble, e.g. diazepam, tricyclic antidepressants, a greater volume.
- Plasma protein levels decrease, allowing more available free active drug at lower doses (Ticehurst, 1990).
- Altered drug elimination is probably the most important change. Reduced kidney function decreases elimination of drugs excreted by this route and the elimination of some drugs metabolised by the liver may also be reduced (Ghodse, 1997).

The overall effect of these changes is to increase the concentration of active drugs and enhance the possibility of toxicity.

REPORTING AND DIAGNOSIS

An under-reported issue

Substance misuse in the elderly is often under-reported, or missed (Naik and Jones, 1994). Historically, attention was diverted from the issue by the influence of Winick's 'maturing out of addiction' theory (Winick, 1962) and the work of Drew (1968). Both drug and alcohol problems were believed to reduce with age. Undeniably there is a general trend towards a decrease in substance abuse over the life span but this should not detract from its continued importance as an issue of later life. Both individual and professional factors may contribute to under-reporting.

The older individual may be more likely to feel that a stigma is attached to their habit, be prone to denial, and reluctant to answer questions. Cognitive problems may preclude them doing so accurately. Ageism and alienation of those who substance abuse lead to the elderly substance misuser being 'doubly stigmatised' (Greenwood, 2000). Relatives may attempt to deny a problem to safeguard the reputation of the family (Dunne, 1994). The elderly may be isolated from typical informants who would bring attention to a problem (Widner and Zeichner, 1991).

Diagnosis of substance misuse

Professionals are accused of a 'lack of enthusiasm', for taking alcohol histories in the elderly (Naik and Jones, 1994). A greater awareness is needed amongst medical staff of both drug and alcohol problems in the elderly. Naik's study showed a significantly less likelihood by the admitting doctor of recording an alcohol history where the patient was of a higher social class and older age. Clinicians need to bear in mind the 'atypical guises', in which the elderly present their abuse problem to medical, social, psychiatric and forensic services (Ticehurst, 1990). The following are all potential clinical presentations:

- frequent falls
- peptic ulceration
- depression
- psychoses
- confusion
- alcohol induced dementia
- incontinence
- poor self care
- nutritional deficiency
- adverse reaction to medication due to drug–drug, or drug–alcohol interaction.

The elderly are not easily considered as substance misusers, resulting in further professional and public bias and increasing their oversight. Professionals may feel 'the person only has a few years left. So let them enjoy themselves' (Dufour and Fuller, 1995), or may have a misguided belief that it is inappropriate to advise older people to change established habits (McInness and Powell, 1994). Adams *et al.* (1996) argue that time constraints and lack of training in screening techniques contribute to the professional neglect.

Screening the elderly

Substance misuse screening should be considered at all times when dealing with the elderly. Professionals need to bear in mind reluctance to divulge information by the patient. A quantitative clinical history should be elicited and, in the case of alcohol, an additional question asked regarding use of alcohol in tea or coffee – often mistakenly considered innocuous by elderly persons (Naik and Jones, 1994).

Standard screening methods

Standard screening tests may have low sensitivity amongst the elderly population (Naik *et al.*, 1995, Adams *et al.*, 1996). Luttrell *et al.* (1997) present a new screening questionnaire for specific use in the elderly as an alternative to these tests which were validated on a younger population. Naik *et al.* (1995) and Luttrell *et al.*'s (1997) studies also showed that the alcohol related laboratory investigations Mean Corpuscular Volume and Gamma GT have a lower sensitivity in older people.

Diagnostic dependence criteria

Diagnostic criteria such as the Diagnostic Statistical Manual (DSM) fail to take into account age-related differences in the pattern and consequences of substance misuse. Tolerance is likely to reduce in the elderly not increase. Tolerance, as a criterion, has thus been dropped from the fourth DSM edition. Disruption of social, occupational and recreational activities, and intoxication when expected to fulfil major role obligations are less obvious indicators of problems in the elderly age group. Atkinson (1990) suggested lowering the 'case' threshold by reducing the number of criteria necessary for diagnosis. A need for specialised operational criteria for the elderly has been identified (King *et al.*, 1994).

SUBSTANCES OF MISUSE

Alcohol

Safe drinking limits may need reconsideration as vulnerability to adverse effects of alcohol can occur even at lower levels of consumption (Dunne, 1994). Two types of elderly alcohol misusers are considered to exist:

1 'Early onset' individuals who begin misuse in young or middle age and continue into old age, are more likely to have a family history of alcohol misuse, history of smoking and a greater alcohol intake.
2 'Late onset' individuals are more likely to have an obvious precipitant for drinking, to be a reactive drinker, have a milder habit and greater psychological stability (Seymour and Wattis, 1992). It is estimated that a quarter to two-thirds of cases have their onset after the age of 60 years.

Atkinson (1994) reviews the question as to whether a different treatment response can be expected between these groups and states that little or no advantage is shown in treatment retention. However, the opinion that the late onset alcohol misuser responds particularly well to treatment is sustained in the literature. As a group the elderly have a good prognosis in treatment and thus an attitude of ageist therapeutic nihilism should be avoided.

Treatment of alcohol misuse

Age should not deter relevant help but is a consideration in planning treatment. In-patient treatment may be required for those with alcohol withdrawal symptoms since studies suggest more frequent complications with alcohol withdrawal in the elderly.

Particular attention should be paid to fluid and electrolyte imbalance and pre-existing medical conditions. Short-acting rather than long-acting benzodiazepines may be a prudent option, avoiding the risk of over-sedation. However, no drugs used in the withdrawal procedure have been studied in the elderly as a specific population (Kraemer *et al.*, 1999). Disulfiram may be dangerous in the elderly.

Treatment may include that of comorbid psychiatric disease. Age-related psychological and social stresses, e.g. grief, social isolation, need consideration. Provided that cognitive functioning does not hamper the intervention there is no reason why approaches such as motivational interviewing, cognitive behavioural therapy, etc. cannot be employed.

Over-the-counter misuse

Over-the-counter (OTC) drugs, frequently (misleadingly) viewed as cheap, accessible, and without harmful effects, are used more commonly in the elderly. Only 10 per cent of the general adult population use regular OTC drugs compared to 69 per cent of the elderly, a consumption pattern seven times greater than the young (Glantz and Backenheimer, 1988; Kofoed, 1985). The elderly are also the largest consumers of prescription medications, so the risk of drug interaction is high (Kofoed, 1985).

Cognitive problems may contribute to inadvertent misuse. The most thorough of doctors may not routinely question their elderly patients about OTC use and abuse may only become evident at a late stage when irreversible organ damage has occurred (e.g. aspirin nephropathy) or when dependence has developed. Clinicians need to maintain an 'index of suspicion', check informants histories, examine multiple sources of information, educate patients and offer proactive counselling to high risk groups, e.g. those with newly developed illness, somatisation disorders, chronic pain or insomnia and patients recovered from other drug dependencies (Kofoed, 1985).

Recently, the issue of potential tolerance and dependence consequent upon long-term use of weak opioid analgesics, e.g. Codydramol, was raised by Edwards and Salib (1999) and the term 'Silent Dependence Syndrome' in old age used to highlight the problem. Other classes of drugs involved in OTC abuse include laxatives, antihistamines, alcohol based liquid medicines and antacids.

Benzodiazepines

Prescription drug related problems are particularly important in the elderly but there is scanty epidemiological data on prescription drug abuse available. Common drugs associated with problems are sedative/hypnotics and opioid analgesics (Jinks and Raschko, 1990; Finlayson and Davis, 1994).

Benzodiazepines are the most frequently prescribed within the sedative/ hypnotic group and the elderly are particularly susceptible to their adverse effects (Juergens, 1993; Closser, 1991). Benzodiazepines are often prescribed on a long-term basis. Populations such as those in residential/ nursing homes receive a high proportion of psychoactive drugs of a sedative nature (Ghodse, 1997). In the elderly, large doses of benzodiazepines are often prescribed with minimal follow up (Shorr *et al.*, 1990), yet related problems of benzodiazepine use are proportionally greater in the elderly.

Increased central nervous system sensitivity to the drugs, less efficient metabolism leading to accumulation, slower washout and persistence of sedation after discontinuation (Closser, 1991) predisposes the elderly person to toxicity. Use or misuse of benzodiazepines may masquerade as age related medical illness. Toxicity may be subtle and defining drug-related problems in those receiving therapeutic doses is more difficult. (Jeurgens, 1993).

Drug related cognitive problems include forgetfulness, altered attention, impaired new learning, sedation and drowsiness (Ghodse, 1997; Jeurgens, 1993; Closser, 1991). Benzodiazepines may exacerbate a dementing illness or cause misdiagnoses of such, so called 'iatrogenic pseudodementia' (Closser, 1991). Withdrawal of benzodiazepines from the elderly has been shown to improve short-term memory in nursing home residents (Salzman *et al.*, 1992). Behavioural disinhibition is more common in the elderly using benzodiazepines (Jeurgens, 1993). Drug related psychomotor problems include ataxia, with resultant increased risk of hip fracture and impaired driving skills (Closser, 1991).

Benzodiazepine withdrawal

Although there is a high prevalence of chronic benzodiazepine use in the elderly, little is known about withdrawal in this population (Schweizer *et al.*, 1989). The limited literature suggests that withdrawal of benzodiazepines in the elderly differs in its intensity and form. Studies show that older, less anxious individuals tolerate gradual withdrawal at least as well as the young, the symptoms of withdrawal are less severe, and depression, anxiety, agitation, irritability and insomnia do not increase in the withdrawal period (Schweizer *et al.*, 1989; Salzman *et al.*, 1992). Abrupt withdrawal, however, in the elderly, has been linked to acute confusional states (Foy *et al.*, 1986). A reduced rate of elimination and consequent slower decline in plasma levels of benzodiazepines ('self-taper') during withdrawal, in association with less rebound reactivity of the neurological system, are speculated to contribute to the clinical differences (Schweizer *et al.*, 1989). Benzodiazepines should only be prescribed with caution, using minimal doses over short periods of time and with adequate medical supervision during the period of use.

Illicit drug misuse

Illicit drug use in the elderly is relatively uncommon. Most cases represent a continuation of a habit from younger age. Young opiate users may die or mature out of addiction, but there is a group that maintains the habit into old age and of which we know little (Ghodse, 1997). A case has been reported of a late onset 'crack' cocaine dependence in a 64-year-old man (Nambudiri and Young, 1991). Illicit drug misuse in the elderly may become more of a problem as existing users graduate into older age groups and as availability increases for all.

Conclusion and recommendations

Within the field of general psychiatry, the elderly are treated as a definite sub-specialty with dedicated services and staff. However, substance misuse services do not make this distinction and have not been planned with attention to the specific needs of this group. Issues surrounding the need of age specific treatment compared to 'mainstreaming' of services remains a topic of debate.

Practitioners working with this client group need to have an awareness of the following issues:

- **Cultural awareness** – practitioners should retain a sensitivity to the elderly person's cultural issues, beliefs and values, recognising that these may differ from other, younger clientele. This may be especially important in relation to the way that health messages are transmitted, i.e. literature and images such as posters, etc. and in the use of language and touch.
- **Self-awareness** – practitioners should reflectively explore their own preconceptions around the elderly. Similarly, there is a need to recognise the elderly person's preconceptions which may influence interaction.
- **Anti-discriminatory practice** – closely linked to self-awareness, there is a need to strive for an anti-discriminatory approach to care both as individual practitioners and on an organisational level.
- **Communication** – good communication skills are needed, especially if the elderly person is hard of hearing, has poor sight, expressive or cognitive difficulties. Comprehension should be checked to ensure the client

understands. It may be appropriate to use written material as well as verbal information given to encourage health messages.

- **Settings** – the place of assessment requires consideration, both in terms of the mix of clientele and the physical surroundings, which may cause an elderly person difficulty. Home visits or visits at an agreed site such as the GP surgery may be preferable for the elderly.
- **Training need** – substance misuse practitioners unused to working with this group may also require assistance or training in other aspects of elderly health such as specific physical or mental health issues. Similarly elderly care practitioners may need training in issues around substance misuse. Awareness raising of services and good working relationships can encourage practitioners to seek appropriate advice and help.
- **The facilitative role of the practitioner** – multiagency working with other statutory and non-statutory agencies may enable the elderly person to access help in other areas of their lives which may ultimately impact on their substance misuse. Voluntary groups such as Alcoholics Anonymous may replace missing social structures and offer a circle of support and friendship. The practitioner has a role in facilitating clients in contacting other agencies and community groups. The practitioner may also have a facilitative and educational role in working with the client's family and other health and social care professionals.

The area of substance abuse within the elderly age group is not a subject that workers in the field of health and social care can afford to ignore. Evidence suggests a growing problem with a need for both greater education to raise awareness and a need for an increase in the recently published literature base. Prudent future organisation and planning of services cannot be achieved without specific regard to the elderly population.

READER INPUT

Questions

(1) What factors may impact on increasing levels of substance misuse in the elderly population?

(2) What reasons might exist for under-reporting of substance misuse in the elderly? How could these be dealt with? (Think not only of the one-to-one clinical relationship but also consider the potential of larger-scale health promotion issues, cultural aspects, the media, etc.)

(3) What physical or psychological symptoms might an elderly substance misuser present to their GP with? What kind of misdiagnoses may occur?

Discussion points

(a) It is suggested that professionals may lack enthusiasm for raising the issue of substance misuse in the elderly. Why might this be the case and how can this be addressed?

(b) What impact might the family have on the assessment, diagnosis and treatment of elderly substance misusers? What issues does this raise and how might these be addressed?

FURTHER READING

Dufour, M. and Fuller, R.K. (1995) 'Alcohol in the elderly', *Annual Review of Medicine* 46: 123–32.

Finlayson, R.E. (1995) 'Misuse of prescription drugs', *The International Journal of Addictions*, 30 (13&14): 1871–901.

REFERENCES

Adams, W.L., Barry, K.L. and Fleming, M.F. (1996) 'Screening for problem drinking in older primary care patients', *Journal of the American Medical Association* 276(24): 1964–7.

Adams, W.L. and Smith Cox N. (1995) 'Epidemiology of problem drinking among elderly people', *The International Journal of the Addictions* 30(13/14): 1693–716.

Atkinson, R.M. (1990) 'Aging and alcohol use disorder: diagnostic issues in the elderly', *International Psychogeriatrics* 2(1): 55–72.

Atkinson, R.M. (1994) 'Late onset problem drinking in older adults', *International Journal of Geriatric Psychiatry* 9(4): 321–6.

Closser, M.H. (1991) 'Benzodiazepines and the elderly. A review of potential problems', *Journal of Substance Abuse Treatment* 8(1–2): 35–41.

Drew, L.R.H. (1968) 'Alcoholism as a self-limiting disease', *Quarterly Journal of Studies on Alcohol* 29(4): 956–67.

Dufour, M. and Fuller R.K (1995) 'Alcohol in the elderly', *Annual Review of Medicine* 46: 123–32.

Dunne, F.J. (1994) 'Misuse of alcohol or drugs by elderly people', *British Medical Journal*, 308 (6929): 608–9.

Edwards, I. and Salib, E. (1999) ' "Silent dependence syndrome" in old age', *International Journal of Geriatric Psychiatry* 14(1): 72–4.

Finlayson, R.E. and Davis, L.J. (1994) 'Prescription drug dependence in the elderly population: demographic and clinical features of 100 inpatients', *Mayo Clinical Proceedings* (12): 1137–45.

Foy, A., Drinkwater, V., March, S. and Mearrick, P. (1986) 'Confusion after admission to hospital in elderly patients using benzodiazepines', *British Medical Journal* 293 (6554): 1072.

Ghodse, A.H. (1997) 'Substance misuse by the elderly', *British Journal of Hospital Medicine*, 58(9): 451–3.

Glantz, M.D. and Backenheimer, M.S. (1988) 'Substance abuse among elderly women', *Clinical Gerontologist* 8(1): 3–26.

Greenwood, J. (2000) 'Stigma: substance misuse in older people', *Geriatric Medicine* 30(4): 43–5.

Jinks, M.J. and Raschko, R.R. (1990) 'A profile of alcohol and prescription drug abuse in a high risk community based elderly population', *Annals of Pharmacotherapy* 24: 971–5.

Juergens, S.M. (1993) 'Problems with benzodiazepines in elderly patients', *Mayo Clinical Proceedings* 68(8): 818–20.

King, C.J., Van Hasselt, V.B., Segal, D.L. and Hersen, M. (1994) 'Diagnoses and assessment of substance abuse in older adults: current strategies and issues', *Addictive Behaviours* 19(1): 44–55.

Kofoed, L.L. (1985) 'OTC drug overuse in the elderly: what to watch for', *Geriatrics* 40(10): 55–9.

Kraemer, K.L., Conigliaro, J. and Saitz, R. (1999) 'Managing alcohol withdrawal in the elderly', *Disease Management* 14(6): 409–25.

Luttrell, S., Watkin, V., Livingston, G., Walker, Z., D'Ath, P., Patel, P., Sukhiwinder, S., Dain, A., Bielawska, C. and Katona, C. (1997) 'Screening for alcohol misuse in older people', *International Journal of Geriatric Psychiatry* 12(12): 1151–4.

McInnes, E. and Powell, J. (1994) 'Drug and alcohol referrals: are elderly substance abuse diagnoses and referrals being missed?', *British Medical Journal* 308: 444–6.

Naik, P.C. and Jones, R.G. (1994) 'Alcohol histories taken from elderly people on admission', *British Medical Journal* 308 (6923): 248.

Naik, P.C., Jones, R.G. and Lilley, J. (1995) 'How can we detect sick elderly excessive drinkers?' *International Journal of Geriatric Psychiatry* 10(12): 1063–6.

Nambudiri, D.E. and Young, R.C. (1991) 'A case of late-onset crack dependence and subsequent psychosis in the elderly', *Journal of Substance Abuse Treatment* 8(4): 253–5.

Patterson, T.L. and Jeste, D.V. (1999) 'The potential impact of the baby-boom generation on substance abuse among elderly persons', *Mental Health and Aging* 50(9): 1184–9.

Salzman, C., Fisher, J., Nobel, K., Glassman, R., Wolfson, A. and Kelley, M. (1992) 'Cognitive improvement following benzodiazepine discontinuation in elderly nursing home residents', *International Journal of Geriatric Psychiatry* 7(2): 89–93.

Schweizer, E., Case, W.G. and Rickels, K. (1989) 'Benzodiazepine dependence and withdrawal in elderly patients', *American Journal of Psychiatry* 146(4): 529–31.

Seymour, J. and Wattis, J.P. (1992) 'Alcohol abuse in the elderly', *Reviews in Clinical Gerontology* 2(2): 141–50.

Shorr, R.I., Bauwens, G.F., Landfeld, C.S. (1990) 'Failure to limit quantities of benzodiazepine hypnotic drugs for outpatients: placing the elderly at risk', *American Journal of Medicine* 89(6): 725–32.

Stoddard, C. and Thompson, D.L. (1996) 'Alcohol and the elderly: special concerns for counselling professionals', *Alcoholism Treatment Quarterly* 14(4): 5969.

Ticehurst, S. (1990) 'Alcohol and the elderly', *Australian and New Zealand Journal of Psychiatry* 24(2): 252–60.

Widner, S. and Zeichner, A. (1991) 'Alcohol abuse in the elderly: review of epidemiology research and treatment', *Clinical Gerontologist* 11(1): 3–18.

Winick, C. (1962) 'Maturing out of narcotic addiction', *Bulletin on Narcotics* 14 (Jan–Mar): 1–7.

CHAPTER 28

ANABOLIC ANDROGENIC STEROID MISUSERS

Precilla Choi

LEARNING OBJECTIVES

After you have studied this chapter you will be able to demonstrate an understanding of:

1 What Anabolic Androgenic Steroids are and how they work.

2 What the physiological and psychological side effects can be.

3 Some of the implications this has for practice.

INTRODUCTION

Although there are many kinds of sporting performance enhancement drugs, the focus of this chapter is on one specific type – Anabolic Androgenic Steroids. Research has revealed that the misuse of Anabolic Androgenic Steroids is not limited to the elite athlete – they are now being misused by recreational exercisers, adults and adolescents, male and female (Choi, 1993).

Steroid use has relevance for practitioners in a variety of fields, from substance misuse to general practice and psychiatry to social work. Physical and psychological effects and side effects may lead to individuals presenting to services with a variety of needs which when investigated may uncover steroid use. Since the late 1980s those working within the field of substance misuse have had significant exposure to this client group.

HISTORY, THEORY AND THE EVIDENCE BASE

Historical background

Historical analysis reveals that the use of substances to improve performance has been prevalent throughout time. From ancient Greek athletes, Roman gladiators and medieval knights and throughout modern history, many examples can be found. Traditionally substances used tended to be stimulants and this continued into the twentieth century with amphetamines and other stimulants (i.e. caffeine and cocaine) used widely, especially in the 1960s. These drugs were usually used on the day of performance. However, in the 1950s, a new class of drugs emerged – Anabolic Androgenic Steroids – that could be used prior to the sporting event giving athletes significant advantages. Predominantly used by strength athletes (weightlifters and bodybuilders) eventually they became popular amongst track and field and other athletes. Their continued popularity is evident from the regular press reports of alleged use by elite level athletes since the Ben Johnson affair at the 1988 Olympics.

What are Anabolic Androgenic Steroids and how are they misused?

Anabolic Androgenic Steroids are a family of drugs comprising the male sex hormone testosterone and various synthetic analogues (not to be confused with corticosteroids prescribed for conditions such as allergic reactions and sports injuries). Developed to promote general body growth (anabolic effect) whilst minimising masculinisation (androgenic effect) and available in both oral and injectable form, Anabolic Androgenic Steroids are generally prescribed to patients with muscle wasting diseases or men unable to produce enough testosterone themselves. In recent years, research into the efficacy of these drugs as a male contraceptive pill has been initiated.

Since the 1950s increasing numbers of athletes have used steroids to increase muscle mass, strength and power. By enhancing the body's use of protein, enabling the muscles to recover more quickly, the athlete can train longer and harder. Taking steroids without taking part in a weightlifting programme and without a diet of adequate protein is unlikely to have the effect athletes desire. In medical disorders for which they are prescribed dosages are within the normal range recommended by the drug manufacturer. In steroid misuse, it is not uncommon for the dosages to be much greater. The amount of androgen (testosterone) produced naturally by male testes is 4–10 mg/day. Some reports suggest that some individuals administer 100 mg/day (Choi *et al.*, 1989). Several steroids may be taken simultaneously, again at high doses – this is known as 'stacking'. Veterinary products are sometimes used too. Misuse tends to be cyclical, continuing for several weeks or months, followed by a period of abstinence in order to give the body a break. This can however be variable from person to person.

Physical effects and side effects

Most, but not all, of the numerous short-term side effects are reversible on cessation. Steroid misuse is known to have effects on the following systems of the male body (Sturmi and Diorio, 1998):

System	Effect
Reproductive	Reduced sperm count, decreased testicular size, changes to libido.
Neuroendocrine	Alterations to various hormone levels, such as pituitary hormones and the body's own testosterone and oestrogen.
Gastrointestinal	Jaundice, other changes to liver function that could lead to liver disorders and cancer.
Cardiovascular	Decreased HDL cholesterol (the good one), elevated blood pressure, changes to heart muscle, all leading to an increased risk of heart disease.
Immune	Poor immune function as a result of reductions in antibodies that are required to fight off viruses.
Dermatology	Acne, hair loss from head.
Musculoskeletal	Alterations to bones, ligaments and tendons.

Gynaecomastia (the growth of breast tissue in men) is not reversible upon cessation but can be corrected surgically. Gynaecomastia develops as a result of the body's own natural production of testosterone shutting down when synthetic testosterone is being taken (also the cause of testicular atrophy and reduced sperm count). As a result the body's natural oestrogen is unopposed leading to breast development. Bodybuilders often use an anti-oestrogen drug called Nolvadex (used to treat breast cancer and infertility in women) whilst taking steroids because it is perceived to prevent gynaecomastia. However, without controlled trials in this client group, it is not yet known how effective Nolvadex is in the prevention of steroid related gynaecomastia.

Infertility has been thought to be reversible but a number of recent case histories indicate otherwise. Lloyd *et al.* (1996) reported five cases of low or absent sperm count still present between six and twelve months after cessation of steroids. Turek *et al.* (1995) reported a case where the patient still had no sperm five years after cessation.

Other long-term effects such as heart disorders, cancers and thrombosis can only be surmised, but recent deaths of known former misusers have been attributed to steroid related disorders. Long-term controlled research studies are required in order to know for sure, but methodologically this is impossible (see discussion below) so we can only continue to speculate.

Women

In women misusers (of whom there are far fewer than men), there are additional side effects, some irreversible. Because women have lower levels of natural testosterone the misuse of steroids can cause masculinisation. This has been seen in clinical studies where female patients on normal doses of therapy have experienced deepening of the voice, facial hair growth, extension of pubic hair and hypertrophy of the clitoris (Strauss *et al.*, 1993). Additionally, menstrual cessation or irregularity and increased libido have been reported (Korkia *et al.*, 1996). Again, however, there has not been enough research on female steroid misusers to be conclusive about the side effects.

Psychological effects

The earliest research concerning the behavioural effects of Anabolic Androgenic Steroids comes from studies where these drugs were used for medical disorders (Kibble and Ross, 1987). Changes such as increased aggressiveness, diminished fatigue, changed libido and mood swings have been reported, all dissipating when drug taking ceases. Such changes are not normally of a serious nature. One cannot, however, extrapolate these findings to steroid misuse because the patients in these studies were taking the normal recommended dose. Since the late 1980s and throughout the 1990s, a large body of scientific evidence has been generated which consistently shows behavioural changes associated with non-medical misuse. These changes can be marked and alarming. Aggression, psychotic episodes, mania and violence (physical assault, attempted murder and murder) have been linked to non-medical steroid misuse (Pope and Katz, 1998). In addition a wide range of other psychological symptoms have been documented including:

Delusions	*Reduced concentration*	*Negativity*
Hallucinations	*Confusion*	*Mood changes*
Suspiciousness	*Forgetfulness*	*Paranoia*
Anxiety	*Depression*	*Increased sex drive*

Methodological difficulties and research limitations

It must be emphasised that whilst research is consistent in finding that behaviour change accompanies steroid misuse, it is not conclusive that the drugs cause these changes. Firstly, a small number of studies have found no changes and secondly, and most importantly, the vast majority of studies have not been double-blind placebo controlled trials (the gold standard of medical science). To conduct such a trial using the huge doses that most misusers employ would be ethically difficult.

Most studies have been retrospective self-report studies with participants asked to recall how they felt at the time of taking steroids. Such memories may not be reliable. Respondents may also have lied. Because of the social undesirability of some behaviours, particularly in relation to violence towards wives/girlfriends (Choi and Pope, 1994) under-reporting might have resulted. It is possible that reported aggression reflects the normal behaviour of the research participants. However, this was not found to be the case by Choi and Pope (1994) who reported that of those who were violent towards their wife/girlfriend while on steroids, half were also violent off-drug, though to a lesser degree. The other half had not been violent at all. This implies that it is not just those individuals who are usually aggressive who behave violently on steroids.

Other limitations identified in Choi and Pope's study are that as the participants were knowingly taking steroids within a gymnasium subculture their expectations may have influenced behaviour. It was not possible to document accurately which steroids and what dosages were taken by the participants as they are obtained illicitly. This has several implications:

1 Participants may be taking steroids different from those they believe they purchased (Choi, *et al.*, 1990).
2 Unknown to the participants, counterfeit preparations will almost certainly have been taken (Malone *et al.*, 1995; Pope and Katz, 1994).
3 The effects of other drugs will not have been accounted for. Most misusers take other substances to enhance performance (Perry *et al.*, 1992).

In summary, there is now substantial evidence that shows behaviour change accompanying steroid misuse that is not present when steroids are not and which shows that behaviour tends to be more pervasive when the misuser is stacking high doses. However, research cannot *conclusively* tell us that these changes are *caused* by steroids although there are indications that they play a part. For example, high dose animal studies have found increased aggression (Rubinow and Schmidt, 1996; Melloni *et al.*, 1997). One recent double-blind placebo controlled human study of fairly high (but not 'misuse') doses has also shown significant effects (Pope *et al.*, 2000). However, another similar study did not find psychological changes (Tricker *et al.*, 1996). Further research is needed to ascertain the reliability of findings. Also needing consideration are the contexts and situations in which associated violence and aggression might occur. Sharpe and Collins (1998) point out it is probably through a biopsychosocial interaction that behavioural effects occur – that is, the pharmacological effect of the drug, the psychology of the individual and the social context/environment operating together.

Misuse of other drugs

Steroid misusers may take other substances, including diuretics to enhance muscle definition and counteract fluid retention (a side effect of steroids), Thyroxine to speed up metabolism and aid fat loss, and Nolvadex to prevent gynaecomastia (Perry *et al.*, 1992). There have been reports of dependency on the opiate 'Nubain' (nalbuphine hydrochloride) amongst bodybuilding steroid users (McBride *et al.*, 1996).

In addition to the above polypharmacy, two other non-steroid drugs need to be mentioned as they are, or have been, also popular with steroid misusers: Human Chorionic Gonadotropin (hCG) and Human Growth Hormone (hGH). hCG mimics the action of two pituitary hormones known as follicular stimulating hormone (FSH) and lutenising hormone (LH) – chemical triggers that tell the (male) body to release natural testosterone. In women hCG triggers ovulation. hCG is popular amongst steroid misusing athletes (including bodybuilders) as it is undetectable by the drug tests employed by sporting federations. It is often taken at the end of a steroid cycle to boost the body's natural testosterone production that will have been shut down by steroids.

hGH is one of the major hormones influencing growth and development, interacting in complex ways with many other hormones and brain chemicals. Because of this, its precise effect is difficult to specify and evaluate. The most obvious action is that it stimulates growth in pre-adolescents. A deficit will result in dwarfism. It is also thought to have effects on muscle growth hence the interest in it by strength athletes. More recently this drug has fallen out of favour as it has not been found to be as effective as Anabolic Androgenic Steroids.

PRACTICAL IMPLICATIONS

A 'different' client group

Coincidental with the growth in steroid misuse in the 1980s was the establishment of needle exchange schemes to prevent the spread of HIV amongst intravenous drug users. A large number of needle exchange clients (anecdotal evidence indicates between one-third and one-half) were steroid misusers. Whilst this was (and is) to be encouraged as equipment sharing amongst injecting steroid misusers carries risks of HIV, Hepatitis B and C, it did provide challenges for those not trained to work with this client group, the major challenge being that steroid misusers do not see themselves as similar to intravenous drug users. Indeed, they are often less informed about injecting technique. Steroids are injected intramuscularly, not intravenously, and clients require larger needles/syringes suitable for injecting oil based steroids.

Steroid misusers are also different to 'traditional' drug users in that they lead healthy lifestyles with high levels of physical exercise, careful diet and low levels of other (legal and illegal) drug use. As a result, they tend to look and feel fit and healthy. Looking and feeling healthy can mean a denial of the potential health risks of misuse. Perry *et al.* (1992) suggest that in addition to counselling on potential side effects, liver function tests, cholesterol, urea and electrolytes, full blood count and blood pressure measurements should be taken so that:

> If the individuals concerned can then see the biochemically adverse effects, it may assist in future abstinence or reduction of dosage or the number of drugs in the stack at any one time. Doctors should stress that because the individual feels and looks well, this does not necessarily equate with total body health.
>
> (Perry *et al.*, 1992: 261)

Another implication of self-perceived difference is that the steroid misuser does not accept that they are drug abusing. The oft heard reply to questioning is: 'I don't take drugs' (Choi, 1993). As a result of this attitude, there can be a reluctance to go to a needle exchange because it means associating with 'traditional' clientele. This is an important issue for needle exchange schemes whose philosophy is harm minimisation.

McBride *et al.* (1998) suggest a variety of aspects pertinent to service provision and practice including:

1 **Philosophy** – based around harm reduction, user friendliness and staff willingness to learn.
2 **Staffing** – a tripartite service including primary care, substance misuse services and sports medicine may provide the optimum response.
3 **Setting** – gym based settings may not be appropriate. Existing service settings may be utilised, perhaps using specific times separate from other clinics.
4 **Information and needle exchange** – there is a need for accurate, contemporary information. This requires close working with clients to identify trends and staff who are proactive in enhancing their knowledge base. Information on safer injecting and needle exchange facilities, particularly for intramuscular steroid use should be available, along with safer sex information.
5 **Psychological tests** – self-completion tests for aggression, anxiety and depression may provide objective feedback on psychological changes during times 'on' steroids and 'off'.
6 **Physiological measures and laboratory testing** – again for objective feedback and monitoring of deleterious effects and to enable timely responses to physical disorder.
7 **Training and dietary advice** – steroids work best for those who eat and train appropriately. Clients should be directed towards clear, expert, advice relevant to their sport and alternatives to drug use considered.

The above can be combined with a motivational interviewing approach (see Chapter 6) enabling the client to make informed decisions around their steroid misuse. Other interventions which may be useful include anger management, social skills/relationship work and work around self-image and esteem.

Dependency

One final issue which has important implications for treatment is the addictive potential of steroids. Whether or not dependence can occur has been the subject of considerable scientific debate and the answer often varies according to the definition of dependence that is used. However, a number of case histories have demonstrated that withdrawal symptoms can result upon cessation. These tend to be depressive in nature and accompanied by cravings (Brower, 1993a). Other evidence such as surveys and self-report studies of strength athletes have shown that many steroid misusers do meet DSM criteria for dependence and experience withdrawal symptoms (Brower, 1993a). These studies suffer from the same methodological issues mentioned earlier concerning the behavioural effects of misuse. Nonetheless, for the clinician the potential mechanisms of dependence are important considerations. These could be through positive reinforcement (perceived positive consequences such as improved body image) or negative reinforcement (avoidance of withdrawal symptoms) or a combination of both involving physiological and psychological features together. Discussions of treatment issues can be found in Brower (1992), Brower (1993a) and Brower (1993b).

Conclusion

The misuse of Anabolic Androgenic Steroids amongst recreational exercisers has grown over the last two decades with considerable public health implications. It is generally accepted that steroid misuse has wide-ranging medical effects. In addition, evidence indicates that substantial behaviour change can accompany misuse, although the causal mechanisms for this remain inconclusive. Undoubtedly biopsychosocial interactions are central in determining the behavioural effects and addictive potential of steroids, but determining the nature of these interactions remains a major challenge for the biomedical, health and social sciences. In the meantime, the challenge for practitioners is to meet the needs of this client group in a proactive and responsive way.

READER INPUT

Case scenario

Joe is a 24-year-old bodybuilder who has recently started attending the needle exchange. He has been training regularly for three years and this year has decided to enter a few competitions. He has used anabolic steroids previously but in tablet form only. Now he's decided to try using injectables. You notice he has a black eye, the result of a fight last weekend. He admits he has got into a few fights recently and has received a written warning from his employer at the night-club where he works as a doorman. He is a little worried about this: 'I don't know why but I just lost it. I'm not normally like that.' He puts some of his irritation down to relationship difficulties with his partner, Gail. Their sexual relationship has deteriorated of late: 'I'm just too tired these days with working late and everything'. He strongly suspects Gail may be having an affair though she vehemently denies this. He admits he has taken to listening in on her phone calls and occasionally following her when she goes out. His physical health is usually good though lately he's had a few days' sickness – nothing much, just feeling generally unwell, dizzy and slightly light-headed at times. Joe puts this down to fighting off a virus. You think his skin tone and the whites of his eyes look a little yellow/orange in colour. He's got few stains on the front of his sweatshirt. 'Had a nosebleed when I was training', he explains.

(1) What kind of advice could you give along with the injecting equipment that Joe has come to collect?
(2) What might the implications of Joe's dizzy spells and nosebleeds be and how could you check this out?

(3) What kind of questions could you ask Joe about his steroid use?
(4) Why might Joe's relationship problems be connected with his steroid use?
(5) Why should you be concerned about Joe's sallow complexion and discoloured eye whites and what should you do to explore this further?
(6) What are the indications that Joe might be experiencing psychological side effects?
(7) What interventions could you employ in working with Joe in the future?
(8) You are aware that the local gym has several steroid misusers, how could you develop the service to encourage more steroid misuers to get in contact with you? Do you see how Joe could play a part in this?

FURTHER READING

Choi, P.Y.L. (1993) 'The alarming effects of anabolic steroids', *The Psychologist* 6 (pt 6): 258–60.
Choi, P.Y.L., Pope, H.G. (1994) 'Violence towards women and illicit Androgenic-anabolic steroid use', *Annals of Clinical Psychiatry* 6, 21–5.
Mottram, D.R. (1996) *Drugs in Sport* (2nd edn) London: E&FN Spon.
Sharp, M. and Collins, D. (1998) 'Exploring the "inevitability" of the relationship between anabolic-Androgenic steroid use and aggression in human males', *Journal of Sport & Exercise Psychology* 20: 379–94.
Sturmi, J.E. and Diorio, D.J. (1998) 'Anabolic agents', *Sports Pharmacology* 17(2): 261–82.
Yesalis, C.E. (1993) *Anabolic Steroids in Sport and Exercise*, Champaign, IL: Human Kinetics.

REFERENCES

Brower, K.J. (1992) 'Clinical assessment and treatment of anabolic steroid users', *Psychiatric Annals* 22: 35–40.
Brower, K.J. (1993a) 'Anabolic steroids: potential for physical and psychological dependence', in C.E. Yesalis (ed.) *Anabolic Steroids in Sport and Exercise*, Champaign, IL: Human Kinetics.
Brower, K.J. (1993b) 'Assessment and treatment of anabolic steroid withdrawal', in C.E. Yesalis (ed.) *Anabolic Steroids in Sport and Exercise*, Champaign, IL: Human Kinetics.
Choi, P.Y.L. (1993) 'The alarming effects of anabolic steroids', *The Psychologist*, 6 (pt 6): 258–60.
Choi, P.Y.L, Parrott, A.C. and Cowan, D. (1989) 'Adverse behavioural effects of anabolic steroids in athletes: a brief review', *Clinical Sports Medicine* 1: 183–7.
Choi, P.Y.L., Parrott, A.C. and Cowan, D. (1990) 'High dose anabolic steroids in athletes: effects upon hostility and aggression', *Human Psychopharmacology* 5: 349–56.
Choi, P.Y.L. and Pope, H.G. (1994) 'Violence towards women and illicit Androgenic-anabolic steroid use', *Annals of Clinical Psychiatry* 6: 21–5.
Kibble, M. and Ross, M.B. (1987) 'Anabolic steroids drug review', *Clinical Pharmacy* 6: 686–92.

Korkia, P., Lenehan, P. and McVeigh, J. (1996) 'Non-medical use of androgens among women', *Journal of Performance Enhancing Drugs* 1: 71–6.

Lloyd, F.H., Powell, P., Murdoch, A.P. (1996) 'Anabolic steroid abuse by bodybuilders and male subfertility', *British Medical Journal* 313: 100–1.

McBride, A.J., Williamson, K. and Petersen, T. (1996) 'Three cases of nalbuphine hydrochloride dependence associated with anabolic steroid use', *British Journal of Sports Medicine* 30: 69–70.

McBride, A.J., Petersen, T. and Williamson, K. (1998) 'Working with Androgenic anabolic steroid users', in M. Bloor and F. Wood (eds) *Addictions and Problem Drug Use: Issues in Behaviour, Policy and Practice. Research Highlights in Social Work 33*. London: Jessica Kingsley.

Malone, D.A., Diemeff, R., Lombardo, J.A. and Simple, B.R.H. (1995) 'Psychiatric effects and psychoactive substance use in anabolic Androgenic steroid users', *Clin J Sports Med* 5: 25–31.

Melloni, R.H., Connor, D.F., Xuan Hang, P.T., Harrison, R.J. and Ferris, C.F. (1997) 'Anabolic-androgenic steroid exposure during adolescence and aggressive behaviour in golden hamsters', *Physiology & Behaviour* 6(3): 359–64.

Perry, H.M., Wright, D. and Littlepage, B.N.C. (1992) 'Dying to be big: a review of anabolic steroid use', *British Journal of Sports Medicine* 26(4): 259–61.

Pope, H.G. and Katz, D.L. (1994) 'Psychiatric effects of anabolic steroids: a controlled study', *Archives of General Psychiatry* 51: 375–82.

Pope, H.G. and Katz, D.L. (1998) 'Psychiatric effects of exogenous anabolic-androgenic steroids', in O.M. Wolkowitz and A.J. Rothschild (eds) *Psychoneuroendocrinology for the Clinician*, Washington DC: American Psychiatric Association.

Pope, H.G., Kouri, E.M. and Hudson, J.I. (2000) 'Effects of supraphysiologic doses of testosterone on mood and aggression in normal men', *Archives of General Psychiatry* 57: 133–40.

Rubinow, D.R. and Schmidt, P.J. (1996) 'Androgens, brain and behaviour', *American Journal of Psychiatry* 153(8): 974–84.

Sharp, M. and Collins, D. (1998) 'Exploring the "inevitability" of the relationship between anabolic-androgenic steroid use and aggression in human males', *Journal of Sport & Exercise Psychology* 20: 379–94.

Strauss, R.H. and Yesalis, C.E. (1993) 'Additional effects of anabolic steroids on women', in C. E. Yesalis (ed.) *Anabolic Steroids in Sport and Exercise*, Champaign, IL: Human Kinetics.

Sturmi, J.E. and Diorio, D.J. (1998) 'Anabolic agents', *Sports Pharmacology* 17(2): 261–82.

Tricker, R., Casaburi, R., Storer, T.W. *et al.* (1996) 'The effects of supraphysiological doses of testosterone on angry behaviour in healthy eugonadal men: a clinical research centre study', *Journal of Clinical Endocrinology and Metabolism* 81: 3754–8.

Turek, P.J., Williams, R.H., Gilbaugh J.H. and Lipshultz, L.I. (1995) 'The reversibility of anabolic steroid-induced azoospermia', *Journal of Urology* 153: 1628–39.

PART V

CASE STUDIES

CHAPTER 29

CASE STUDIES

Andrew McBride and Trudi Petersen

NICKY

Nicky is a 25-year-old single woman who works from time to time in unskilled cleaning and bar work. She presents to acute psychiatric services in an over-aroused, agitated and distressed state having been picked up by police and taken to a place of safety under the Mental Health Act. She says that there is nothing wrong with her, but that the police and her neighbours are in a conspiracy against her and people have been following her everywhere she goes on foot and by car. She says that this has been going on for some weeks. She says that there are people in camouflaged clothing hiding in her garden and that she can hear them talking about her at night. She has been very distressed by these experiences and has taken to carrying a knife for her own protection and has seriously considered killing herself with the knife when the plot against her becomes too much for her to take.

Nicky was picked up by the police wandering on a busy road threatening passing motorists with her knife. She says that she would only injure others if they threatened her first. She refuses to describe what the people in the garden are saying about her, but indicates that they are talking about what fate they have in store with her.

Nicky has never been seen by psychiatric services before. She says that she has been using amphetamine by injection for three or four years in gradually increasing amounts. She says that she has not slept for some weeks and has spent the last few nights wandering around the town because she is too frightened to go back to her own flat.

A comprehensive assessment reveals no family history of mental illness or substance misuse problems. One of three children, Nicky was raised locally and attended local schools. She obtained two GCSEs and left school to work for the same cleaning company as her mother. Heterosexual, she has had a number of partners but is currently single. She has no children. There is no past medical history of relevance. She takes the contraceptive pill but is on no other medication.

At the time of her presentation she lives alone in a housing association flat and has a large circle of friends, some of whom are closely involved with drug use, others of whom have no such connection.

At the time of assessment Nicky appears thin, exhausted with widely dilated pupils and multiple injection sites on her arms. She is anxious and fearful and as the interview proceeds becomes irritable and suspicious that you might also be involved in the plot.

QUESTIONS

- What factors in the history do you consider of importance to the risk assessment?
- Where should Nicky be cared for in the immediate future?
- Could the Mental Health Act be used to detain Nicky in hospital for assessment and/or treatment in the event that she refused the offer of such help?
- What other elements should be incorporated in a management plan?

Nicky agrees to be admitted to hospital voluntarily and agrees to take some anti-psychotic medication on the understanding that this will help her to relax and sleep. After five days Nicky's psychotic symptoms have largely resolved. She complains of low mood, irritability, difficulty in sleeping, and maintains that although no longer happening, the events that she had described were true.

QUESTION

- What treatment options might be tried to help Nicky with her withdrawal symptoms?

After two weeks in hospital Nicky is no longer complaining of withdrawal symptoms, but is anxious about going home. She now recognises that her amphetamine use has contributed to her breakdown, but is uncertain that she will be able to resist amphetamine if it is offered to her.

QUESTIONS

- What approaches might be taken to try to ensure that Nicky remains in contact with services after discharge?
- What psychosocial interventions might be helpful in reducing the risk of rapid relapse to amphetamine use, and the risk of a recurrence of psychotic symptoms?

JANET

Background

Janet is a 38-year-old woman who is a single unemployed mother of two children aged 14 and 6. She lives alone. She was referred to social services by an anonymous neighbour who has concerns about the safety of the 6-year-old. She says that Janet is often drunk and that the younger child is left to fend for herself. She has seen the child out wandering the streets. On one occasion the neighbour took her home only to be met at the door by an intoxicated Janet who became abusive and slammed the door in her face, after roughly pulling the child inside.

Janet was visited at home by Maggie, a social worker. Janet was clearly intoxicated, she was smelling of alcohol and her speech was slurred. She appeared dishevelled. The children, she said, were in school. Initially Janet was quite hostile towards Maggie, refusing to let her in the house but eventually the social worker was able to convince Janet that the situation would be better dealt with indoors, rather than on the doorstep in full view of everyone.

On entering the house Maggie noted that the environment was generally clean, though there was a strong smell of alcohol pervading the house and mounds of unwashed clothes and dishes were heaped on the kitchen drainer.

Maggie spent some time with Janet, developing rapport with her and breaking down the barriers. Janet eventually admitted that things had got a little 'out of hand' and that she was drinking 'a fair bit'. Maggie asked her exactly what she meant by this to which Janet admitted to drinking two bottles of wine every day, usually starting in the morning, just after the children had left for school. Maggie asked her what happened if she did not drink and Janet described a range of withdrawal symptoms.

After an hour Janet admitted that she was worried about her alcohol intake but that she had put off getting any help as she was worried that she would be seen as an unfit mother and her children taken into care. Her drinking had escalated in the last six months since her husband left. She did not want to go to her GP as he was a personal friend of her ex-husband. 'I don't know what to do?' she said tearfully.

Decision

The social worker liaised with the GP and the school with a view to ensuring the safety and well being of the children as outlined in the Children Act. She called a case conference about Janet's situation where it was agreed that the situation would be monitored and that Janet would be referred urgently to the local specialist alcohol service for help with her drinking. Janet's referral was received by the team the following week . She was categorised as a priority client because of her children and was allocated a key worker who was able to arrange an appointment for a few days after this.

QUESTIONS

- What skills did Maggie use to develop a rapport with Janet and enable her to develop some trust?
- What could Maggie have done if Janet had denied alcohol use or refused to let her in?
- What might Janet's main concerns be when she first attends the alcohol service and how might these be dealt with?

Assessment

Janet attended for her appointment where she met Linda, her keyworker. Janet was anxious and apprehensive about what might happen.

QUESTIONS

- What can Linda do to help Janet feel more at ease during the assessment?
- What kind of questions could Linda ask in relation to the following:
  - (a) Janet's current level and pattern of drinking?
  - (b) Janet's drinking history?
  - (c) Her mental health?
  - (d) Her physical health?
  - (e) Her family and social circumstances?
  - (f) Her motivation?
  - (g) Janet's previous attempts to cut down or stop?
- What tools or investigations might be used to:
  - (a) Give more detailed information on Janet's drinking pattern?
  - (b) Explore her physical health in more detail and enable Linda to give her some objective feedback regarding this?
- What confidentiality issues exist and how might these be dealt with?
- Are there any factors that should be taken into account when arranging appointment times with Janet?

Plan

Janet's assessment indicated that she had developed a dependency on alcohol. She had blood taken for a liver function test which came back as being outside the normal range. Janet was asked to keep a drink diary for a week which identified some specific stressors related to her drinking and demonstrated a consistent pattern of consumption. Her main social support was her parents who lived seventy miles away, and a close friend, James, who lived nearby. At first Janet was unwilling to let the team share information with her GP but after discussing confidentiality she felt reassured that details about her situation would not be discussed with her ex-husband though she was aware that if it was considered that her children may be at risk then social services would need to take action and confidentiality may need to be breached.

Janet and Linda discussed the option of controlled drinking but Janet felt she would prefer to detox and attain abstinence, for the time being at least. She did not want to detox in hospital. It was decided that this may not be the best option as there was a waiting list for detox of several weeks and it would make it difficult for her to manage with the children. The summer holidays were approaching and it was agreed that this may be a good time to detox at home. Janet's parents were able to have the children for the first week of the holidays, her ex-husband had already arranged to take them away for a few days the week after. For the final part of the detox James and his sister were able to help out. It was arranged that James would move into Janet's spare room during the detox and help supervise her medication. Linda and Debbie, one of the team care assistants, would be able to visit daily to monitor the detox.

QUESTIONS

- What other kinds of input might be helpful for Janet during this time and post-detox?

Outcome

Janet detoxed successfully. She remained abstinent for a further six months before returning to occasional social drinking. A year after this her mother died unexpectedly and Janet again started drinking heavily but was able to identify this as problematic early on and sought help. She obtained bereavement counselling and support from a voluntary sector group. This time she reduced her alcohol use with no input from the statutory sector team.

QUESTIONS

- What might have happened if her drinking had escalated severely?
- What might help Janet avoid developing a pattern of drinking in the future?

WAYNE

Background

Wayne is a 19-year-old unemployed man who lives with his parents and younger sister in a flat in a run down area of the city. Until last year his drug history consisted of occasional amphetamines, a brief period of solvent abuse in his teens, regular cannabis use and occasional dihydrocodeine and benzodiazepine misuse (which he took from his grandmothers prescription). Last year he was introduced to heroin by his friend, Del. He and Del began smoking heroin at weekends. This increased until they were smoking most days. Del began injecting a month ago, initiating Wayne into this by injecting him. Wayne was too nervous to try and inject himself at that time but now Del has gone into prison and Wayne will need to inject himself if he wants to continue doing this. He knows a few other people who inject, including the person he and Del originally obtained their heroin from but there is no one that he trusts to inject him.

Errol is an experienced voluntary worker based in the needle exchange. He meets Wayne for the first time when he presents himself asking for needles.

QUESTIONS

What, why and how should Errol ask Wayne about his current injecting practice in relation to:

- Wayne's knowledge of injection sites.
- His technique – how he actually plans to inject.
- His knowledge of first aid?
- The setting he injects in, where and with whom?

Assessment

Errol observes Wayne's injection sites. He is careful to ask this specifically, asking Wayne to simply show him his arms may not reveal all his IV sites. Wayne is injecting mainly into his left anteriocubital fossae (The crook of his elbow). It is clear that Wayne has a poor injecting technique, there are several traumatised areas and a swelling which looks red and sore. There are a couple of track marks and bruises on the inside of his wrist.

Outcome

Errol is able to advise Wayne on his choice of injection sites. He suggests he tries to avoid the inside of his wrists and informs him of more appropriate areas. He uses appropriate literature to demonstrate to Wayne where his arteries and nerves are and the importance of avoiding these. He also informs him of how to avoid hitting an artery and what to do if he does hit one. He suggests Wayne seeks medical advice in relation to the swelling as it may be infected and advises him on technique, explaining how to feel for a vein and what depth and angle to put the needle in at. He also talks to him about the risks of sharing injecting equipment as Wayne has admitted to sharing needles and syringes with Del as well as sharing other equipment used in drug preparation and administration such as spoons, filter and water for flushing his works through. Wayne is not concerned about sharing with Del as he had told him he underwent HIV and Hepatitis C test which was clear. Wayne said he also washed the used works out with water and bleach.

QUESTIONS
What should Errol inform Wayne about in relation to:

- Sharing injecting equipment?
- Transmission of HIV and Hepatitis C and B?
- Cleaning used works with bleach?
- What would help Wayne gain greater protection against Hepatitis B?
- Why is it important that Wayne is given written and visual information as well as verbal information? Why is it important to check before giving him any written information?
- How could Errol check that Wayne has understood what he has told him, both now and in future visits?
- What should Errol inform Wayne about in relation to disposal of his used injecting equipment and what should he give him to enable him to do this more safely? Why is this of particular importance in relation to Wayne's home situation?
- Could Wayne be discouraged from further injecting? What alternatives might Errol suggest? Do you think a brief intervention or short motivational interviewing approach might be helpful?

Follow-up

Wayne continued to inject. He did not share needles and syringes again, managing to keep an 'emergency' pack in the bottom of his bag. He did share spoons and filters however. He started on a Hepatitis B vaccination programme at his GP's. With Errol's encouragement Wayne managed to reduce his injecting, smoking whenever he felt able to. He began to rotate his injection sites, resting each area in order to keep the veins in good condition. Errol retained a good relationship with Wayne and kept him aware of the potential for change and the types of services which were available locally that might help him.

Several months later Wayne decided to have a blood test for Hepatitis C. Unfortunately he proved to be positive for the virus and he was referred to a hepatologist. He was very distressed by this and went on a month long 'binge', injecting several times a day. He also shared injecting equipment with another person, also Hepatitis C positive. Things did improve after this. He has joined a community-based hepatitis self-help group which he attends regularly. He has asked his GP to refer him to the statutory sector drugs team and is awaiting a date for a liver biopsy which will tell him more about the nature and impact of his hepatitis infection. Though he still injects at present, Wayne hopes he will be able to stop injecting in the future and obtain treatment for his hepatitis.

DAVID

Background

David has been on a methadone prescription with another drug service for the last four years. He has recently moved into a new area and has been referred to the local drug service by the team who have been prescribing. It has been agreed, in principle, that the team will take over prescribing. The information obtained from David's previous prescriber is scanty. David is a long-standing client of their service. He was put onto a methadone prescription initially as he was injecting large amounts of heroin. He has a drug history going back to the age of 16; his first heroin use was at the age of 20. There is some brief forensic history. He has served several prison sentences for assault. He was also seen by forensic services when he was 20 following an assault on one of his previous school teachers who he had harboured a grudge against for years. He was at that time diagnosed as having an antisocial personality disorder but was never followed up.

David has been on 55 mls of methadone for the last two years; this was increased from his initial starting dose of 50 mls. His previous prescriber saw him in person monthly. There were no urine results included with his referral letter.

Assessment

Kim was allocated as David's keyworker. She carried out an assessment of David's history and current situation. There appeared to be some discrepancy between the forensic history he told her and the one his previous agency had furnished the team with. David admitted to spending time in prison but downplayed this, saying that in each of the circumstances he had been acting in self-defence. It was, he said, purely bad luck that he had been the one arrested. He readily admitted to using on top of his prescription and provided a urine sample that was positive for opiates and methadone. He said he felt really relieved that he was finally able to tell someone he was using on top. He'd been 'having a bit of a crisis' recently and he'd fallen in with 'a bad crowd'; this was one of his reasons for moving away.

Plan

The team took over David's prescribing and his prescription was increased to 60 mls. He was placed on a daily supervised consumption in the chemists. David said that he appreciated this but the daily pick-up would cause him problems as he was actually working. He had a job as a security guard which entailed long hours and shift work. Could he possibly have his prescription to pick up weekly? Kim was firm, reiterating the team's policy that methadone prescriptions should be supervised. David was very unhappy about this. David rang and cancelled his next appointment but agreed to attend in a fortnight. He did attend that one but was unable to produce a urine sample. Kim let it go but felt uncomfortable about this. David attended his next few appointments on time producing urine samples that were positive for methadone only. However, on one of these occasions Kim suspected that something was amiss. His urine felt cold and he had been very quick in producing the sample. She suspected it was not his, but David was adamant that it was. Kim arranged for a male staff member to supervise David's next urine sample. On this occasion David broke down and admitted he had been using on top again. He was very worried that his prescription would be stopped. He admitted to giving samples of someone else's urine. 'I didn't want to disappoint you. I know you're on my side. Not like my last keyworker, I never saw them and they didn't care. They weren't like you.'

QUESTIONS

How should Kim respond to this 'manipulative' behaviour?

Should David's prescription be increased?

A couple of days later David's chemist rang to say that he was concerned that David was not sticking to his prescription. He had missed a couple of days the week before and on one occasion had persuaded a locum pharmacist to dispense it to him to take home rather than consume on the premises. His supervised urine sample came back as positive for opiates, methadone, benzodiazepines and cocaine. David was informed that persistent on top use would result in him possibly losing his prescription. 'You can't do that – I've been on it for four years' he said.

David did not attend his next appointment and Kim withheld his next prescription. Eventually David turned up. He was clearly intoxicated and was verbally abusive. He threatened to smash the clinic up and punched the wall before leaving. Kim was left shaken and upset by the incident.

QUESTIONS

What should Kim do in this situation?

What should happen following this?

What kind of support should be available for Kim?

Outcome

Following team discussion, Kim wrote to David informing him that his behaviour had been unacceptable and why this was so. It was agreed that he would be discharged. A reducing prescription was arranged to run over a one-week period. He was informed of options for the future which included an outline of referral, as this was felt appropriate. His GP and previous service provider were informed of this.

Kim was able to receive support from the team and to request supervision quickly. She was also encouraged to review the situation reflectively. Her positive actions were reinforced and she was able to learn from the incident, identifying how she might deal with a similar situation in the future. She was encouraged to seek help if she required it at any point following the incident.

QUESTIONS

What should Kim have included in the initial assessment that should be included in any future assessment?

Follow-up

The team reviewed its policy on risk management and risk assessment and changes were made to practise following this.

ARSHAD

Arshad is a 14-year-old school student. He has been brought to see you by his mother, who has found a small quantity of what Arshad says is cannabis. Arshad inadvertently left the substance in a pocket which he then put in the laundry. There is no family history of relevance, his school achievements are average, he has good peer and family relationships and a number of constructive recreational activities. Arshad and his mother appear anxious and miserable but there is no evidence of significant health problems in any member of the family.

What are Arshad and his mother most likely to be concerned about?

What is the best way to approach the interview? Mother and son together or individually? How do you decide?

Arshad's mother is concerned that cannabis may act as a gateway drug to other problems. She has read that cannabis in itself is associated with difficulties that may affect his education and may get him into trouble with the police. Arshad says that he has used the drug occasionally with friends, but it is no big deal and it helps him to chill out. Arshad's mother wants him referred for specialist treatment and is considering taking him to the police to be cautioned for his behaviour.

What skills will you need to display in dealing with the seemingly irreconcilable views of Arshad and his mother?

What would you say if Arshad's mother asks your advice about her proposed course of action?

What outcomes would you consider to reflect success for your discussion?

BILLY

Billy is a 52-year-old twice divorced man in receipt of health related state benefits. He lives in a bedsit in a shared house with four other men, all of whom are unemployed and have a history of alcohol problems. Billy is referred for specialist help by hospital medical services after he has been admitted as an emergency because of vomiting blood and abdominal pain.

Billy's main problem is of high alcohol intake: usually between 9 and 12 litres of 6 per cent ABV cider per day, or its equivalent in lager or spirits. He drinks from waking to sleeping and if unable to obtain alcohol takes benzodiazepine tranquillisers bought on the black market. If Billy stops drinking he suffers severe withdrawal symptoms including a recent history of fits and delirium tremens. He has a past history of pancreatitis, peptic ulceration, liver disease and peripheral neuropathy, which has now impaired his walking to the extent that he frequently trips and falls when intoxicated. He complains of low mood, high levels of anxiety and an inability to meet people unless he has been drinking. He gives a history of having taken a number of overdoses, always whilst intoxicated, the last having been two weeks before his recent admission to hospital.

Billy's father, a maternal uncle and two brothers have a history of severe alcohol problems. Billy has no contact with his two ex-wives, three adult children or two younger step-children. His only social network is his group of acquaintances from the house in which he lives, with whom he drinks.

Between the time of his leaving the hospital and attending for assessment he has started drinking again in a similar way to before. Although it is difficult to assess, because he has been drinking, there is some evidence during your interview that his memory may be impaired.

He asks for help to stop drinking because he is scared that he is going to die if he does not address his drink problem now.

What factors in the history and mental state would you consider relevant to a risk assessment?

Where would be the most appropriate for a detoxification?

Prior to a further detoxification what steps should be taken to manage the risks identified?

What steps should be taken before detoxification to improve the chances of Billy making progress after detoxification has been completed?

One year after first being seen Billy has been detoxified in hospital twice. He has attended Alcoholics Anonymous from time to time, but never with a consistent pattern. He has twice been resident in dry houses and rehabilitation facilities. He has tried Acamprosate, always refused Disulfiram and been reluctant to engage in any form of individual or group psychological treatment.

How can you optimise the likelihood of this time being different?

How best can you maintain therapeutic optimism in the face of Billy's difficulties?

How best would you negotiate a treatment plan and what would you hope such a treatment plan will look like?

It transpires on testing that Billy does indeed have short-term memory problems which persist after detoxification. What implications does this have for the treatment package provided?

MIKE

Mike is a 25-year-old single student, who lives in rented private accommodation. He attends his local Accident and Emergency Department complaining of abdominal cramps, flu-like symptoms, restlessness and irritability. On examination he is clammy and unwell-looking, with dilated pupils. He has injection sites on his arms.

What is the most likely explanation for this combination of symptoms and signs?

What information and advice should be given at this point?

Mike is referred to, and later attends local Community Drug Service. He gives the following story.

Mike experimented with smoking tobacco in his teens, but never became a regular smoker. He began drinking modestly in his late teens, but when he first went to university at the age of 18 began drinking heavily because of symptoms of home sickness and anxiety. At around the same time he began smoking cannabis, and taking ecstasy and stimulants when out clubbing. After about a year of this pattern of alcohol and drug use, he began to be aware that after week-ends of ecstasy use (when he would use up to 10–15 tablets) he noticed his mood fall during the week, with impaired concentration, and posed difficulty in coping with work. A friend introduced him to smoking heroin, which he began to do one or two days a week. During holidays when he returned home, he discontinued all drug use, but in his second year at university, now aged 20, he began using heroin in preference to other drugs, and began to run up debts as his heroin use increased. To try to save money he began injecting the heroin, and after a few months his debts led him to give up his academic career, and return to his home town. He has successfully stopped using heroin on two occasions, but since returning to university he has begun using again to cope with the pressures of work. He says that he was using half a gram per day. If heroin is unavailable, he either drinks heavily or takes dihydrocodeine or benzodiazepines.

The youngest of three children, all Mike's family are professional people, with no history of mental or physical illness. Mike's father went through a period of heavy drinking in his forties. There is no other relevant history of substance misuse.

Mike was a healthy infant and child, and enjoyed a stable, happy family upbringing. He attended local state schools, obtaining good qualifications which enabled him to attend university, after a year travelling around Europe at the age of 19. He had no particular career in mind. He is a socially anxious young man, and has had only two short relationships with women. He had no children. He had a few close friends from school who know nothing of his heroin use, and a larger circle of acquaintances in the town where he is now a student. His university friends drink and smoke and take ecstacy but never use heroin. In addition to university, he works in the evening as a barman, and has a student loan. His parents also give him additional money when times are hard, but know nothing of his heroin use.

Mike has always been extremely careful to use sterile injecting equipment, and not share any materials with anybody else. He has recently been tested anonymously for Hepatitis B and C and HIV, and the tests were all negative. He has never suffered any significant medical problems and is on no medication.

Mike has never seen a psychiatrist or attended his GP or any other helping agency because of mental health problems. His social anxiety is not a great handicap to him, and since discontinuing ecstasy use, he has not suffered episodes of depression.

Mike was cautioned for possession of cannabis, but has never otherwise been in trouble with the police. he has a clean driving licence and sometimes has use of his parents' cars.

Mike says that he has come for help now because he is worried about failing the second year of his course. He does not want history to repeat itself. He does not want his family to know of his heroin use, although they are aware that he has been struggling with his course work recently. He does not want the university to know, but is happy for his GP to be involved.

Mike says that he would like to stop using heroin now as quickly as possible, and then stay off. He is worried about withdrawal symptoms as they have become more severe recently and make his social anxiety and ability to cope with his university work more difficult. He has never been on a prescription before and will not consider any residential treatment options, whether this is in-patient detoxification or residential rehabilitation.

What treatment options would you discuss with Mike to help him achieve his aims? Consider what psychological help might be of benefit, what social support needs to be considered and what prescribing might be most appropriate?

Mike does not want his house-mates to find out about his heroin use, and is therefore reluctant to consider a short-term supported detoxification in the community. He decides to try to withdraw using methadone, and after assessment has been completed, he stabilises and stops injecting on a dose of 35 mg methadone daily over the course of two weeks. His track marks heal up; he puts on weight and his levels of anxiety return to normal. He is able to continue with his studies, and although disgruntled at attending the Community Pharmacist every day, has no shortage of time in which to do this. He attends for weekly supportive counselling and makes plans to pay off his drug debts, sever his links with his drug-using friends, and reconnect with a different group of friends that he has dropped since his heroin use began again.

The methadone is gradually reduced from 35 mg to 10 mg without significant ill effects. Mike then learns that his father has inoperable cancer with a very poor prognosis and begins using heroin again, on top of the methadone. He only smokes the heroin, but he is using between half a gram and 1 gram per day.

What options are available now? The initial plan was for abstinence, but Mike now thinks that he can't cope with his father's illness, his forthcoming examinations, and with discontinuation of his opioid use.

Six months pass since Mike was first started on methadone, his father has now died, he passed his end of year exams, but was only able to discontinue heroin use when taking 65 mg methadone daily. He has completed a course of Hepatitis B vaccinations. He is working through his grief with the support of his family and his life circumstances are now stable. He decides that he does not want to discontinue methadone, and asks to be left on it for at least the next few months.

How should Mike's request be dealt with? What are the most important things to discuss with him about moving into a phase of methadone maintenance? If maintenance is decided to be the best alternative for him, what risks and problems might follow? What risks are associated with trying to persuade Mike that discontinuing methadone would be the best course to pursue?

JANE

Jane is a 32-year -old former general nurse who has taken a career break to bring up three children who are all under five years of age. Her husband works away a good deal having recently changed jobs. The family has only recently moved into the area. Jane presents complaining of anxiety and low mood of modest severity with sleep disturbance, irritability and poor concentration, particularly in the mornings. Jane doesn't smoke or take illegal drugs but has taken to drinking up to a litre of 9 per cent ABV white wine, a glass or two at lunchtime the rest in the evening after the children have gone to bed. She suffers no significant physical withdrawal symptoms but is able to see a possible link between the stresses in her life, her consumption of alcohol and her symptoms of depression and anxiety.

What risk factors can you identify in the story?

What further assessment would you want to carry out?

What role might the husband play in helping to address the problem as identified?

What brief interventions might be helpful for Jane?

Jane is found on testing to have slightly abnormal liver function tests.

How should the results of her blood tests be fed back to her?

What would be a reasonable target for Jane to aim for in terms of reducing her drinking?

The GP arranges to repeat the blood tests in three months' time. Jane agrees to see the primary care counsellor for three sessions in the first instance and to keep a drinks diary. Jane arranges some additional support for childcare, works on establishing a new social network, picking up on social activities that she has abandoned since giving up work for her children and moving house. Her GP offers antidepressant treatment which she declines.

MARY

Mary is a 46-year-old widowed mother of three children, now aged 16, 19 and 22 years. She lives alone with her youngest child, in the house she inherited from her parents. She lives on State benefits. She has been on the same prescription of 80 mg of injectable methadone for the past ten years. Before this she had been on oral methadone intermittently for a further ten years, and before this had used heroin from the age of 19 years. She injects the methadone into her femoral vein without difficulty. She smokes cannabis to sleep, and takes a specific Serotonin re-uptake inhibitor antidepressant because of complaints of low mood.

Mary is the second child of her mother's relationship with her father. She has four other half brothers and sisters, all with different fathers. Her mother died of cirrhosis of the liver when in her late forties. She has had no contact with her father throughout her life. One brother died of a heroin overdose, and two of her sisters have alcohol and drug problems.

Mary's family upbringing was overshadowed by her mother's drinking, which resulted in several periods in local authority residential care. Mary says that she was physically and sexually abused by one of her step-fathers, between the ages of 8 and 13 years. She says that her mother never believed that this happened, and no charges were ever brought against the perpetrator.

Mary attended local schools, where she was frequently in trouble for disruptive behaviour. After several suspensions, she was expelled from secondary school at the age of 14 years for assaulting a member of staff. She never returned to school. She is literate and numerate but has no qualifications.

Mary met her husband when she was 16; he was four years older. He introduced her to heroin use and spent much of their marriage in prison for drug related offences of burglary and theft, possession with intent to supply and similar offences. The marital relationship was turbulent and sometimes violent. Her husband's death was drug related. Since his death twelve years ago, Mary has had only transient occasional sexual relationships, which were sometimes abusive. Mary has never worked. As the children have grown older she has lived an increasingly reclusive life, her closest relationships being with one of her sisters who does not misuse alcohol or drugs, and another methadone dependent patient of the service with a very similar life history.

Mary has a past history of Hepatitis B and is Hepatitis C positive. She has failed to attend for follow-up regarding her Hepatitis C at the local hospital. Her blood pressure is high and this is managed by her GP. She is on thyroxine because of under-active thyroid. She has the healed scars of multiple abscesses from her early days of injecting opiates and barbiturates.

Mary has a long history of deliberate self-harm, but has not taken an overdose or deliberately cut herself now for eight years. She complains of chronic low mood, low self-esteem, sleep disturbance, erratic eating pattern, and occasional nightmares about the death of her husband and early abuse. She has taken a range of antidepressants, antipsychotic and other pharmacological attempts to treat her emotional distress over the years, but it is not clear that any treatment has been of benefit. When younger she was frequently hospitalised because of self-harm and threats of suicide. She has not been in a psychiatric in-patient unit for nine years.

Mary has a past history of shoplifting, but her husband took responsibility for all the criminal activity that went on in her younger days, and she has avoided any time in prison. She has no driving licence.

Of Mary's three children, the oldest daughter trained as a cook and lives abroad. The younger son is in school, and the middle son is frequently in trouble with the police for minor, probably drug related, property offences.

Mary began smoking at the age of around 10 years, and drinking cider prodigiously at around the same age. She continues to smoke twenty cigarettes a day, but no longer drinks alcohol because of her Hepatitis C and because it makes her aggressive. She has used all the drugs that are available at different times in her life, but from the age of 16, when she met her husband, her main drug of misuse was heroin, backed up by occasional amphetamine binges.

What factors would you consider relevant in conducting a risk assessment on Mary's current circumstances?

What help should Mary now be receiving, and who should provide it?

Is there any scope for interventions to move Mary into a process of change. What would be the first priorities?

How would you try to evaluate the impact of treatment to date, in Mary's life?

How would you evaluate future treatment, in terms of her physical and mental health, and social well-being?

INDEX